LEGAL ISSUES IN MEDICAL PRACTICE
Medicolegal Guidelines for Safe Practice

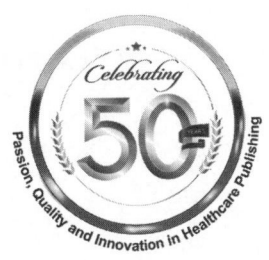

LEGAL ISSUES IN MEDICAL PRACTICE
Medicolegal Guidelines for Safe Practice

Second Edition

Editor

VP Singh MD (Forensic Medicine) LLB
Professor
Department of Forensic Medicine
Dayanand Medical College and Hospital
Ludhiana, Punjab, India

Foreword
SM Kantikar

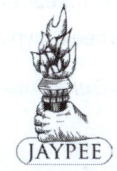

JAYPEE BROTHERS MEDICAL PUBLISHERS
The Health Sciences Publisher
New Delhi | London

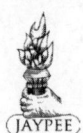 **Jaypee Brothers Medical Publishers (P) Ltd**

Headquarters

Jaypee Brothers Medical Publishers (P) Ltd
4838/24, Ansari Road, Daryaganj
New Delhi 110 002, India
Phone: +91-11-43574357
Fax: +91-11-43574314
Email: jaypee@jaypeebrothers.com

Overseas Offices

J.P. Medical Ltd
83 Victoria Street, London
SW1H 0HW (UK)
Phone: +44 20 3170 8910
Fax: +44 (0)20 3008 6180
Email: info@jpmedpub.com

Website: www.jaypeebrothers.com
Website: www.jaypeedigital.com

© 2020, Jaypee Brothers Medical Publishers

The views and opinions expressed in this book are solely those of the original contributor(s)/author(s) and do not necessarily represent those of editor(s) of the book.

All rights reserved. No part of this publication may be reproduced, stored or transmitted in any form or by any means, electronic, mechanical, photocopying, recording or otherwise, without the prior permission in writing of the publishers.

All brand names and product names used in this book are trade names, service marks, trademarks or registered trademarks of their respective owners. The publisher is not associated with any product or vendor mentioned in this book.

Medical knowledge and practice change constantly. This book is designed to provide accurate, authoritative information about the subject matter in question. However, readers are advised to check the most current information available on procedures included and check information from the manufacturer of each product to be administered, to verify the recommended dose, formula, method and duration of administration, adverse effects and contraindications. It is the responsibility of the practitioner to take all appropriate safety precautions. Neither the publisher nor the author(s)/editor(s) assume any liability for any injury and/or damage to persons or property arising from or related to use of material in this book.

This book is sold on the understanding that the publisher is not engaged in providing professional medical services. If such advice or services are required, the services of a competent medical professional should be sought.

Every effort has been made where necessary to contact holders of copyright to obtain permission to reproduce copyright material. If any have been inadvertently overlooked, the publisher will be pleased to make the necessary arrangements at the first opportunity. The **CD/DVD-ROM** (if any) provided in the sealed envelope with this book is complimentary and free of cost. **Not meant for sale.**

Inquiries for bulk sales may be solicited at: jaypee@jaypeebrothers.com

Legal Issues in Medical Practice: Medicolegal Guidelines for Safe Practice / VP Singh

First Edition: 2016

Second Edition: 2020

ISBN: 978-93-89776-05-8

Printed at: Sterling Graphics Pvt. Ltd.

Dedicated to

*All those who strongly feel that
Medicolegal awareness is a must for all involved in patient care
and to all the Medical Practitioners who want to practice their
professional skills conscientiously and fearlessly and are ambitious to
promote quality in healthcare*

Contributors

Editor

VP Singh MD (Forensic Medicine) LLB
Professor
Department of Forensic Medicine
Dayanand Medical College and Hospital
Ludhiana, Punjab, India

Contributing Authors

Ajay Kumar MD (Forensic Medicine)
Associate Professor
Department of Forensic Medicine
and Toxicology
Government Medical College and
Hospital
Chandigarh, India

Akashdeep Aggarwal
MD (Forensic Medicine)
Associate Professor
Department of Forensic Medicine
and Toxicology
Government Medical College
Patiala, Punjab, India

Amandeep Singh
MD (Ophthalmology)
Consultant
Department of Ophthalmology
Amandeep Eye Hospital
Kharar, Punjab, India

Amrita Ghosh MBBS
MD (Biochemistry) MSc (Medical Biochemistry)
Faculty (Demonstrator)
Medical College
Kolkata, West Bengal, India

Archana Kumari MS
Assistant Professor
Department of Obstetrics and
Gynaecology
All India Institute of Medical
Sciences
New Delhi, India

Arun Mavaji Seetharam
MD (Hospital Administration)
Assistant Professor
Department of Hospital
Administration
Kasturba Medical College and
Hospital
Manipal, Karnataka, India

Arvind Kumar Singh
MD (Anesthesiology) LLB
Senior Advisor (Anesthesiology)
Director
MS PS IHQ
Ministry of Defence (Army)
Director General Medical Services
(DGMS) (Army)
New Delhi, India

Chandrashekhar A Sohoni
DNB (Radiodiagnosis)
Consultant
Department of Radiology
NM Medical
Pune, Maharashtra, India

Charu Mittal MD DNB
Consultant
Department of Obstetrics and
Gynecology
Sahara Multispeciality Hospital
Gwalior, Madhya Pradesh, India
Ex-Assistant Professor
Baroda Medical College
Vadodara, Gujarat, India

Christopher Barry MD PhD FACS
Advisory Board Member
Mohan Foundation
(NGO to Promote Organ
Donation)
Chennai, Tamil Nadu, India

Dasari Harish MD (Forensic Medicine)
Professor and Head
Department of Forensic Medicine
and Toxicology
Government Medical College and
Hospital
Chandigarh, India

Debashis Sinha BA LLB
Advocate
Honourable High Court at
Calcutta and Counsel
Honourable Supreme Court of
India
Kolkata, West Bengal, India

Dinesh Verma MD (Ophthalmology)
DO (Lond) FRCS (Edin) FRCOphth (UK)
Founder President, i4vision
Diagnostics Pvt Ltd
New Delhi, India
Visiting Professor, Doheny Eye
Institute
University of Southern California
Los Angeles, USA
Medical Director, Netcare
Healthcare
London, UK

Gautam Biswas MD (Forensic Medicine)
Professor and Head
Department of Forensic Medicine and Toxicology
Dayanand Medical College and Hospital
Ludhiana, Punjab, India

Hemal Kanvinde MSc PhD
Quality Assurance Officer
Mohan Foundation
(NGO to Promote Organ Donation)
Chennai, Tamil Nadu, India

Joseph Thomas MS MCh (Urology) DNB MNAMS FRCS PGMLE PGDBE
Professor, Department of Urology
Kasturba Medical College and Hospital
Manipal, Karnataka, India

Krishnadutt H Chavali MBBS MD DNB PGDHA MNAMS FIMSA
Professor and Head
Forensic Medicine and Toxicology
AIIMS
Raipur, Chhattisgarh, India

Lakesh Anand MD FIMSA FCCS MAMS FCCP
Professor
Department of Anesthesiology and Intensive Care
Government Medical College and Hospital
Chandigarh, India

Manpreet Singh MD FACEE FCCP FIMSA FCCS MAMS
Assistant Professor
Department of Anesthesiology and Intensive Care
Government Medical College and Hospital
Chandigarh, India

Manu Shankar MS DNB (Surgery) FNB (Minimal Access Surgery) FIAGES FICS
Senior Consultant
Department of Minimal Access and General Surgery
Fortis Escorts Hospital
NIT, Faridabad, Haryana, India

MC Gupta MD (Medicine) MPH LLM
Advocate and Medicolegal Consultant Member
Supreme Court Bar Association
New Delhi, India

Mukesh Yadav MD MBA (HCA) LLB PGDHOQM PGDHR
Professor and Head
Department of Forensic Medicine and Toxicology
Rama Medical College
Hapur, Uttar Pradesh, India

Pardeep Singh MD (Forensic Medicine)
Professor and Head
Department of Forensic Medicine and Toxicology
Gold Field Institute of Medical Sciences and Research
Faridabad, Haryana, India

Parmod Goyal MD (Forensic Medicine)
Professor and Head
Department of Forensic Medicine
Adesh Institute of Medical Sciences and Research
Bathinda, Punjab, India

Piyush Ranjan MD
Additional Professor
Department of Medicine
All India Institute of Medical Sciences
New Delhi, India

PS Mittal MD
Consultant
Department of Obstetrics and Gynecology
Sahara Multispeciality Hospital
Gwalior, Madhya Pradesh, India
Ex-Assistant Professor
Baroda Medical College
Vadodara, Gujarat, India

Pradeep Sreevastava MHA (AIIMS) DHA MBA
Brigadier Incharge Administration (Brig IC Adm)
Army Medical Corps (AMC)
Centre and College
Lucknow, Uttar Pradesh, India

VJ Purushotham MBBS D'Ortho MS Ortho
Professor of Orthopaedics
Bangalore Medical College and Research Institute
Bengaluru, Karnataka, India

Rahul S Kamble MBBS MD
Consultant Microbiologist And Infection Control Officer
Lilavati Hospital And Research Centre
Mumbai, Maharashtra, India

Rajendra S Bangal MD DNB (Forensic Medicine) LLB PGDLPO
Professor and Head
Department of Forensic Medicine and Toxicology
Smt Kashibai Navale Medical College and General Hospital
Pune, Maharashtra, India

Rajesh K Sinha PhD
Deputy Director and Professor
Amity Medical School
Amity Education Valley
Amity University Haryana
Manesar, Haryana, India

Ranabir Pal MD PhD MBBS (Honours) DCH MBA FAIMER FELLOW MNAMS MNASc
Professor and Chair (Head)
Department of Community Medicine
MGM Medical College and Hospital
Kishanganj, Bihar, India

Rashmi Datta MD (Anesthesiology and Critical Care) DNB (General Medicine) DNB (Aviation Medicine)
Consultant and Head
Department of Anesthesiology and Critical Care Base Hospital,
Delhi Cantonment and
Army College of Medical Sciences
New Delhi, India

Sameer Mehta Post Graduate Diploma (Hospital Management)
Director
Hosmac India Private Limited
Mumbai, Maharashtra, India

Shilpa Pharande MDS (Orthodontics and Dentofacial Orthopedics) PGDMLS PGDHM
Member
World Association for Medical Law, Belgium
Consultant (Dentist)
Pharande Multispeciality Dental Clinic
Pune, Maharashtra, India

Shrayan Pal MBBS (Hons) PGT JR2 MD (Dermatology, Venereology and Leprosy)
Post Graduate Trainee (PGT JR2)
Department of Dermatology, Venereology and Leprosy
MGM Medical College and Hospital
Kishanganj, Bihar, India

Sujatha Niranjan MSW
Manager
Department of Information Systems
Mohan Foundation
(NGO to Promote Organ Donation)
Chennai, Tamil Nadu, India

Sumana Navin MBBS PGD Hospital Management
Course Director
Mohan Foundation
(NGO to Promote Organ Donation)
Chennai, Tamil Nadu, India

Sundeep Mishra MBBS MD DM FACC FSCAI
Professor
Department of Cardiology
All India Institute of Medical Science (AIIMS)
New Delhi, India

Sunil Shroff MS FRCS (G) DURO (London)
Managing Trustee
Mohan Foundation
(NGO to Promote Organ Donation)
Professor
Department of Urology
Sri Ramachandra Medical College and Research Institute
Chennai, Tamil Nadu, India

Swapnil S Agarwal MD DNB MNAMS
Professor
Department of Forensic Medicine and Toxicology
Pramukhswami Medical College and Shree Krishna Hospital
Gujarat, India

Utsav Parekh MD
Associate Professor
Department of Forensic Medicine and Toxicology
Pramukhswami Medical College and Shri Krishna Hospital
Gujarat, India

VP Singh MD (Forensic Medicine) LLB
Professor
Department of Forensic Medicine
Dayanand Medical College
Ludhiana, Punjab, India

Vivekanshu Verma MD (Forensic Medicine)
Senior Resident and Fellow
Emergency Medicine
Medicolegal Advisor
Medanta–The Medicity
Gurugram, Haryana, India

Yogesh Dave MD DPED DCS PGDHHM PGDMLS CFN QM-AHO Tele Health Diploma Naco Specialist in Children MBA (HRM)
Editorial Board Member
Indian Journal of Pediatrics Education and Research,
Bhavsinhji District Hospital
Porbandar, Gujarat, India

Foreword

Dr SM Kantikar
MD (Path) LLB PGDMLE

Member
National Consumer Disputes
Redressal Commission, New Delhi

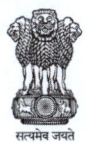

Upbhokta Nyay Bhawan
F-Block, General Pool Office Complex
INA, New Delhi-110023
Tel/Fax: 011-24608811, 24651505
Mobile: 9999110833
E-mail: smkantikar@gmail.com

It is my great pleasure to go through this authoritative treatise on medicolegal issues commonly encountered by the doctors in their day-to-day clinical practice.

Doctors are known to use their skills to solace the sufferings of their patients; but, sometimes, they are unable to do the full justice and become liable to face medicolegal conflicts on account of medical mistakes. Currently, doctors as well as healthcare establishments are facing numerous litigations related to medical malpractice. The doctors must understand that ignorance of law is no excuse, and medicolegal awareness is extremely important.

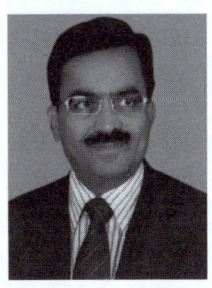

Legal Issues in Medical Practice: Medicolegal Guidelines for Safe Practice has presented essential medicolegal information that can be used as guidelines for safe clinical practice. Chapters on various medicolegal issues are written by the specialists who are well experienced in clinical as well as medicolegal domains. Most of the pertinent issues such as medical ethics, informed consent, medical documentation, medical negligence, and various laws applicable to the medical professionals have been elaborated in the book. A separate section on medicolegal issues related to various specialties has presented *practice management strategies* for safe clinical practice.

VP Singh has used his academic and research experience to edit the detailed views of the authors and presented a reliable medicolegal book with a problem-solving approach. The guiding principles recommended in the book are well supported by relevant judgments from Indian Courts. I am sure that medical fraternity would find the book very handy allaying their unfolded fears about legal implications and more particularly Consumer Protection Act.

SM Kantikar MD LLB
Member
National Consumer Disputes
Redressal Commission
New Delhi, India

FOREWORD

Dr. SM Kantikar
MD MNAMS LLM DHHM

Member,
National Consumer Disputes
Redressal Commission, New Delhi

Upphokta Nyay Bhawan
F Block, General Pool Office Complex,
INA, New Delhi-110023.
Tel.: 011-24608801, 24658543
Mobile: 99811 10803
E-mail: smkantikar@gmail.com

It is my great pleasure to go through this authoritative treatise on medicolegal issues commonly encountered by the doctors in their day-to-day clinical practice.

Doctors are bound to face the results, to solace the sufferings of their patients, but sometimes, they are unable to do the full justice and become liable to face medicolegal conflicts on account of medical mistakes. Nowadays, do not visualise, healthcare establishments are facing numerous litigations related to medical malpractice. The doctors must understand that ignorance of law is no excuse, and medicolegal awareness is extremely important.

I appreciate Dr SM Shah that, clinical scenarios outlining as to safe practices presented as initial medicolegal foundation that can be used as guidelines for safe clinical practice. It caters on various medicolegal domains. Most of the pertinent issues such as medical ethics, informed consent, medical records, medical negligence, and various laws applicable to the various organisations have been elaborated in the book. A separate section on medicolegal issues related to various specialities has presented the practice modalities that assist in safe clinical practice.

Dr Shah has used his academic and research experience to edit the detailed views of the author, and presented as a simple medicolegal book with a problem-solving approach. The guiding principles recommended in the booklets will supported by relevant judgment, from various Courts. I am sure that medical fraternity would find the book very useful, alleviating their unbiased fears about legal implications, and more particularly Consumer Protection Act.

SM Kantikar, MD
Member
National Consumer Disputes
Redressal Commission
New Delhi, India

Endorsements

Legal Issues in Medical Practice: Medicolegal Guidelines for Safe Practice is a valuable gift to Indian doctors to help them practice confidently without fear of medicolegal problems. The valuable tips doled out, bring in the impeccable knowledge and vast practical experience of the authors and editorial team. Dr VP Singh, an authority in medical law, as Editor of the book has ensured that it remains useful in day-to-day practice. This book is a must-have for all doctors today.

Shri Mahendrakumar Bajpai, Advocate, Supreme Court of India
Hon Director, Institute of Medicine and Law, Mumbai, Maharashtra, India
(*www.imlindia.com*)
Editor, Medical Law Cases—For Doctors (*www.mlcd.in*)

Legal Issues in Medical Practice: Medicolegal Guidelines for Safe Practice provides valuable tips and information on various medicolegal aspects involved in day-to-day practice. It gives facets of medical laws, ethical aspects of dealing with patients as well as ways to exercise abundant caution while dealing with patients.

Dr Suganthi Iyer MBBS DHA LLB PGDMLE PDCR
Assistant Director (Legal and Medical Services)
Hinduja Hospital, Mahim, Mumbai, Maharashtra, India

Legal Issues in Medical Practice: Medicolegal Guidelines for Safe Practice is well-written and contains useful information on medicolegal issues, which have become very relevant today. I recommend this book to all medical practitioners, for empowering themselves for difficult situations.

Dr PK Kohli MBBS MS MNAMS PhD LLB PGDMLS PGDHHM
Senior Surgeon and Medicolegal Expert, Editor
Indian Journal of Healthcare Quality and Management

Legal Issues in Medical Practice: Medicolegal Guidelines for Safe Practice deals with the medicolegal and complex ethical issues encountered by clinicians during their day-to-day practice. I firmly believe that the book will promote the good medical practice leading to patient-centred approach. In nutshell, this book is a must read for every healthcare professional who is ambitious to deliver high standards of care for patients.

Dr Arvind Arora MBBS MRCP (UK)
Consultant Medical Oncologist
Nottingham University and Hospitals
NHS Trust, Nottingham, UK

Preface to the Second Edition

Today, medicine has become a prevailing and complex part of our society. The patient–doctor relationship has become more formal and structured. Doctors are no longer regarded as infallible, and are exposed to more liabilities and restrains, than privileges. However, in spite of all the vicissitudes, the practice of medicine is capable of healing the ailing mankind, provided it is practiced with due care, sincerity, and efficiency. Anyone who practices medicine must be aware that there are unique ethical and legal issues which evolved relative to the recent time. Medical laws have emerged as a vast specialization that regulates the practice of medicine. As law evolves with time, we need to understand and follow the medicolegal principles applicable in the practice of medicine. Providing best possible care is not enough. Even the best care provided will be considered inadequate, if the applicable legal principles are not followed. As law is never static, physicians must *learn, unlearn,* and *relearn* the up-to-date medicolegal principles.

For a busy clinician, this book is a handy guidance for effective management of medicolegal conflicts confronted in day-to-day clinical practice. In this book distinguished subject experts have provided the evidence-based guiding principles to tackle with such issues. I hope medical practitioners will find this book very useful in their practice.

In the 4 years since the first edition of this book was published, I have received numerous messages from readers discussing various aspects of the book. I have also built up ideas based on my experiences in reading, writing, and editing. With the aid of all this information all chapters have been thoroughly revised and updated. The most obvious change in the current edition is addition of six new chapters.

New chapters added:
1. *Medicolegal Aspects of Discharge against Medical Advice*
2. *Violence against Doctors and Hospitals*
3. *Patient Safety and Risk Management in Healthcare*
4. *Healthcare Associated Infections: A Preventable Threat to Patient Safety*
5. *Communication Skills in Healthcare: A Tool to ensure Patient Satisfaction*
6. *Documentation in Healthcare: Standards and Guidelines*

I express my gratitude to all the contributors and to the publisher for their support. I am also grateful to all our readers for placing their reliance on us and for sharing our optimism. Feedback and suggestions from the esteemed readers are welcome.

VP Singh
MD (Forensic Medicine) LLB

Preface to the First Edition

"The illiterate of 21st century will not be those who cannot read and write, but those who cannot learn, unlearn and relearn"
—**Alvin Toffler**

In the modern world of consumerism, the status of a physician has changed from savior to service provider. The privilege of being a physician has bestowed more liabilities than immunity. Providing best possible care to the patient is not enough. Physicians must regain the faith of their patients, without whom they could never transform from a disciple to a master of the noble medical profession.

Medical laws have emerged as a vast specialization that regulates the practice of medicine. A physician, ignorant toward the medical laws is an illiterate in the eyes of law, though he may be the master in his profession. Quality healthcare is incomplete without adapting to the legal principles. A physician must always be willing to *learn, unlearn* and *relearn*.

For a busy medical practitioner, who finds legal language to be perplexing, *Legal Issues in Medical Practice: Medicolegal Guidelines for Safe Practice* is a humble presentation of the medicolegal principles in a lucid and easily understandable language. The book has thoroughly discussed all essential medicolegal issues and has provided the evidence-based guiding principles to tackle the actual medicolegal issues. This authoritative treatise is written by 38 distinguished experts who are authorities in their fields of specialization. I am confident that medical practitioners will find this book useful to prevent as well as solve the medicolegal conflicts.

I express my gratitude to all the authors and to the publisher for their cooperation. I am also grateful to all our readers for placing their reliance on us and for sharing our optimism. Feedback and suggestions from the esteemed readers is welcome, and will be a boon to further improve the quality of this treatise.

VP Singh

Contents

Section 1: Ethics in Healthcare: The Guiding Values!

1. **The Ethics of Medical Practice** 3
   VP Singh, Parmod Goyal
   Medical Ethics 3
   Autonomy 4
   Beneficence 4
   Nonmaleficence 4
   - Conflict Between Autonomy and Beneficence/Nonmaleficence 5
   - Justice 5
   - Paternalism versus Autonomy: What Serves the Patient Best? 5
   - Does Paternalism Really Serve the Purpose? 6
   - Changing Ethos: Paternalism to Patient Autonomy 6
   - Should Physicians do Whatever Patients say? 7
   - What Serves the Patient Best? 7
   - Ethical Guidelines for Medical Practitioners 8

   Indian Medical Council (Professional conduct, Etiquette and Ethics) Regulations 8
   - Chapter 1: Code of Medical Ethics 8
   - Chapter 2: Duties of Physicians to their Patients 9
   - Chapter 3: Duties of Physician in Consultation 10
   - Chapter 4: Responsibilities of Physicians to Each Other 10
   - Chapter 5: Duties of Physician to Public and Paramedical Profession 11
   - Chapter 6: Unethical Acts 11
   - Chapter 7: Misconduct 14
   - Chapter 8: Punishment and Disciplinary Action 16

2. **Confidentiality and Disclosure in Medical Practice** 18
   VP Singh, Akashdeep Aggarwal
   When Confidentiality may be Breached? 19
   - Legal Requirement/Administration of Justice 19

   Guidelines on Medical Confidentiality 20
   - Medical Council of India Regulations 20
   - Right to Information Act and Medical Confidentiality 21
   - RTI and Medicolegal Cases 22
   - Medical Confidentiality and HIV Status 23
   - NACO Guidelines on Confidentiality in HIV-positive Individuals Operational Guidelines for ICTCs: (July 2007) 23
   - Guidelines on HIV Testing (March 2007) 24
   - Judicial Decisions on Medical Confidentiality and HIV Status 25
   - Mandatory HIV Screening 25
   - HIV Testing of Patients Prior to Surgery 25

Section 2: Medicolegal Menace: Let's Face The Truth, Now!

3. Disclosing Medical Errors: Why, When and How? 31
VP Singh, Gautam Biswas
Medical Errors *31*
Disclosure of Medical Errors *32*
   How did it Start? *32*
   Ethics, Law and Policy *33*
Consequences of Disclosing Medical Errors *33*
   Benefits of Disclosure to the Patient *33*
   Harms of Disclosure to the Patient *34*
   Harms of Disclosure to the Medical Practitioner *34*
   Benefits of Disclosure to the Medical Practitioner *34*
Guidelines on Disclosing Medical Errors *34*
   How to Handle Medical Errors in Practice? *34*
   When Disclosure should Take Place? *35*
   Timing of Disclosure *35*
   Stages of Disclosure *35*
   What to Say? *36*

4. End of Life Care Decisions: Ethical and Legal Issues 40
Rashmi Datta, Pradeep Sreevastava, Arvind Kumar Singh
Palliative Care at the End of Life *40*
Magnitude of the Problem *41*
Medical Futility *41*
Withholding or Withdrawal of Life Support *43*
Advanced Directives and Do-not-resuscitate Orders *43*
Euthanasia *44*
   Active Euthanasia *44*
   Passive Euthanasia *44*
   Voluntary Euthanasia *44*
   Nonvoluntary Euthanasia *44*
Implications to Human Organ
Transplantation Act *45*
   Legal Aspects of End of Life Issues in India *45*

5. Medicolegal Aspects of Discharge Against Medical Advice 49
Krishnadutt H Chavali, Swapnil S Agarwal, VP Singh
How Prevalent is Dama? *49*
Causes and Predictors of Dama *50*
   Why Patients Leave Against Medical Advice? *50*
   Who is at Risk of DAMA? *50*
Legal Status of DAMA *51*
   Dissolution of the Therapeutic Relationship *51*
   Is there any Protection Against Future Litigation? *51*
   Validity of DAMA *52*
   Duty of Doctor in DAMA *52*
Consequences of DAMA *52*
   Risk to the Patient *52*
   Risk to the Doctor/Hospital *53*

    Managing DAMA: A Practical Approach *54*
        Assess Decision-making Capacity 54
        If Patient Lacks Capacity 54

6. **Violence Against Doctors: Causes, Effects, and Solutions**   60
    Sundeep Mishra
    Definition *61*
    Factors Predisposing to Violence *61*
    Situation Unique to India *62*
    What Leads to Violence by Attendants/Relatives? *62*
        Physician Related Factors 62
        Patient Related Factors 62
        Hospital Related Factors 63
        Role of Community 63
        Role of Media 64
    How to Anticipate Violence in Healthcare Setting? *64*
    Managing Violence in Healthcare Setting *65*
        At the Time of Violence 65
    Preventing Violence in Healthcare Setting *65*
        Preventive Tips for the Physicians 65
        Preventive Tips for the Hospital Administrators 67
    Strong and Effective Laws: Essential in Fight Against Violence *67*
        Strengthening the Law Against Violence 67
        Implementation of Effective Laws 69
        Role of Media in Preventing Violence 69
        Health Related Literacy 69
        Insurance Schemes 69

Section 3: Patient Safety Initiatives: A Key to Medicolegal Safety

7. **Patient Safety and Risk Management**   73
    Sameer Mehta
    Strategies for Safety in Healthcare *74*
        Emergency Care and Patient Safety 74
        Possible Solutions 74
    Radiology and Imaging *75*
    Counseling Rooms—Informed Consent *76*
    Isolation Rooms *77*
    Medical Records *77*
    Patient Accessibility *78*
    Patient Handling and Movement Assessment *79*
    Infection Control *79*
        Monitoring Differential Pressure 81
    Medical Gases *82*
        Safety Measures Related to Medical Gases 82
        Storage of Cylinders 83
    Smart Hospitals *83*
    Risk Management *83*
        The Process of Risk Management 83

8. **Healthcare-associated Infections: A Threat to Patient Safety** 87
   Rahul S Kamble
   What is Healthcare-associated Infection? *88*
      What are the Sources of Healthcare-associated Infections? *88*
      Important Facts Related to Healthcare-associated Infection *88*
      Which Infections are not Healthcare-associated *89*
      Common Healthcare-associated Infections *89*
      Ventilator-associated Condition *90*
   Transmission of Infection *91*
      Source of Microorganisms *91*
      Susceptible Host *91*
      Means of Transmission *92*
   The Burden of Hospital-acquired Infection *92*
   Preventing Hospital-acquired Infection *92*
   Infection Prevention Initiatives *94*
      Recommendations by Agency for Healthcare Research and Quality *94*
      Initiative by the World Health Organization *94*
      The Joint Commission's National Patient Safety Goals *94*
      Active Surveillance Culture *95*
   Indicators of Healthcare-associated Infections *96*
   Management of Healthcare-associated Infections *97*
      Strategies for Management of Healthcare-associated Infections *97*
      Principles of Empiric Therapy *97*
      Specific Empiric Situations *97*
      Initial Antibiotic Therapy *97*
      Therapeutic Strategies of Documented Healthcare-associated Infections *97*
      Gram-negative Organisms *98*
      Gram-positive Organisms *98*
   Newer Research Related to Healthcare-associated Infection *98*
   Medicolegal Aspects Related to Healthcare-associated Infection *99*
      All Healthcare-associated Infections are not Preventable! *100*
   Medical Negligence Cases Related to Healthcare-associated Infection *101*
      Case 1: Patient Suffered Hepatitis C Infection *101*
      Case 2: Patients Lost Vision due to Eye Infection *102*
   Legal Provisions Applicable to Healthcare-associated Infection *103*
      Section 304A IPC (Causing Death by Negligence) *103*
      Section 337 IPC (Causing Hurt by Act Endangering Life or Personal Safety of Others) *103*
      Section 338 IPC (Causing Grievous Hurt by Act Endangering Life or Personal Safety of Others) *104*
      Section 269 IPC (Negligent Act Likely to Spread Infection of Disease Dangerous to Life) *104*
      Section 270 IPC (Malignant Act Likely to Spread Infection of Disease Dangerous to Life) *104*

9. **Communication Skills in Healthcare: A Tool to Ensure Patient Satisfaction** 107
   Archana Kumari, Piyush Ranjan
   What is Communication *108*
      Types of Communication *108*
   Communication in Healthcare *109*
      Importance of Communication Skills for Doctors *109*
   Basic Principles of Good Communication *110*
   Tips for Good Communication in OPD Setting *110*
      The Medical Interview with Patient *110*

Tips for Good Communication in an Indoor and ICU Setting *111*
    Communicating with the Attendants 111
Barriers to Communication *113*
Consequences of Ineffective Communication *113*
How to Assess the Communication Skills of Healthcare Workers? *114*
Breaking Bad News *114*
Teaching Communication Skills and Medical Curriculum *115*
    AETCOM: An Initiative by Medical Council of India 115

Section 4: Medical Records: A Double-edged Sword

10. Medicolegal Aspects of Informed Consent   121
VP Singh, Dasari Harish
Evolution *122*
    Judicial Decisions Introducing the Concept of Informed Consent 122
Objectives *123*
Meaning *123*
    Implied Consent 124
    Express Consent 124
What makes the Consent Legally Acceptable? *124*
    Conditions for a Valid Consent 125
    Age for Consent 125
    Duty to Warn a 'Material Risk' 127
Exceptions *128*
Obtaining Consent: The Procedure *128*
    Documentation of Informed Consent 128
Judicial Decision on Informed Consent *129*
    Samira Kohli Case: Landmark Judgment on Informed Consent 129
    Extracts from the Supreme Court's Judgment (Samira Kohli's Case) 129

11. Medicolegal Aspects of Medical Records   132
Joseph Thomas, Arun Mavaji Seetharam, Rajesh Kumar Sinha
Component of Medical Records *132*
Electronic Health Records: An Emerging Trend In India *133*
    Ownership of Data 134
    Data Access and Confidentiality 134
    Electronic Health Records Preservation 134
    Data Privacy and Security 134
Confidentiality of Medical Records *135*
Categories of Medical Records *135*
Guidelines on Medical Record *136*
    Medical Council of India Guidelines 136
    NABH Guidelines 136
Medicolegal Aspects of Medical Records *141*
    Preservation of Records 141
    Ownership of Medical Records 142
    Summoning Medical Records by Courts 142
Judicial Decisions Related to Medical Records *143*

12. **Documentation in Healthcare: Standards and Guidelines**   145
    Utsav Parekh
    Medical Documentation *145*
       Documentation not Directly Related to the Patient *146*
    Legal Importance of Documentation *146*
       Key Role in Litigation Process *146*
       Standard of "Continuum of Care" *146*
       Regulation Governing Medical Records *147*
       Cases Compelling Medical Documents *147*
    Benefits of Good Quality Documentation *147*
    Errors in Documentation *148*
       Vacuum in Clinical Documentation *148*
       Failing to Write a Complete Note *148*
       Failing to be Concise *149*
       Illegible Medical Documentation *149*
       Medical Council of India Guidelines on Prescription Writing *150*
       Use of Unsafe Abbreviations *150*
    Clinical Documentation Guidelines *150*
       Guiding Principle 1: Comprehensive and Complete Record *151*
       Guiding Principle 2: Patient Centered and Collaborative *151*
       Guiding Principle 3: Ensure and Maintain Confidentiality *152*
    Key Points for Good Medical Documentation *152*
    Critical Issues in Medical Documentation *154*
       Discharge Notes *154*
       Written Feedback from Patient/Attendants *155*
       Issuing Medical Certificate *155*
       Documenting Adverse Events *155*
       Documenting Instructions to the Patient *157*
       Documenting Patient's Refusal *157*

Section 5: Litigation Against Medical Practitioners: Let's Take the Bull by the Horns

13. **Medical Negligence: Meaning, Scope and Legal Interpretation**   161
    VP Singh, Vivekanshu Verma
    What is Medical Negligence? *161*
    Essential Components of Medical Negligence *161*
       Duty of Care *162*
       Dereliction in Duty of Care *162*
       Damage *163*
       Direct Causation *163*
    Types of Medical Negligence *163*
       Medical Negligence as a Tort *163*
       Medical Negligence as a Crime *163*
       Negligence Per Se *164*
    Vital Issues in Medical Negligence *164*
       Burden of Proof of Medical Negligence *164*
       Reasonable Care *166*
    Criminal Liability of Medical Professionals *167*
       Guidelines: Prosecution of Doctors for Criminal Rashness or Criminal Negligence *167*

14. **How to Defend a Medical Negligence Lawsuit?**   169
    VP Singh, MC Gupta
    Pattern of Complaints Against Medical Practitioners *169*
    Complaints under Consumer Protection Act: Step-by-step Approach *170*
      The Complaint *170*
      Inform the Insurance Company *170*
      Selection of Defence Lawyer *170*
      Preparing the Written Statement *171*
      Rejoinder and Affidavits *171*
      Examination of Witnesses *172*
      Arguments *172*
      The Order *172*
      Appeal *172*
    Facing the Court: Medicolegal Tips and Advice *173*
      Avoid Talking to the Complainant or his Advocate *173*
      Avoid Fingerpointing *173*
      Avoid Alteration or Destruction of Medical Records *173*
      Appearing in a Criminal Case *173*

15. **Compensation in Medical Negligence: How much is Justified?**   176
    VP Singh, Mukesh Yadav
    Compensation in Medical Negligence *176*
      Multiplier Method: Can it be Used in Medical Negligence Cases? *177*
      Multiplier's Method is not Applicable in Medical Negligence Cases *178*
    How much Compensation is Just and Adequate? *179*
    Impact of High Quantum of Compensation *180*
    Medical Liability—A Future Crisis: Learning from the Other Countries *180*
      The Crisis *180*
    Crisis Reform Models *181*
      Caps on Noneconomic Damages *181*
      No-fault Compensation *182*
      Health Courts *182*

16. **Professional Indemnity Insurance: Better Safe than Sorry**   185
    Rajendra S Bangal
    Professional Indemnity Insurance *185*
      What does it Cover? *186*
      What it does not Cover? *186*
      Factors Influencing the Amount of Insurance *187*
    Some Important Information *188*
      AOO: AOY Ratio *188*
      Premium Rates (Individuals) *189*
      Premium Rates (Clinical Establishments) *189*
    Retroactive Date *189*
      An Ideal Indemnity Insurance Policy: Proposed Components *190*

Section 6: Medical Laws and Judgments: A Ray of Hope!

17. Landmark Judgments Related to Medical Professionals — 195
VP Singh, Krishnadutt Chavali
Dr Suresh Gupta's Case *195*
   Facts of the Case *195*
   Patient's Allegation *196*
   Doctor's Defence *196*
   Relevant Sections of Indian Penal Code *196*
   Findings of the Court *197*
   Supreme Court's Observation on Criminal Negligence *197*
Jacob Mathew's Case *198*
   Facts of the Case *198*
   Patient's Allegation *198*
   Doctor's Defence *198*
   Findings of the Court *198*
Supreme Court's Observation on Negligence *199*
   Negligence as a Tort *199*
   Negligence as a Tort and as a Crime *199*
   Negligence by Professionals *199*
   Standard of Care Required by a Medical Practitioner *200*
Martin D'Souza's Case *200*
   Facts of the Case *200*
   Patient's Allegation *201*
   Doctor's Defence *201*
   Findings of the Court *201*
   Supreme Court's Observation *201*
V Kishan Rao's Case *202*
   Facts of the Case *202*
   Patient's Allegation *202*
   Doctor's Defence *202*
   Findings of the Court *202*
   Supreme Court's Observation on Expert Medical Opinion *203*
   Supreme Court's Observation on Martin D'Souza's Case *203*

18. Medicolegal Outlook on Transplantation of Human Organs Act — 204
Sunil Shroff, Sumana Navin, Hemal Kanvinde, Sujatha Niranjan, Christopher Barry
Transplantation of Human Organs and Tissues Rules 2014 *204*
   Medicolegal Aspects of Living Donation and Transplantation *207*
   Medicolegal Aspects of Deceased Organ Donation and Transplantation *208*
Future Challenges *209*

19. Medicolegal Outlook on Bio-Medical Waste Management Act — 212
VP Singh, Pardeep Singh
Bio-medical Waste *212*
Law on Bio-medical Waste Management *213*
Bio-medical Waste Management Rules, 2016 *213*
   Application of the Rules *213*
   Important Definitions *214*
   Duty of an Occupier *214*
   Prescribed Authority *216*

Procedure for Authorization *216*
　　　Advisory Committee *216*
　　　Monitoring of Implementation of the Rules in Healthcare Facilities *217*
　　　Annual Report *218*
　　　Appeal *218*
　　　Liability of the Occupier, Operator of a Facility *218*
　　　Treatment and Disposal *218*
　　　Segregation, Packaging, Transportation, and Storage *218*
　　Salient Features of Bio-medical Waste Rules 2016 *222*
　　　Name of the Rules *222*
　　　The Categories of Bio-medical Waste *223*
　　　Widened Scope of the Rules *223*
　　　The Authorization *223*
　　　Duties and Responsibilities *223*
　　　Phasing out the Use of Chlorinated Plastic Bags *223*
　　　Tracking the Bio-medical Waste Bags *223*
　　　Newer Technologies Incorporated *224*
　　　Occupational Safety of Healthcare Workers *225*
　　　Records of the Bio-medical Waste *225*
　　Penalties Under the Environment Protection Act *225*
　　　Penalties for Offences *225*
　　　Who can File a Complaint Under the Act? *225*
　　　If the Violation is also an Offence Under any Other Legislation *226*

20. **Medicolegal Outlook on PC-PNDT Act**   227
　　Chandrashekhar A Sohoni
　　Preconception and Prenatal Diagnostic Techniques Act in a Nutshell *227*
　　　Registration of Ultrasound Machine *227*
　　　Record Keeping *228*
　　　Monitoring and Implementation *229*
　　　Offences and Penalties *230*
　　　PC-PNDT Act–Controversies and Practical Difficulties: Safety Measures to be taken by the Doctors *230*

Section 7: Medicolegal Issues in Various Specialties: Eagle's Eye and Lion's Heart!

21. **Medicolegal Issues in Obstetrics and Gynecology**   239
　　Charu Mittal, PS Mittal
　　Medicolegal Issues in Obstetrics *240*
　　　Obstetric Cases Vulnerable to Malpractice Lawsuits *240*
　　　Errors in Antenatal Care: Medical and Legal Implications *241*
　　　Wrongful Birth *241*
　　　Wrongful Life *241*
　　　Wrongful Conception *242*
　　　Wrongful Death *242*
　　　Ectopic Pregnancy *242*
　　　Premature Baby *242*
　　　High-risk Pregnancy *243*
　　　Medical Disorders in Pregnancy *243*
　　　Cesarean Section *243*

       Vaginal Birth After Cesarean 243
       Intrauterine Fetal Death/Stillbirths 243
       Ultrasonography in Obstetrics: Legal Issues 244
       Obstetric Anesthesia 244
   Medicolegal Issues in Gynecology 245
   Medicolegal Issues in Perioperative Patient Care 245
       Hysterectomy 245
       Retained Surgical Objects 246
       Sterilization/Family Planning Operation 247
   Surgical Complications: Medical and Legal implications 248
       Role of Consent 248
   Specialist as an Expert Witness in a Court of Law 248
   General Precautions During Day-to-day Practice: Avoiding Malpractice Lawsuits 249

22. **Medicolegal Issues in Surgery**   **252**
   Manu Shankar
   Preoperative Period in Surgery 253
       Document Preoperative Status 253
       Document the Shared Decision Making Process 253
       Involve Other Specialties 253
       Give Sufficient Time to Patient 254
   Peroperative Period 254
       Unexpected Peroperative Findings 254
       Deviation from Planned Surgery 254
       Need to Call Other Specialists During Surgery 255
   Postoperative Period 255
       Postoperative Complications 255
       Repeat Surgery 255
   Consent in Surgery 256
   Role of Anesthesia 256
   Surgical Complications 256
   'Never Events' in Surgery 258
       Retained Surgical Items 258
       Wrong Site Surgery 258
   Take Home Message for the Surgeons 259

23. **Medicolegal Issues in Orthopedics**   **261**
   VJ Purushotham
   Medicolegal Risks in Orthopedics 262
       Morbid Results are Easily Noticeable 262
       Lack of Proper Rapport with the Patients 262
       Scope of Consent in Orthopedics 263
       Reasons of Litigation Against Orthopedic Surgeons 263
       Wrong-site Surgery 264
   Tips on Preventing Medicolegal Conflicts 265
       Good Communication and Rapport 265
       Documentation and Informed Consent 265
       Advocating Treatment Options 266
       Avoid Medical Jousting Please! 266

      Practice Evidence-based Orthopedics *266*
      Safe Operation Theater Setup *266*
  Orthopedist in the Court of Law *267*

24. Medicolegal Issues in Ophthalmology   269
Dinesh Verma, Amandeep Singh

  Vulnerable Domains in Ophthalmic Practice *270*
      Laser Assisted In Situ Keratomileusis Complications
      (Suboptimal Visual Outcome) *270*
      Cataract Surgery *271*
      Ocular Trauma *272*
      Retinal Conditions *272*
      Missing Serious Systemic Diseases *273*
      Organ Donation *273*
  Managing the Risk of Lawsuits *274*

25. Medicolegal Issues in Pediatrics   277
Yogesh dave

    Who is a Child? *277*
    Who is a Pediatrician? *278*
    Why Study Medicolegal Issues in Pediatrics? *278*
    Informed Consent in Pediatrics *278*
    Age for Consent in Pediatrics *279*
    Error in Diagnosis During Emergencies *280*
    Avoidable Surgeries *280*
    Patient Safety in Pediatrics *280*
    Neonatal Intensive Care: Vulnerable to Malpractice Lawsuits *281*
    Parental Refusal to Medical Treatment *282*
    Communication Skills—Key Role in Pediatrics *282*
    Legal Risks of Ineffective Communication *283*
    Communicate Well with Children and Families *283*

26. Medicolegal Issues in Radiology   285
Chandrashekhar A Sohoni

  Why Radiology is Vulnerable to Medicolegal Conflicts? *287*
      Nature of the Specialty *287*
      Radiological Opinion as 'Written and Signed' Document *287*
      Commercialization of Healthcare *287*
      Unclear Baseline for Standard of Practice *287*
      Expectation vis-à-vis Performance: A Mismatch *288*
      Emotional Facet of the Disease *288*
      Ignorance About the 'Diagnostic' Limitations of Radiology *288*
      Easy to Accept Cause-effect Relationship *289*
      Judicial Decisions on Radiological Errors *289*
  Avoiding Litigation in Radiology *290*
      Being Alert *290*
      Communication with the Referring Doctor and the Patient *290*
      Role of Informed Consent *291*
      Publishing Diagnostic Errors Regularly *291*
      Errors in Radiology: The Way Ahead *291*

27. **Medicolegal Issues in Blood Transfusion Practice**   294
Ranabir Pal, Amrita Ghosh, Debashis Sinha, Shrayan Pal
- Current Scenario in India *295*
  - National Blood Policy *295*
- Scenario of Legal Framework *295*
  - Drugs and Cosmetics Rules *296*
- Medicolegal Aspects *297*
  - Façade of Non-remunerated Blood Donation *297*
  - Code of Ethics Relating to Transfusion Medicine *298*
  - Ethical Principles Relating to Patients *298*
  - Ethical Principles Relating to Donors *299*
  - Stewardship of Blood Supply *299*
  - The Informed Consent in Blood Donation *301*
  - Challenges of Blood Screening *301*
  - Donor Screening: A Concept to be Conceptualized *302*
  - Who will Bell the Cat? *303*
- Alternatives to Blood Transfusion: Newer Research *303*
  - Stem Cell-derived Blood Cells *303*
  - Placental Umbilical Cord Blood Transfusion *303*
- Blood Transfusion Safety *304*
  - WHO Recommendation for Blood Safety and Availability *304*
  - Guidelines for Administration of Blood and Blood Components *304*
  - Training and Competency Assessment *306*
- Adverse Effects of Transfusion *308*
  - Noninfectious Hazards of Transfusion *308*
  - Infectious Hazards of Transfusion *309*
- Documentation of Blood Transfusion Practice *309*
  - Blood Collection Records *309*
  - Laboratory Records *309*
  - Blood Issue and Usage Records *310*
  - Storage of Records *310*
  - Disposal of Records *310*
- Clinician's Guidelines in Case the Patient Needs Transfusion *310*
  - Collecting Blood Prior to Transfusion *311*
  - Storing Blood Products Prior to Transfusion *311*
  - Administering Blood *311*
  - Checking the Blood Pack *312*
  - The Final Patient Identity Check *312*
  - Documenting the Transfusion Process *312*
  - Transfusion Reactions: What Every Physician Should Know *313*
- Litigation Related to Blood Transfusion Practice *313*
  - HIV Infection by Blood Transfusion *313*
  - Wrong Blood Group Transfusion *314*
- Take Home Message *314*
- World Blood Donor Day, 14th June 2018 *315*

28. **Medicolegal Issues in Dentistry**   319
Shilpa Pharande
- Medicolegal Aspects of Dental Practice *319*
  - Temporomandibular Disorders *319*
  - Root Resorption *320*

Medical Emergencies in Dentistry 320
    Inhalation/Ingestion of Foreign Objects 320
    Incidental Findings on Pretreatment Screening 321
    Diagnosis of Malignancy in Dentistry 321
    Esthetic Dentistry 322
    Negligence in Dentistry 322
    'No Negligence' Occasions in Dental Practice 323
  Protection Against Litigation 323
  How to Avoid Litigation? 324
    Steps at Personal Level 324
    Interpersonal Behavior 324
    Academic and Technical Update 324
    Awareness of Medical Laws 325
    Reasonable Skills and Care 325

29. **Medicolegal Issues in Anesthesiology** 328
  Manpreet Singh, Ajay Kumar, Lakesh Anand
  Standard of Care 328
  Duty of Care and Liability 329
  Medicolegal Issues in Anesthesiology 329
    Death on Operation Table 329
    Witnessed Death on Operation Table: Recommendations for Doctors 329
    Anesthesia Deaths 331
    Awareness During Anesthesia 331
  Error of Judgment 333
  Mistake 333
  Burden of Proof 334
  Res Ipsa Loquitur 334
  How to Decrease the Likelihood of a Lawsuit? 335
  Accepted Practices and Procedures 336
  Accidents, Misadventures, and Mishaps 336
  Inherent Risks 336
  Choice of Treatment 337
  Keeping the Professional Knowledge and Skill up-to-date 337
  Cases to Observe 337

Index 341

SECTION 1
Ethics in Healthcare: The Guiding Values!

Chapter 1 The Ethics of Medical Practice
Chapter 2 Confidentiality and Disclosure in Medical Practice

CHAPTER 1

The Ethics of Medical Practice

VP Singh, Parmod Goyal

"Justice consists not in being neutral between right and wrong, but in finding out the right and upholding it, wherever found, against the wrong."
—Theodore Roosevelt[1]

■ INTRODUCTION

Medicine is a profession that incorporates science and technology for caring the sick. In twentieth century with advancement in medical science, patient care has become more effective with better medications having fewer side effects. Surgery has moved towards less invasive modes of management, with lesser morbidity and faster recovery. With so much advancement in the field of *medicine*, the medical fraternity is becoming dependent on technology. Market forces also tend to influence decision making by the doctors. Amidst all these developments, the medical practitioners often face ethical and legal challenges in their clinical practice. Keeping in mind the recent trends of medicolegal issues, the importance of ethical standards in practice of medicine becomes even more relevant.

■ MEDICAL ETHICS

Medical ethics is a system of moral principles that apply values and judgments to the practice of medicine. It guides the medical practitioners in their behavior and decision making related to their relationship with patients, colleagues and society. A physician is expected to be compassionate towards his patient, willing to take time to explain all the aspects of illness. The fundamental values of medicine insist that every physician has an obligation to keep the patient's interest above everything else. The basic principles of medical ethics that guide the medical practitioners in clinical decision making are:
- Autonomy
- Beneficence
- Nonmaleficence
- Justice.[2]

■ AUTONOMY

Autonomy literally described as self-rule, is the principle that recognizes the rights of individuals to self-determination. In medical profession, respecting the patient's autonomy requires the medical practitioners to give full information and get permission before doing anything to the patient, i.e., *informed consent* prior to treatment. Apart from ethical concerns, informed consent is also a legal duty. Another implication of respecting the patient's autonomy is *medical confidentiality*. Medical practitioner impliedly promises his patients that he will keep confidential the information confided to him. Keeping promises is a way of respecting people's autonomy. Every effort should be made to ensure that confidentiality is maintained. However, in medical practice absolute confidentiality cannot exist. Often, it becomes necessary to share patient's information with other healthcare providers, so as to provide appropriate patient care. In healthcare system, safeguarding confidentiality is far more challenging. With the advent of electronic health records, the risk of misuse of patient's confidential information has increased manifold. While discussing the patient's condition at the bedside where other patients are also present, confidentiality is not protected. There are occasions when law mandates disclosure of the confidential information, like informing to the police about medicolegal cases, reporting certain notifiable diseases, disclosing professional secrets to the court if asked to do so. While treating the patients suffering from mental illness, physician has a duty to disclose and warn others if the patient threatens to be violent.

Respect for patient's autonomy obligates the physicians not to deceive patients, and tell the truth about their diagnosed illness, unless they clearly wish not to be told about the illness. In the practice of medicine, sometimes there are situations where telling the absolute truth may not be the best option. Medical professionals often have to give bad news of poor prognosis or impending death to the patients. They should weigh the benefit against the detriment before disclosing the truth as it may be more ethical to withhold the truth partially for the time being and disclose it in bits over time to avoid overwhelming the patient or relatives. In medical practice, there are situations that challenge the principle of autonomy and create ethical dilemmas in decision making.

■ BENEFICENCE

Beneficence refers to the actions that promote wellbeing of others. It is the moral obligation to do good for others and to help them in active way. In medical practice, it means taking actions that are beneficial to the patients based on the patient's point of view as well.

■ NONMALEFICENCE

Nonmaleficence is a concept of *not causing harm* to others. This principle is well expressed in the Latin phrase, *primum non nocere* which means *first do no harm*.[3] It is not enough to just prevent intentional harm, but, one must be appropriately cautious not to cause harm. In the practice of medicine, however, almost all treatments carry some risk of harm. It is important to know how likely it is, that the proposed treatment will cause harm to the patient. This needs empirical information from the reliable medical research about the probabilities of various harms and benefits possible with the proposed intervention. This concept also explains the need for practicing 'evidence based medicine'. The obligation to provide net benefit over harm requires the medical professionals to be clear about the risks present and their probability, when they make assessments of benefit over harm. The medical practitioner, must therefore, consider the principles of beneficence and non-maleficence together and try to produce net benefit over harm. A single action may have combined implications of beneficence and nonmaleficence, which in medical ethics is referred to as *double effect*. A classic example of the double effect is administration of high dose of morphine to relieve pain in a patient suffering from advanced stage of malignancy. Such an act has combined effect of beneficence (relieving the pain) and maleficence (respiratory suppression leading to death of the patient).

Conflict Between Autonomy and Beneficence/Nonmaleficence

Sometimes the patient may disagree with the proposed treatment, which the physician believes to be the best for the patient, on the basis of medical literature. This usually occurs when patient's interest clashes with patient's welfare leading to conflict between the principles of autonomy and beneficence. For example, a Jehovah patient may refuse blood transfusion due to religious or cultural views. Also, the patient may want unnecessary treatment which may cause medically unnecessary potential risks as in case of hypochondria or cosmetic surgery. In such ethical dilemmas, usually the physician, just to nurture healthy physician-patient relationship, submits to the principle of autonomy and acts as per the patient's desires. In such a situation, the physician must do his best efforts to balance the patient's welfare with interest. In such cases, if complication/undesired outcome occurs, the chances of allegation of medical malpractice is higher and it is far more challenging for the treating medical professional to defend his actions. He must get the written informed consent signed by the patient; documenting in detail the treatment to be followed and the probability of risks involved.

Justice

Justice is the moral obligation to act on the basis of fairness. In simplistic sense, justice refers to equality. However, it does not mean treating all individuals the same. It is important to treat equals equally and to treat unequals unequally, in proportion to their morally relevant inequalities. Medical practitioner must recognize the competing moral concerns and take fair decisions. In the context of healthcare resources, justice requires providing sufficient healthcare to meet the needs of all who need it and if this is impossible, to provide healthcare resources in proportion to the extent of individual's need for healthcare.

Paternalism versus Autonomy: What Serves the Patient Best?

Paternalism

Paternalism comes from the Latin word, *pater* which means *to act like a father* or to *treat another person like a child*. Paternalism propounds that someone can better protect the interests of others, based on the value that *father knows what is best for the children*. Paternalism has a long history in the medical profession. From the days when the *Hippocratic* principles were developed, the physician has been recognized as a guardian who uses his specialized knowledge and experience to decide the patient's benefit. The primary theory behind the *Hippocratic Oath* is the principle of beneficence which clearly reflects in the original oath as the resolve to serve 'for the benefit of the sick, according to the physician's ability and judgment'. The relation between physician and the patient resembled that between a caring father and his child, hence the term *paternalism*. Such father-child relationship stood firm and unchallenged for centuries. Until much of the twentieth century, the society acknowledged that the physicians were in the best position to make medical decisions on behalf of the patients.

Does Paternalism Really Serve the Purpose?

Medical ethics obligates the medical practitioner to do what is in the best interest of the patient? The real challenge is the interpretation: *What is the best interest of the patient?* In patient-physician interaction, there is asymmetric information, as the physician has access to technical knowledge and skill which the patient lacks, and the patient has access to personal preferences that are at times difficult to express. This bifocal vision may result in different perceptions and the physician's opinion may not coincide with the patient's view. The physician's efforts to do the best for the patient may advertently or inadvertently disregard the patient's wishes.

When the patient is not in a position to act voluntarily or autonomously, the paternalistic approach to prevent the patient from doing harm to himself, seems justified. For instance, emergency treatment to save the life of a dying patient at the critical time when there is no time to wait for patient's autonomy, termed as *weak paternalism*, might be morally justified. On the other hand, *strong paternalism*, which overrides the clearly voluntary action, is difficult to justify.

Paternalism is argued on the notion that, 'It is the patient's life or health which is at stake, not the physician's...so it must be the patient, not the physician, who must be allowed to decide whether the game is worth the candle."[4] John Stuart Mill, a British philosopher expressed that a competent person's freely made decision should never be over-ridden, even for that person's own good. He wrote: *"The only purpose for which power can be rightfully exercised over any member of a civilized community, against his will, is to prevent harm to others. His own good, either physical or moral, is not a sufficient warrant. He cannot rightfully be compelled to do or forbear because it will be better for him to do so, because it will make him happier, because in the opinion of others, to do so would be wise or even right."*[5]

Changing Ethos: Paternalism to Patient Autonomy

The paternalistic philosophy has a long history from the time of Hippocrates well into the twentieth century until 1960s. After this long era of unchallenged and well accepted paternalism, tremendous changes occurred that transformed the predominantly paternalistic ideology: Doctor knows the best to patient autonomy or self-determination. In present era, the medical paternalism has come under criticism through the concept of patient's authority to take decision on his medical needs. The concept of patient autonomy or self-determination has emerged as dominant ethos in the medical practice.[6] While taking the medical decisions; it requires that medical benefits be weighed, not only against medical risks, but nonmedical values as well. For illustration, a medical decision that advises a couple to refrain from reproduction due to the genetic risks they may face in having children, has not addressed the ethical issue from the couple's perspective. In such a situation patient autonomy empowers the couple, after receiving all the necessary medical information, to take the final decision to have their children or not.

Supporters of paternalism may criticize that, offering full information and allowing patients to take crucial medical decisions may lead to unwise and irrational decisions even by technically competent patients. However, this criticism does not offer any explanation, why a person is presumed as requiring protection from his so called unwise decisions once they become medical patients, and yet are otherwise thought entitled to take decisions outside the medical set-up (like choosing a life partner, selecting a career). There are situations that challenge the principle of pure autonomy and make it complicated to follow on a consistent basis. For example, children, mentally incapacitated patients and patients who are otherwise incompetent to take decisions will be unable to exercise autonomy.

Should Physicians do Whatever Patients say?[7,8]

The principles of autonomy providing moral right to the patients to control their own treatment, may be conceived as imparting obligation to the physicians to respect the medical decisions of their patients. Does that mean, physicians have an obligation to do whatever patients say? Nonetheless, a physician should keep in mind that the obligation towards patient's decisions is not absolute as the same is to be weighed upon with other ethical values deserving commitment from the physician. Physicians are bound by their obligation to the medical profession which may supersede the duty to respect patient's choice. For example, patient's wish to be helped to die cannot be fulfilled as it violates the values of medical profession. A more challenging situation may arise when a dying patient (or his family) asks for continuing treatment which is futile as per physician's opinion. In continuing treatment that will do no good to the patient may be viewed as contrary to the values of medical profession particularly in the backdrop of limited resources and does not obligate the physician to respect the patient's wishes. Obligation to practice patient autonomy cannot be taken as simplistic directive to comply with all the expressed wishes of the patient, as the same may come into conflict with other moral values of the medical values.

What Serves the Patient Best?[9,10]

Acting in the patient's best interest is one of the most fundamental convictions of the medical profession. But, *what serves the patient best*? is sometimes an ambiguous decision indeed. Although it is the patient who has to bear the consequences of medical decisions, absolute freedom of patient without necessary deliberations can be counterproductive in patient care. There are many factors that affect even the competent person's ability to make rational choices. Instead of evaluating the choices simultaneously people in reality evaluate them in succession and in this process they often choose the first option that they consider to offer satisfactory outcome, even though that choice may not be the most rational outcome. These limitations have been called 'bounded rationality'. Decisions of a competent patient which are rational within the constraints of this 'bounded rationality' may not appear rational to the physician without considering these constraints. The exercise of autonomy may fulfil the patient's desire but may not necessarily serve the patient best.

Having said all this, a primary concern remains here, i.e., *what serves the patient best?* One thing is clear that to serve the patient best, patient's involvement in decision making is inevitable, rather the most accepted concept in the current scenario. Generally accepted and much referred concept of *shared decision making* lays emphasis on 'active participation from both patient and professional in decision making process, and agreement on decision'. Both patient and physician discuss the preferences and facts into the decisional process to reach a shared decision. This decision might involve a compromise between the parties as they may not consider it to be the best decision, yet both accept it as treatment to be followed. Trying to find a compromise, which both parties are committed to agree on, will nurture the patient-physician relationship, than simply allowing the patient to make the decision on his own.

Ethical Guidelines for Medical Practitioners

In India ethical guidelines for medical practitioners were framed by Medical Council of India (MCI) in the year 2002, titled Indian Medical Council (Professional conduct, Etiquette and Ethics) Regulations, 2002. An abridged form of the *Code of Ethics* has been provided below. (The full version may be downloaded from *www.mciindia.org*).

■ INDIAN MEDICAL COUNCIL (PROFESSIONAL CONDUCT, ETIQUETTE AND ETHICS) REGULATIONS

Chapter 1: Code of Medical Ethics

- A physician shall uphold the dignity and honor of his profession. Reward or financial gain will be a subordinate consideration.
- Only the doctors having qualification recognized by MCI and registered with MCI/State Medical Council(s) are allowed to practice Modern system of Medicine or Surgery.
- A physician should affiliate with associations of allopathic medical professions.
- Physicians should attend CMEs for at least 30 hours every 5 years.

Maintenance of Medical Records

- Physicians shall maintain the medical records of their indoor patients for 3 years from the date of start of the treatment in a standard proforma. If any request is made for medical records by the patients/authorized attendant or legal authorities, the same may be duly acknowledged and documents shall be issued within 72 hours.
- A physician shall maintain a register of medical certificates giving full details of certificates issued. When issuing a medical certificate enter the identification marks of the patient and keep a copy of the certificate.
- Try to computerize medical records for quick retrieval.

Display of Registration Numbers

- Physician shall display their registration numbers in his clinic and in all his prescriptions, certificates, money receipts given to his patients.
- Physicians shall display as suffix to their names only recognized medical degrees or such certificates/diplomas and memberships/honors which confer professional knowledge or recognizes any exemplary qualification/achievements.

Use of Generic Names of Drugs

Every physician should, as far as possible, prescribe drugs with generic names and he shall ensure that there is a rational prescription and use of drugs.

Highest Quality Assurance in Patient Care

Physician shall not employ any attendant who is neither registered nor enlisted under the Medical Acts in force and shall not permit such persons to attend, treat or perform operations upon patients wherever professional discretion or skill is required.

Exposure of Unethical Conduct
A physician should expose incompetent or corrupt, dishonest or unethical conduct of members of the profession.

Payment of Professional Services
Physician should announce his fees before rendering service and not after the operation or treatment is under way. It is unethical to enter into a contract of "no cure no payment." Physician rendering service on behalf of the state shall refrain from anticipating or accepting any consideration.

Evasion of Legal Restrictions
The physician shall observe the laws of the country in regulating the medical profession and shall also not assist others to evade such laws. He should cooperate in observance and enforcement of sanitary laws and regulations in the interest of public health.

Chapter 2: Duties of Physicians to their Patients

Obligations to the Sick
- Though a physician is not bound to treat each and every person asking his services, he should be ever ready to respond to the calls of the sick and the injured.
- A physician should try to make his visits at the hour indicated to the patients.
- A physician advising a patient to seek service of another physician is acceptable; however, in case of emergency a physician must treat the patient. No physician shall arbitrarily refuse treatment to a patient.
- When a patient is suffering from an ailment which is not within the range of experience of the treating physician, he may refuse treatment and refer the patient to another physician.

Secrecy
- Confidences entrusted by patients to him should never be revealed unless it is a legal requirement.
- Physician must determine whether his duty to society requires him to disclose confidential information to protect a healthy person against a communicable disease.

Prognosis
Physician should neither exaggerate nor minimize the gravity of a patient's condition. He should ensure that the patient or his family have such knowledge of the patient's condition as will serve the best interests of the patient and the family.

Never Neglect the Patient
- Physician should not neglect the patient, nor should he withdraw from the case without giving adequate notice to the patient and his family.
- Physicians shall not willfully commit an act of negligence that may deprive his patients from necessary medical care.

Engagement for an Obstetric Case

When a physician engaged to attend an obstetric case is absent and another is sent for and delivery accomplished, the acting physician is entitled to his professional fees, but should secure the patient's consent to resign on the arrival of the physician engaged.

Chapter 3: Duties of Physician in Consultation

Unnecessary Consultations should be Avoided

In case of serious illness and in doubtful or difficult conditions, physician should request consultation. Such consultation should be in the interest of the patient only. Consulting pathologists/radiologists or other diagnostic laboratory investigations should be done judiciously.

Statement to Patient after Consultation

All statements to the patient/representatives should take place in presence of the consulting physicians, except as otherwise agreed. Differences of opinion should not be divulged unnecessarily but when there is irreconcilable difference of opinion the circumstances should be frankly and impartially explained to the patient/representative.

Treatment after Consultation

- Attending physician may make subsequent variations in the treatment if any unexpected change occurs. At the next consultation, reasons for such variation should be discussed/explained. Same privilege and obligations belong to the consultant who treats patient in emergency, during the absence of attending physician.
- The attending physician may prescribe medicine at any time for the patient, whereas the consultant may prescribe only in case of emergency or as an expert when called for.

Patients Referred to Specialists

When the attending physician refers the patient to a specialist, a case summary should be given to the specialist, who should communicate his opinion in writing to the attending physician.

Fees and Other Charges

- Physician shall display his fees and other charges on the board of his chamber and/or the hospitals he is visiting. Prescription should make clear if the physician himself dispensed any medicine.
- Physician shall write his name and designation in full along with registration number in his prescription letterhead. (In government hospital where the patient load is heavy, name of the prescribing doctor must be written below his/her signature).

Chapter 4: Responsibilities of Physicians to Each Other

Conduct in Consultation

No insincerity/rivalry should be indulged in during consultations. No statement/discussion should be carried on, which would impair the confidence reposed in physician in charge of the case.

Consultant not to take Charge of the Case
- When a physician has been called for consultation, he should normally not take charge of the case, especially on the solicitation of the patient.
- The consultant shall not criticize the referring physician and shall discuss the diagnosis treatment plan with the referring physician.

Appointment of Substitute
- If a physician requests another physician to attend his patients during his temporary absence, professional courtesy requires the acceptance of such appointment only when he has the capacity to discharge the additional responsibility along with his other duties.
- The physician acting under such an appointment should give the utmost consideration to the interests and reputation of the absent physician and all such patients should be restored to the care of the latter upon his return.

Visiting Another Physician's Case
- When it becomes the duty of a physician occupying an official position to see and report upon an illness or injury, he should communicate to the physician in attendance so as to give him an option of being present.
- The physician occupying an official position should avoid remarks upon the diagnosis or the treatment that has been adopted.

Chapter 5: Duties of Physician to Public and Paramedical Profession
- Physicians should disseminate advice on public health issues. They should play their part in enforcing the laws of the community.
- Physicians, especially those engaged in public health work, should enlighten the public concerning quarantine regulations and measures for the prevention of epidemic and communicable diseases.
- The physician should notify the communicable disease under his care, in accordance with the laws, rules and regulations. When an epidemic occurs a physician should not abandon his duty for fear of contracting the disease himself.

Chapter 6: Unethical Acts
Physician shall not aid or abet or commit any of the following unethical acts.

Advertising
- Soliciting of patients directly or indirectly, by a physician, group of physicians or institutions or organizations is unethical. A physician shall not make use of him (or his name) as subject of any form of advertising or publicity through any mode either alone or in conjunction with others which tantamount to invite attention to him or to his professional position, skill, qualification, achievements, attainments, specialities, appointments, associations, affiliations or honors and/or of such character as would ordinarily result in his self-advertisement.

- A physician shall not give to any person, whether for compensation or otherwise, any approval, recommendation, endorsement, certificate, report or statement with respect of any drug, medicine, nostrum remedy, surgical, or therapeutic article, apparatus or appliance or any commercial product or article with respect to any property, quality or use thereof or any test, demonstration or trial thereof, for use in connection with his name, signature, or photograph in any form or manner of advertising through any mode nor shall he boast of cases, operations, cures or remedies or permit the publication of report thereof through any mode.

A physician is permitted to make a formal announcement in press regarding the following:
- Starting practice
- Change of type of practice
- Changing address
- Temporary absence from duty
- Resumption of another practice
- Succeeding to another practice
- Public declaration of charges.

Printing of self-photograph, or any such material of publicity in the letter head or on sign board of the consulting room or any such clinical establishment shall be regarded as acts of self-advertisement and unethical conduct on the part of the physician. However, printing of sketches, diagrams, picture of human system shall not be treated as unethical.

Patent and Copyrights

A physician may patent surgical instruments, appliances and medicine or copyright applications, methods and procedures. However, it shall be unethical if the benefits of such patents or copyrights are not made available in situations where the interest of large population is involved.

Running an Open Shop (Dispensing of Drugs and Appliances by Physicians)

- A physician should not run an open shop for sale of medicine for dispensing prescriptions prescribed by doctors other than him or for sale of medical or surgical appliances. It is not unethical for a physician to prescribe or supply drugs, remedies or appliances as long as there is no exploitation of the patient.
- Drugs prescribed by a physician or brought from the market for a patient should explicitly state the proprietary formulae as well as generic name of the drug.

Rebates and Commission

- A physician shall not give, solicit, or receive nor shall he offer to give solicit or receive, any gift, gratuity, commission or bonus in consideration of or return for the referring, recommending or procuring of any patient for medical, surgical or other treatment.
- A physician shall not directly or indirectly, participate in or be a party to act of division, transference, assignment, subordination, rebating, splitting or refunding of any fee for medical, surgical or other treatment.

Abovementioned provisions shall apply to the referring, recommending or procuring by a physician or any person, specimen or material for diagnostic purposes or other study/work. However, there is no prohibition on payment of salaries by a qualified physician to other duly qualified person rendering medical care under his supervision.

Secret Remedies

The prescribing or dispensing by a physician of secret remedial agents of which he does not know the composition, or the manufacture or promotion of their use is unethical and as such prohibited. All the drugs prescribed by a physician should always carry a proprietary formula and clear name.

Human Rights

The physician shall not aid or abet torture nor shall he be a party to either infliction of mental or physical trauma or concealment of torture inflicted by some other person or agency in clear violation of human rights.

Euthanasia

- Practicing euthanasia shall constitute unethical conduct. However, the question of withdrawing supporting devices to sustain cardiopulmonary function even after brain death shall be decided by a team of doctors and not merely by the treating physician alone.
- A team of doctors shall declare withdrawal of support system. Such team shall consist of the doctor in charge of the patient, Chief Medical Officer/Medical Officer in charge of the hospital and a doctor nominated by the in-charge of the hospital from the hospital staff or in accordance with the provisions of the Transplantation of Human Organ Act, 1994.

Code of conduct for Doctors and Professional association of doctors in their relationship with Pharmaceutical and allied Health sector industry.

In dealing with Pharmaceutical and allied health sector industry, a physician shall follow the stipulations given below:

- *Gifts*: A physician shall not receive any gift from any pharmaceutical or allied health care industry and their sales people or representatives.
- *Travel facilities*: A physician shall not accept any travel facility inside the country or outside, from any pharmaceutical or allied healthcare industry or their representatives for self and family members for vacation or for attending conferences, seminars, workshops, CMEs, etc., as a delegate.
- *Hospitality*: A physician shall not accept individually any hospitality like hotel accommodation for self and family members under any pretext.
- *Cash or monetary grants*: A physician shall not receive any cash or monetary grants from any pharmaceutical and allied healthcare industry for individual purpose in individual capacity under any pretext. Funding for medical research, study, etc., can only be received through approved institutions by modalities laid down by law/rules/guidelines adopted by such approved institutions, in a transparent manner. It shall always be fully disclosed.
- *Medical research*: A physician may carry out or participate in research projects funded by pharmaceutical and allied healthcare industries. A physician is obliged to know that the fulfilment of the following items (i) to (vii) will be an imperative for undertaking any research assignment/project funded by industry-for being proper and ethical.

    A physician shall ensure that:
    i. Research proposal(s) has the due permission from the competent concerned authorities.
    ii. Research project(s) has the clearance of national/state/institutional ethics committees/bodies.
    iii. It fulfills all the legal requirements prescribed for medical research.
    iv. Source and amount of funding is publicly disclosed at the beginning itself.

v. Proper care and facilities are provided to human volunteers, if they are necessary for the research project(s).
vi. Undue animal experimentations are not done and when these are necessary they are done in a scientific and a humane way.
vii. While accepting such an assignment a medical practitioner shall have the freedom to publish the results of the research in the greater interest of the society by inserting such a clause in the MoU or any other document/agreement for any such assignment.

- *Maintaining professional autonomy*: In dealing with pharmaceutical and allied healthcare industry, a medical practitioner shall always ensure that there shall be no compromise either with his/her own professional autonomy and/or with the autonomy and freedom of the medical institution.
- *Affiliation*: A physician may work for pharmaceutical and allied healthcare industries in advisory capacities, as consultants, as researchers, as treating doctors or in any other professional capacity. In doing so, physician shall always ensure that:
  - His professional integrity and freedom are maintained.
  - Patient's interests are not compromised in any way.
  - Such affiliations are within the law.
  - Such affiliations/employments are fully transparent and disclosed.
- *Endorsement*: A physician shall not endorse any drug or product of the industry publicly. Any study conducted on the efficacy or otherwise of such products shall be presented to and/or through scientific bodies or published in scientific journals in a proper way.

Chapter 7: Misconduct

The following acts of commission or omission on the part of a physician shall constitute professional misconduct rendering him/her liable for disciplinary action.

Violation of the Regulations

If a physician commits violation of any of these regulations.

Adultery or Improper Conduct

Abuse of professional position by committing adultery or improper conduct with a patient or by maintaining an improper association with a patient will render a physician liable for disciplinary action.

Conviction by Court of Law

Conviction by a Court of Law for offences involving moral turpitude/Criminal acts.

Sex Determination Tests

- Sex determination test shall not be undertaken with intention to terminate a female fetus, unless there are other absolute indications for termination of pregnancy as specified in the MTP Act, 1971.
- Any act of termination of pregnancy of normal female fetus amounting to female feticide is a professional misconduct by the physician leading to penal erasure besides rendering him liable to criminal proceedings as per the provisions of this Act.

Signing Professional Certificates, Reports and Other Documents

- Physicians may be required to give certificates, notification, reports and other similar documents in their professional capacity for subsequent use in the courts or for administrative purposes, etc.
- Any physician who is shown to have signed or given under his name and authority any such certificate, notification, report or similar document which is untrue, misleading or improper, is liable to have his name deleted from the Register.
- Physicians shall not contravene the provisions of the Drugs and Cosmetics Act and regulations made there under. Prescribing steroids/psychotropic drugs when there is no absolute medical indication or selling Schedule H and L drugs and poisons to the public except to his patient; in contravention of the above provisions shall constitute gross professional misconduct on the part of the physician.
- Performing or enabling unqualified person to perform an abortion or any illegal operation for which there is no medical, surgical or psychological indication. A physician shall not issue certificates of efficiency in modern medicine to unqualified or nonmedical person.
- A physician should not contribute to the lay press articles and give interviews regarding diseases and treatments which may have the effect of advertising himself or soliciting practices; but is open to write to the lay press under his own name on matters of public health, hygienic living or to deliver public lectures, give talks on the radio/TV/internet chat for the same purpose and send announcement of the same to lay press.
- An institution run by a physician for a particular purpose such as a maternity home, nursing home, private hospital, rehabilitation center or any type of training institution, etc., may be advertised in the lay press, but such advertisements should not contain anything more than the name of the institution, type of patients admitted, type of training and other facilities offered and the fees.
- It is improper for a physician to use an unusually large sign-board and write on it anything other than his name, qualifications obtained from a University or a statutory body, titles and name of his speciality, registration number including the name of the State Medical Council under which registered. The same should be the contents of his prescription papers. It is improper to affix a sign-board on a chemist's shop or in places where he does not reside or work.
- Physicians shall not disclose the secrets of a patient that have been learnt in the exercise of their profession except: (1) In a court of law under orders of the Presiding Judge; (2) In circumstances where there is a serious and identified risk to a specific person and/or community; and (3) notifiable diseases. In case of communicable/notifiable diseases, concerned public health authorities should be informed immediately.
- The physicians shall not refuse on religious grounds alone to give assistance in or conduct of sterility, birth control, circumcision and medical termination of pregnancy when there is medical indication, unless the medical practitioner feels himself/herself incompetent to do so.
- Before performing an operation the physician should obtain in writing the consent from the husband or wife, parent or guardian in the case of minor, or the patient himself as the case may be. In an operation which may result in sterility the consent of both husband and wife is needed.

- Physicians shall not publish photographs or case reports of his/her patients without their permission, in any medical or other journal in a manner by which their identity could be made out. If the identity is not to be disclosed, the consent is not needed.
- In the case of running of a nursing home by a physician and employing assistants to help him, the ultimate responsibility rests on the physician.
- Physician shall not use touts or agents for procuring patients. Physician shall not claim to be specialist unless he has a special qualification in that branch.
- In vitro fertilization or artificial insemination shall not be undertaken without informed consent of the female patient and her spouse as well as the donor. Such consent shall be obtained in writing only after the patient is provided, at her own level of comprehension, with sufficient information about the purpose, methods, risks, inconveniences, disappointments of the procedure and possible risks and hazards.

Chapter 8: Punishment and Disciplinary Action

The offences and misconduct given above do not constitute a complete list of the infamous acts which calls for disciplinary action. MCI or State Medical Councils can also deal with any other form of professional misconduct on the part of a registered practitioner.

- Any complaint with regard to professional misconduct can be made to the appropriate Medical Council for Disciplinary action. Upon receipt of any complaint, the appropriate Medical Council would hold an enquiry and give opportunity to the registered medical practitioner to be heard in person or by pleader.
- If the medical practitioner is found to be guilty of committing professional misconduct, the appropriate Medical Council may award such punishment as deemed necessary or may direct the removal altogether or for a specified period, from the register of the name of the delinquent registered practitioner. Deletion from the Register shall be widely publicized in local press as well as in the publications of different Medical Associations/Societies/Bodies.
- In case the punishment of removal from the register is for a limited period, the appropriate Council may also direct that the name so removed shall be restored in the register after the expiry of the period for which the name was ordered to be removed.
- Decision on complaint against delinquent physician shall be taken within 6 months. During the pendency of the complaint the appropriate Council may restrain the physician from performing the procedure or practice which is under scrutiny. Professional incompetence shall be judged by peer group as per guidelines prescribed by MCI.
- Where either on a request or otherwise the MCI is informed that any complaint against a delinquent physician has not been decided by a State Medical Council within 6 months from the date of receipt of complaint by it and further the MCI has reason to believe that there is no justified reason for not deciding the complaint within the said prescribed period, the MCI may: (1) Impress upon the concerned State Medical council to conclude and decide the complaint within a time bound schedule; (2) May decide to withdraw the said complaint pending with the concerned State Medical Council straightaway or after the expiry of the period which had been stipulated by the MCI in accordance with para (1) above, to itself and refer the same to the Ethical Committee of the Council for its expeditious disposal in a period of not >6 months from the receipt of the complaint in the office of the MCI.

- Any person aggrieved by the decision of State Medical Council on any complaint against a delinquent physician, can appeal to MCI within 60 days from the date of receipt of the order passed by the said Medical Council. If MCI is satisfied that the appellant was prevented by sufficient cause from presenting the appeal within the aforesaid 60 days, may allow it to be presented within a further period of 60 days.

CONCLUSION

With the advances in medical sciences as well as changing moral principles of the community at large, clinicians are frequently facing dilemmas in many facets of daily medical practice. Besides, there is anxiety amongst the medical practitioners regarding increasing trends of complaints and lawsuits, many of them are due to inability to comprehend and resolve ethical dilemmas in clinical settings. In addition to moral obligations, clinicians are also bound by legal framework regulating medical practice. It is now well-accepted that legal and ethical considerations are inseparable part of good medical practice. The clinician should remain attentive to the patient's perspective and control their behavior so that the patient's best interest is taken care of at all times.

REFERENCES

1. Theodore Roosevelt. The strenuous life: essays and addresses. Dover Publications. 2009.
2. Raanan Gillon. Medical Ethics: four principles plus attention to scope. BMJ. 1994;309:184-8.
3. Dana JL. The four principles of biomedical ethics: a foundation for current bioethical debate. J Chiropr Humanit. 2007;14: 34-40.
4. Mathews E. Can paternalism be modernized? Journal of Medical Ethics. 1986;12:133-5.
5. Mill JS. On liberty. 1869. Library of economics and liberty. Available: http://www.econlib.org/library/Mill/mllbty.html.
6. Rothman DJ (1991). Strangers at the Bedside: A history of how law and bioethics transformed medical decision making, 1992, Basic Books.
7. Leng S. Who's in control? Why both doctors and patients are frustrated. Available: http://www.kevinmd.com/blog/2013/11/control-doctors-patients-frustrated.html.
8. Blustein J. Doing what the patient orders: maintaining integrity in the doctor-patient relationship. Bioethics. 1993;7(4):290-314.
9. Charles C, Gafni A, Whelan T. Shared decision-making in the medical encounter: What does it mean? (or it takes at least two to tango). Social Science and Medicine. 1997;44(5):681-92.
10. Charles C, Whelan T, Gafni A. What do we mean by partnership in making decisions about treatment? BMJ. 1999;319: 780-2.

CHAPTER 2

Confidentiality and Disclosure in Medical Practice

VP Singh, Akashdeep Aggarwal

> "What I may see or hear in the course of treatment or even outside of treatment in regard to the life of men, I will keep to myself."
>
> —Hippocrates[1]

■ INTRODUCTION

Confidentiality is essential to the trusting relationship between patient and the physician. All the information related to the patient, received by a physician during the course of treatment are considered as professional secret. Such information has to be kept confidential and must not be divulged without patient's consent. It is a physician's duty to refrain from disclosing voluntarily to any third party, the information which he has learned directly or indirectly in his professional relationship with the patient. The purpose of medical confidentiality is to enable the patient to make full revelation of the information with assurance that the physician will guard the confidential nature of the information disclosed. Full revelation of the information facilitates the physician to treat the patient appropriately.

Medical privacy involves informational privacy (e.g., confidentiality, anonymity, secrecy and data security); physical privacy (e.g., modesty and bodily integrity); associational privacy (e.g., intimate sharing of death, illness and recovery); proprietary privacy (e.g., self-ownership and control over personal identifiers, genetic data, and body tissues); and decisional privacy (e.g., autonomy and choice in medical decision-making).[2] Patient has a right to privacy which is protected by code of medical ethics. If the healthcare provider breaches the confidentiality of patient, he may face professional and legal sanctions.

However during the course of treatment, information related to patient is to be shared with other clinicians and healthcare workers involved in the treatment. As such, it is justifiable so long as precautions are taken to restrict the access of confidential information to persons not involved in the treatment process. In addition, patient must be informed the ways in which the confidential information will be shared for the purpose of treatment only.

■ WHEN CONFIDENTIALITY MAY BE BREACHED?

The obligation of medical confidentiality is not absolute as there are certain exceptions to the rule of confidentiality, where disclosure of personal health information is permissible.

Legal Requirement/Administration of Justice

A doctor has to disclose the professional secrets when required by law to do so. He may be compelled to divulge the confidential information by a Court order, while giving evidence in a Court of law. In such situations, patient's consent is not required and the doctor can easily justify the breach in confidentiality. A doctor has to disclose the health information for the purpose of administration of justice (e.g., malpractice cases, consumer protection cases, workman's compensation cases, demanded by the police on a written requisition, etc.).

Patient's Interest

A doctor may disclose the patient's confidential information, if he believes it to be in patient's best interests. Such situations may arise when patients are incapable of making their own decisions. The information regarding a patient's health is given to a relative or other appropriate person in circumstances where the doctor believes it undesirable on medical grounds, to reveal the information to the patient. While referring a patient to another doctor, confidential health information may be shared with healthcare professionals involved in patient care during the transit and also to the doctor to whom the patient is being referred.

Medical Research

Confidential information of the patient may be disclosed for the purpose of research or experiment strictly as per the guidelines issued by some authoritative body like Indian Council of Medical Research (ICMR). Identity and records of the human participants of the research or experiments are as far as possible kept confidential. No details about identity of said human participants are disclosed without valid scientific and legal reasons which may be essential for the purpose of therapeutics or other interventions, without the specific consent in writing of the human participant concerned, or someone authorized on their behalf. It must also be ensured that the said human participant does not suffer from any hardship, discrimination or stigmatization due to the research or experiment.[3]

Health Insurance Purpose

Medical practitioners may disclose the health information of his patient, when demanded by insurance companies as provided by the Insurance Act, when the patient has relinquished his rights on taking the insurance.

Public Safety

Physician has to disclose confidential health information related to communicable/notifiable diseases as a statutory requirement. A physician can divulge confidential information of his patient, without consent, if he believes it to be in favor of public interest. Before disclosing the confidential information of his patient, physician has to balance the public interest against his patient's interest. If the public interest is at significant risk due to non-disclosure of patient's health information, and at the same time, public interest outweighs the patient's interest, then physician may be justified in disclosing the information.

■ GUIDELINES ON MEDICAL CONFIDENTIALITY

Medical Council of India Regulations

In exercise of the powers conferred under Sec 20A read with Sec 33(m) of the Indian Medical Council Act, 1956, the Medical Council of India with the previous approval of the Central Government, made the regulations namely *Indian Medical Council (Professional conduct, Etiquette and Ethics) Regulations.* These regulations have addressed the important issue of medical confidentiality.

Regulation 1.3.2

If any request is made for medical records either by the patients/authorized attendant or legal authorities involved, the same may be duly acknowledged and documents shall be issued within the period of 72 hours. Thus it is clear that no doctor can refuse to handover the patient's medical record to the authorized person under the garb of *breach of confidentiality*.

Regulation 2.2: Patience, Delicacy and Secrecy

Confidences concerning individual or domestic life entrusted by patients to a physician and defects in the disposition or character of patients observed during medical attendance should never be revealed unless their revelation is required by the laws of the State. Sometimes, however, a physician must determine whether his duty to society requires him to employ knowledge, obtained through confidence as a physician, to protect a healthy person against a communicable disease to which he is about to be exposed. In such instance, the physician should act as he would wish another to act toward one of his own family in like circumstances.

Regulation 5.2: Public and Community Health

At all times, the physician should notify the constituted public health authorities, of every case of communicable disease under his care, in accordance with the laws, rules and regulations of the health authorities.

Regulation 7.6: Sex Determination Tests

On no account, sex determination test shall be undertaken with the intent to terminate the life of a female fetus developing in her mother's womb, unless there are other absolute indications for termination of pregnancy as specified in the Medical Termination of Pregnancy Act, 1971. Any act of termination of pregnancy of normal female fetus amounting to female feticide shall be regarded as professional misconduct on the part of the physician leading to penal erasure besides rendering him liable to criminal proceedings as per the provisions of this Act.

Regulation 7.14

The registered medical practitioner shall not disclose the secrets of a patient that have been learnt in the exercise of his/her profession except:
- In a court of law under orders of the Presiding Judge.

- In circumstances where there is a serious and identified risk to a specific person and/or community, and notifiable diseases.
- In case of communicable/notifiable diseases, concerned public health authorities should be informed immediately.

Regulation 7.17

A registered medical practitioner shall not publish photographs or case reports of his/her patients without their permission, in any medical or other journal in a manner by which their identity could be made out. If the identity is not to be disclosed, the consent is not needed.

Right to Information Act and Medical Confidentiality

The Right to Information Act (RTI), 2005 entitles the citizens to access information that is publicly available and related to public interest. The demands for information in medical records are increasing. All the information requested through RTI need not be disclosed. The request for information from the third party about a patient does not come under the definition of information provided under Sec 2 (f) of the RTI Act.

Sec 8 of the Act provides certain exemptions from disclosure of information:
- *Information which would impede the process of investigation or apprehension or prosecution of offenders. [Sec 8(1)(h) RTI Act, 2005]*
  This provision is especially relevant to the medicolegal cases. In such cases, the Public Information Officer would be entitled to have clearance from the police or other investigating agency before releasing the information.
- *Information available to a person in his fiduciary relationship* need not be disclosed unless, the competent authority is satisfied that the larger public interest warrants the disclosure of such information. [Sec 8(1)(e) RTI Act, 2005]*
  *Fiduciary is a person who occupies a position of trust in relation to someone else, therefore requiring him to act for the latter's benefit within the scope of that relationship. In business or law, it generally means someone who has specific duties, such as those that attend a particular profession or role, e.g., doctor, lawyer, financial analyst or trustee.
- *Information which relates to personal information the disclosure of which has no relationship to any public activity or interest, or which would cause unwarranted invasion of the privacy of the individual need not be disclosed unless the Central Public Information Officer or the State Public Information Officer or the appellate authority, as the case may be, is satisfied that the larger public interest justifies the disclosure of such information. [Sec 8(1)(j) RTI Act, 2005]*

In a physician-patient relationship, it is the most important duty of a physician to maintain professional secrecy. Physicians cannot disclose to any other person, the information regarding his patient, which he has gathered during the course of treatment. The medical practitioners and administrators must be well versed with the provisions of RTI Act so as to decide, whether to provide or not, the information requested under RTI Act.

The confidentiality required to be maintained of the medical records of a patient, considering the regulations framed by the Medical Council of India cannot override the provisions of the Right to Information Act. If there be inconsistency between the regulations and the RTI Act, the provisions of the Act will prevail and the information will have to be made available under the Act.

Decision regarding disclosure of personal information of an individual may vary from case to case depending upon the circumstances of the case. In *Secretary General, Supreme Court of India* vs. *Subhash Chandra Agarwal*,[4] Delhi High Court held that personal information including tax returns, medical records, etc., cannot be disclosed in view of Sec 8(1)(j) of the RTI Act. The court, however, further stated that, *if it can be shown that sufficient public interest is involved in disclosure, the bar (preventing disclosure) would be lifted and after duly notifying the third party (i.e., the individual concerned with the information or whose records are sought) and after considering his views, the authority can disclose it.*

Maharashtra State Information Commission permitted disclosure of medical records of former Minister Mr Surupsinh Naik, who had been imprisoned and it was alleged that he used his political influence to falsify medical symptoms to stay in a hospital rather than a prison during his 1 month sentence. The RTI Act request was filed in the public interest to expose this political corruption. The Commission held:

Public Information Officer can disclose personal information, since there is a feeling in the minds of people that highly placed people and people with money power can spend their jail term not in the prison but in the hospital, public interest will be better served, if this information about hospitalization is disclosed even though this information is of a 3rd person and of a personal nature. The information about hospitalization, medication and discharge report of a patient in the government hospital, if required by the legislature cannot be denied to them.[5]

RTI and Medicolegal Cases[6]

Large number of requests are received by health authorities under the RTI Act to provide information related to medicolegal cases such as copies of postmortem reports, medicolegal reports, etc. Public Information Officers (PIOs) should be well versed with the provisions of RTI Act so that they are able to decide whether the information requested is to be provided or not.

If an FIR has been registered in a case and investigation is in progress, the PIO can claim exemption under clause (h) of Sec 8(1) on the ground that providing copy of PMR or MLR would impede the investigation and/or apprehension or prosecution of offenders. Similarly, in cases where the disclosure of information may endanger the life and safety of any person (potential witnesses, victim, etc), exemption can be claimed under Sec 8(1)(g). In case of doubt whether an FIR has been registered in a case, the PIO may officially write to the Police and ascertain the status. Time limit of 30 days for providing information under the RTI Act is sufficient for this purpose.

Issuing Copy of MLR/PMR to Other Persons (Other than the Patient and the Police Officer Investigating the Case)[6]

Delhi High Court in State vs. Gian Singh held that, a medicolegal report or postmortem report is a confidential document and not a public document.[7] As per the medicolegal manual prepared by Health Department Haryana, copy of PMR/MLR may be provided, subject to fulfilment of the following three conditions:
1. Applicant shall submit a written application addressed to the concerned Medical Officer clearly stating his/her relationship with the patient/deceased person.
2. Applicant shall pay the fee prescribed by the State Government with the Health department and enclose the receipt for the same along with the application, and
3. The Applicant shall furnish NOC from concerned Police Station (investigating the matter) clearly stating that the issuance of copies of MLR/PMR will not hinder the investigation.

Alternatively, the applicant shall produce order of the Court directing the Medical Officer concerned to provide him/her copy of the PMR/MLR.

Medical Confidentiality and HIV Status

Confidentiality in HIV-positive patients is a sensitive issue in medical practice due to its interrelated ethical and legal repercussions. In India, most public health policies dealing with HIV infection encourage individuals to come forward voluntarily for testing, counseling and treatment. Many public health authorities have argued that failure to maintain confidentiality could threaten the cooperation of HIV-positive individuals.

The right of HIV-positive individual to confidentiality comes in conflict with the right of the partner to be informed about the risk of infection, known as partner notification. Persons unknowingly placed at risk of HIV infection, have a moral right to information so as to protect them, seek testing and commence treatment, if necessary. The dilemma between individual rights of HIV-positive patients and social control over them has led to controversies all over the globe.

In medical practice, physicians may face clinical situations when they know the identity of the person deemed to be at risk. The ethical and legal issues related to breach in confidentiality due to partner notification were examined in detail in *Tarasoff case*. In this case, Prosenjit Poddar, a student of the University of California, told his psychiatrist about his intention to kill a girl named Tatiana Tarasoff. Realizing the seriousness of his intention, the therapist concluded that Poddar should be detained for observation. Concerned about the breach of confidentiality, the therapist's supervisor rejected the recommendation and ordered that all records relating to Poddar's treatment be destroyed. The police released Poddar on his assurance that he would *stay away from the girl*. Two months later, he killed Tatiana. The girl's parents sued the University for negligence. The court held that the physician could be held liable for failing to take adequate steps to protect a known intended victim of his patient. It was considered ethically permissible for the physician to notify the person whom the physician believed was endangered. Many States in the USA legislated that physicians are legally obliged to notify subjects who are at risk of infecting third parties. However, civil liberty groups demanded proper guidelines for the physicians in relation to disclosure decisions. This resulted in formulation of the *policy on privilege to disclose* which included the criteria for disclosure:

- The physician reasonably believes that notification is medically appropriate and that there is a significant risk of infection.
- The patient has been counseled regarding the need to notify partners.
- The physician has reason to believe that the patient will not notify his/her partners.
- The patient has been informed of the physician's intent to notify partners and has been given the opportunity to express a preference as to whether the partners should be notified by the physician directly or by a public health officer.[8]

NACO Guidelines on Confidentiality in HIV-positive Individuals Operational Guidelines for ICTCs: (July 2007)

Operational guidelines for Integrated Counseling and Testing Centres (ICTCs) by National AIDS Control Organization (NACO)[9] aim to ensure uniformity in counseling and testing services across the country. These guidelines suggest that, *information gathered during counselling must not be shared with others. The HIV test result must be reported only to the client* unless the client states the desire to share the test result with a family member, partner or close friend. HIV testing is to be done after obtaining the informed consent from the client. This permission is entirely the choice of the person submitting for the test and can never be implied or presumed. Except in circumstances when disclosure to another person is required by law or ethical considerations, the HIV-positive person has the right to privacy, and also the right to exercise informed consent in all decisions about disclosure in respect of his/her status. The operational guidelines for ICICs also suggest about partner notification that an HIV-positive person should be encouraged to share the positive test result with his/her spouse, sexual or needle sharing partner(s). This process of encouraging the client to share the test result might take multiple visits. If after multiple visits the counselor feels that the client* is not ready to share his/her status and the regular sexual partner of the HIV-positive individual is deemed to be at risk, the partner can be notified of the person's positive status.

*Client is a person seeking healthcare services, including in an ICTC, is a client and not a patient. Patients are considered passive recipients of treatment/care/hospitalization, whereas clients are consumers who make a choice whether or not to avail of a certain service.

Guidelines on HIV Testing (March 2007)

The NACO published *Guidelines for HIV testing*[10] in March 2007. The manual provides comprehensive document that guides on all the aspects related to HIV testing as well as training. NACO discussed issues related to confidentiality and informed consent for HIV testing under the chapter titled *Legal and ethical issues of HIV/AIDS* as follows:

Confidentiality and HIV/AIDS

The patient has the right to confidentiality. The physician should not reveal confidential communications or information, without the consent of the patient, unless provided for by law or the need to protect the welfare of the individual or public interest. Civil and criminal penalties may ensue for unlawful disclosure of HIV-positive status. However, the principle of confidentiality is never absolute and has always been subject to limits in the interest of society, public welfare and the rights of the other individuals.

Exceptions to confidentially are appropriate when necessary to protect public health or when necessary to protect individuals, including healthcare workers, who are endangered by persons infected with HIV. If a physician knows that a seropositive individual is endangering a third party, the physician should within the constraints of the local law: (i) Attempt to persuade the infected patient to cease endangering the third party; (ii) If persuasion fails, notify authorities, and (iii) If the authorities take no action, notify the endangered third party.

Informed Consent for HIV Testing

Informed consent applies to HIV testing and it is real informed consent and not implied consent. Full disclosure of the nature of HIV disease, nature of the proposed test, implications of a positive and a negative test result and the consequences of treatment must be made prior to taking consent. The consent must be voluntary and patient must be able to understand and competent to refuse. Testing should always be accompanied with counselling. Informed consent for testing and disclosure must be in writing.

Human immunodeficiency viruses testing in a minor and an incompetent patient can be undertaken with a guardian's consent. HIV testing should not be undertaken without written informed consent because of the issues of confidentiality, discrimination, victimization and psychological harms and burdens raised by an HIV-positive result.

Judicial Decisions on Medical Confidentiality and HIV Status

In India, till date, there is no legislation exclusively dealing with issues of medical confidentiality and partner notification in HIV-positive individuals. However, law on confidentiality in *people living with HIV/AIDS* (PLHA) may be construed from the Court decisions on the issue.

In Mr X vs. Hospital Z,[11] the Supreme Court of India allowed for disclosure of a person's HIV status to their partner. Mr X donated blood for his uncle's surgery at Hospital Z. After few months, Hospital Z informed the uncle that Mr X's blood had tested positive for HIV. Meanwhile, Mr X was to be married to Ms Y, but he himself called off the wedding when he heard about his HIV status. Several people including members of Mr X's family had been made aware of his HIV-positive status. He was completely ostracized by the community. Mr X approached the Supreme Court for damages against Hospital Z, on the grounds that they disclosed confidential information. The Supreme Court held that:

> *An HIV-positive patient who may transmit the disease to his or her prospective spouse is not entitled to the maintenance of confidentiality, since the life of the spouse has to be saved. Therefore, a hospital can disclose a patient's HIV status to the prospective spouse (partner), and in fact, since acts that are likely to spread communcable diseases are a crime under the Indian Penal Code, the failure of the hospital to inform the spouse of the disease would make them participant criminals.*

The court also ruled that since being infected with a venereal disease (read HIV/AIDS) is ground for divorce under Indian matrimonial laws, a person suffering from such a disease has no right to get married until they are cured. An appeal was filed, seeking clarification, and challenging the judgment of the Supreme Court decision to suspend the right of PLHA to marry when that was not even an issue before it. In the appeal, Mr X vs. Hospital Z (AIR 2003 SC 664), while the Supreme Court rescinded its earlier observations regarding marriage, and restored the right to marry for PLHA, it upheld its previous decision about partner notification maintaining that this disclosure was permissible.

Mandatory HIV Screening

The UNAIDS/WHO support mandatory HIV testing of the blood to be used for transfusion or for manufacture of blood products. Mandatory screening of donors is required prior to all procedures involving transfer of bodily fluids or body parts, such as artificial insemination, corneal grafts and organ transplant. The UNAIDS/WHO do not support mandatory testing of individuals on public health grounds. Many countries require mandatory HIV testing for immigration purposes and for pre-recruitment and periodic medical assessment of military personnel. The UNAIDS/WHO recommend that such testing should be done only when accompanied by proper counselling of the individuals and referral to medical and psychosocial services for those who are tested HIV positive.[12]

The NACO has also opposed mandatory HIV testing for public health purposes. It further said that such mandatory testing on public health grounds could be counterproductive as it may scare away a large number of suspected cases from getting detected and treated.[13]

HIV Testing of Patients Prior to Surgery

The practice of insisting the patients for HIV testing before surgery or routine compulsory pre-surgical HIV testing without informed consent is widespread both in private and government institutions in India. The practice is not legitimized, often secretive and discretionary. A multicenter study on 2200 healthcare providers indicated 67% of respondents reported that they screened patients for HIV before elective surgery, and 92% felt that universal pre-surgical HIV screening was a desirable policy.[14] A survey explored the views of medical practitioners working in 9 hospitals on mandatory *HIV testing of patients prior to surgery*. The survey indicated that the predominant reason for surgeons favoring mandatory tests was their fear of acquiring HIV infection from a patient. This fear appeared to lead them to focus on risk avoidance and self protection, for which they favored mandatory testing rather than the nationally recommended practice of adopting universal precautions.[15] However, the arguments in favor of mandatory HIV tests on the basis of risk of transmission of HIV infection from patients to surgeon are not sustainable on scientific grounds. The documented risk of transmission of HIV infection is reported to be very low, and from scientific perspective, surgeon's apprehensions are overstated.[16] Moreover, if a patient is in 'window period', the pre-surgical test results will be rather misleading and result in false assurance that the test is negative.[17] In spite of scientific evidence indicating the pre-surgical HIV testing as no-essential, the surgeon's insistence on compulsory testing is stringent. To conclude the whole discussion, there is no substitute for universal or standard precaution, and compulsory pre-surgical HIV testing is an unconscionable practice that has no legitimate and scientific basis. Voluntary HIV testing that requires the patient's consent is an appropriate and legally accepted approach.

CONCLUSION

Medical confidentiality remains important both to patients as well as healthcare professionals. Effective treatment requires accurate information. Patients are most likely to provide this information when they are not worried about public exposure. In addition to analyzing medical confidentiality from the physician's perspective as a professional responsibility, it is extremely important to understand that patient interests are at the core of medical confidentiality policy. The obligation of medical confidentiality is not absolute as there are certain exceptions to the rule of confidentiality, where disclosure of personal health information is permissible. In the absence of specific legislation on medical confidentiality, physicians have to maintain a fine balance between maintaining confidentiality and disclosing the health information, on the basis of various ethical guidelines and court decisions available.

REFERENCES

1. Hippocrates, vol I: The oath, in the Loeb classical library, Jones WHS (trans). London and Cambridge, MA, Harvard Univ Press. 1948.
2. Allen A. Privacy and Medicine. In EN Zalta (Ed), The Stanford Encyclopedia of Philosophy. Available:http://plato.stanford.edu/archives/spr2011/entries/privacy-medicine/
3. Ethical guidelines for biomedical research on human participants. ICMR 2006. Available: http://icmr.nic.in/ethical_guidelines.pdf.
4. http://www.indiankanoon.org/doc/1342199/
5. http://sic.maharashtra.gov.in/files/upload/mumbai/hearings%20of%20april%202007.pdf.
6. Haryana Medico Legal Manual 2012. Available: http://www.haryanahealth.nic.in/userfiles/file/pdf/PM%20Branch/Medico%20Legal%20Manual/2.%20Haryana%20Medicolegal%20Manual%202012%2031.1.2012.pdf.
7. 1981 Cri LJ 538.
8. Abraham S, Prasad J, Joseph A, Jacob KS. Confidentiality, partner notification and HIV infection: issues related to community health programs. The National Medical Journal of India. 2000;13(4):207-11.
9. Operational Guidelines for Integrated Counselling and Testing Centres, National AIDS Control Organization, Government of India. 2007. Available: http://naco.gov.in upload/Policies%20&%20Guidelines/20, %2 Operational%20 Guidelines%20for%2 Integrated %20 Counseling%20and%2 Testing %20Centres.pdf.

10. Guidelines on HIV testing: NACO, Govt. of India, 2007. Available: http://www.who.int/hiv/pub/guidelines/india_art.pdf.
11. Mr X vs. Hospital Z. 1998(8)SCC 296.
12. UNAIDS Global Reference Group on HIV/AIDS and Human Rights. Available: http://www.who.int/rpc/research_ethics/hivtestingpolicy_en_pdf.pdf.
13. National AIDS Control Organization (NACO).National AIDS Prevention and Control Policy. New Delhi: NACO; 2003.
14. Kurien M, Thomas K, Ahuja RC, Patel A, Shyla PR, Wig N, Mangalani M, et al. Screening for HIV infection by health professionals in India. Natl Med J India. 2007;20(2):59-66.
15. Kabir Sheikh, John DH Port er. It's 100% for me: Hospital Practitioners' perspectives on mandatory HIV testing. IJME. 2009;6(3):132-37.
16. Narain JP, Pattanayak S, Shah NK. HIV testing policies: an overview. Indian J Med Res. 1993;97:219-22.
17. Pandya SK. Patients testing positive for HIV: ethical dilemmas in India. Issues Med Ethics. 1997;5(2):49-55.

SECTION 2
Medicolegal Menace: Let's Face The Truth, Now!

Chapter 3   Disclosing Medical Errors: Why, When and How?
Chapter 4   End of Life care decisions: Ethical and Legal issues
Chapter 5   Medicolegal aspects of Discharge Against Medical Advice
Chapter 6   Violence Against Doctors: Causes, Effects, and Solutions

CHAPTER 3

Disclosing Medical Errors: Why, When and How?

VP Singh, Gautam Biswas

> *"Confession of errors is like a broom which sweeps away the dirt and leaves the surface brighter and clearer. I feel stronger for confession."*
> —**Mahatma Gandhi**[1]

◼ INTRODUCTION

"I felt a sense of shame like a burning ulcer. This was not guilt: Guilt is what you feel when you have done something wrong. What I felt was shame: I was what was wrong. And yet I also knew that a surgeon can take such feelings too far. It is one thing to be aware of one's limitations. It's another to be plagued by self-doubt."[2]

These lines written by Dr Atul Gawande in his book *Complications*, clearly describe the angst felt by a doctor on discovering that the patient suffered due to medical error. Even a talk on medical errors is like a nightmare, which haunts the conscience of those involved. However, in spite of the best care provided by the safest hands, things may go wrong and patients may be inadvertently harmed as a result of medical errors. This chapter has been devoted to a specific aspect of medical errors which is considered most challenging by the medical practitioners: The issue of disclosure; what and how should patients be told about medical errors?

◼ MEDICAL ERRORS

Institute of Medicine (IOM)[3] of US has defined *medical error* as, *failure of a planned action to be completed as intended or the use of a wrong plan to achieve an aim*. Medical errors are generally considered as preventable events. An error may result in adverse event or iatrogenic injury leading to prolongation of hospital stay, disability at discharge, or death. Many times errors may not result in injury as they may get noticed in time or because of good luck (**Box 1**). National Academy of Sciences, Institute of Medicine estimated that as many as 98,000 people die every year in the US because of mistakes committed by medical practitioners in hospitals.[2] In a Harvard Medical practice study 31,429 medical records were reviewed, and it was found that adverse events occurred in 3.7% of the admitted patients. In 69% of these cases, the adverse events were considered preventable.[4]

Adverse events resulting from medical errors must be distinguished from side effects, which may be anticipated, but unavoidable complications that may occur during the appropriate treatment. Similarly, it is essential to distinguish negligent acts from honest mistakes. Narrow

> **BOX 1 Types of Errors.**
>
> - Diagnostic errors
>   - Error or delay in diagnosis
>   - Failure to employ indicated tests
>   - Use of outmoded tests or therapy
>   - Failure to act on results of monitoring or testing
> - Treatment errors
>   - Error in the performance of an operation, procedure, or test
>   - Error in administering the treatment
>   - Error in the dose or method of using a drug
>   - Avoidable delay in treatment or in responding to an abnormal test
>   - Inappropriate (not indicated) care
> - Preventive errors
>   - Failure to provide prophylactic treatment
>   - Inadequate monitoring or follow-up of treatment
> - Other errors
>   - Failure of communication
>   - Equipment failure
>   - Other system failure
>
> *Source*: Leape, Lucian; Lawthers, Ann G; Brennan, Troyen A, et al. Preventing Medical Injury. Qual Rev Bull. 1993;19(5):144-9.

demarcation exists between a complication due to medical errors and the one due to negligent act. If the standard of care provided by the medical practitioner falls below the standard expected of a reasonably careful and knowledgeable practitioner acting in a similar situation, it will be labeled as medical negligence. Strictly speaking, negligence is to be established in Court of law.

■ DISCLOSURE OF MEDICAL ERRORS

How did it Start?

In 1987, after losing >1.5 million dollars in two malpractice claims, the Veteran Affairs Medical Centre (VAMC) in Lexington adopted a new approach to medical errors: *Disclose, Apologize and Compensate*, which was totally contrary to the earlier response to medical errors: *Deny and Defend*. The risk management committee of VAMC Lexington decided that in case a medical error is identified, the facility had an ethical duty to inform the patient or family of the error. In 1999, the VAMC Lexington reported that this practice continued to be followed because the administration and staff believed that it is the right thing to do, and it resulted in unanticipated financial benefits to the medical center.[5]

In 1999, a report issued by Institute of Medicine (*To Err is Human: Building a Safer Healthcare System*) stated that, healthcare appeared to be a decade or more behind other high-risk industries in ensuring basic safety. The IOM's report received tremendous media coverage and public concern about the safety of healthcare delivery system. Healthcare sector responded to this report with wide range of patient safety measures.[6] IOM and VAMC Lexington reports resulted in a significant culture shift from *Defend and Deny* to *Transparency, Disclosure and Apology*. Disclosure of medical errors has been increasingly accepted by healthcare sector and the gap between acceptability of error to actual disclosure is narrowing.

Ethics, Law and Policy

Medical ethics demand commitment from the medical practitioners to act solely for the patient's best interest. Studies have confirmed that most patients and their relatives want to know if medical error has taken place, and favored that such errors be reported to Government agencies and hospital agencies.[7] Failure to disclose medical errors to patients is likely to be perceived as fraudulent concealment and deception. Modern medical ethics promote involvement of patients in their treatment. For shared decision making by the patient, transparency in healthcare system is a must. To treat a patient who suffered an injury due to medical error, the principle of informed consent requires that the patient must be informed about what transpired during the treatment that led to the injury. However, physician's apprehensions about risk of litigation as a result of admitting medical errors, sometimes compel them to cover up medical errors, thereby preventing them from taking appropriate ethical steps in practice of medicine.

The law recognizes that medical errors may occur without negligence of medical practitioner even if the patient is harmed, in case the practitioner provided due care and skill as expected from him in the given circumstances. However, law does not accept dishonesty and fraudulent acts. In *Dr Neeraj Sardana vs. Rashmi Kakkar*,[8] a dental surgeon did not inform the patient that during tooth extraction her jaw was broken. The patient continued to suffer pain even after tooth extraction, and came to know about her jaw fracture when she got consultation from other dental surgeon. The judge concluded that the dental surgeon was negligent, and breached the duty of disclosure owed to the patient. In another case, an orthopedic surgeon concealed from the patient that he had operated on the wrong disc. He then convinced the patient to undergo second operation by him for the continued pain. This was considered by the Court as fraudulent concealment of relevant information and nullified the validity of consent for second operation.[9] These Court decisions suggest that a medical practitioner has a legal obligation to inform the patient about medical errors.

Disclosure of medical errors to the patients is not explicitly addressed in the Code of Ethics. Most of the professional bodies like Association of Physicians and Surgeons in India have no clear-cut policies requiring the medical practitioners to disclose the medical errors to the patients. However, as a part of quality assurance programs, many hospitals are adopting the policies that encourage the reporting of adverse events. But these policies do not address the specific issue of disclosure of medical errors to the patients: Whether to tell and what to tell?

With the passage of time, healthcare sector is accepting the concept of disclosure of medical errors to the patients, and evolving their policies in favour of error disclosure. The Veteran's Administration Hospital System in New York has an elaborate policy on reporting adverse events that includes instructing practitioners to disclose errors to patients.[10] Canadian Medical Protective Association (CMPA) promotes honesty, and advises the physicians to be accurate and factual in their disclosure to patients. The CMPA also offers assistance to physicians who contact the Association in advance of talking to patients and their relatives about medical errors.[11]

■ CONSEQUENCES OF DISCLOSING MEDICAL ERRORS

Benefits of Disclosure to the Patient

Disclosing the fact that medical error has occurred, gives opportunity to the patients to obtain timely treatment for the harm that has occurred due to the medical error. Timely corrective measures also prevent further harm to the patients. Sometimes, to mitigate the harmful effects of medical errors, close monitoring or certain curative steps (medical or surgical procedure) may be required, which, patients may not allow if they are unaware of the reasons for doing so. Disclosure is also essential to obtain the informed consent for further treatment necessary to treat the harmful effect of medical errors. Disclosure of medical error also helps the patients to have more realistic expectations from the treatment provided, and also promotes patient's trust in healthcare professionals.

Harms of Disclosure to the Patient

Patients may feel anxious and helpless to know that harm occurred due to medical interventions. It may destroy their faith and confidence in medical profession in general. Patients may decline beneficial treatments due to lack of trust on healthcare system. Some patients do not want to be burdened by all the information related to medical care, and the complexities of their illness. American College of Physicians Ethics Manual expressed that, the therapeutic nondisclosure also called therapeutic privilege is withholding the health information from the patient if disclosure is believed to be medically contraindicated. This exception to medical confidentiality can undermine the entire concept of informed consent. Thus therapeutic nondisclosure should be rarely invoked and only after a thorough review of the benefits and harms to the patient and ethical justification of nondisclosure.[12]

Harms of Disclosure to the Medical Practitioner

Clinicians find it difficult, rather, challenging to acknowledge their errors openly before patients and colleagues. Disclosure of errors can damage a medical practitioner's self-esteem, and reputation. When the medical error is revealed, the patient may become angry and aggressive, and such reactions can be highly stressful to the medical practitioners. Medical practitioners remain anxious and fearful that disclosing the medical errors will expose them to increased risk of malpractice lawsuit. However, the fear of lawsuits and professional sanctions seems exaggerated and misplaced.[14]

Benefits of Disclosure to the Medical Practitioner

The medical practitioner may feel relieved of the emotional stress by admitting the mistake. Probably the disclosure may strengthen the patient's trust, appreciating the physician's honesty. Disclosing errors may help the medical practitioners to make the constructive changes in their practice.[13] Sincere disclosure of a medical error may decrease the chance of legal liability. Moreover, if the medical error is concealed and the patient comes to know about the mistake from some other source, the medical practitioner will be at a greater risk of law suit.[14] It has been accepted by the healthcare sector that disclosure of medical errors to the patients in a structured manner is the right thing to do.

■ GUIDELINES ON DISCLOSING MEDICAL ERRORS

How to Handle Medical Errors in Practice?

Although clinicians generally support disclosure, multiple barriers prevent them from actually telling the patients about medical errors, such as apprehension of legal action, feeling of shame, and lack of disclosure training, etc.[16-18] Disclosure guidelines are presented below for healthcare providers and healthcare organizations as guiding principles for developing their own disclosure policies.

When Disclosure should Take Place?

Unfortunately, in spite of following all patient safety measures, an event or circumstance may arise which could have resuled, or did result in unnecessary harm to a patient. Multiple factors may be responsible for the harm, viz. natural progression of the disease, risks inherent in the investigation or the treatment, system failure, healthcare provider failure or combination of any or all of these. Whatever may be the reason, if a patient suffers harm, it becomes obligatory for the medical practitioner to inform the patient about the harm. In case of near miss incidents, decision regarding disclosure is discretionary. In such cases disclosure may be made if there is a residual safety risk, and patient would be benefited from knowing the incident of near miss. **Flowchart 1** demonstrate the circumstances, when disclosure should take place.[21]

Timing of Disclosure

If any unintended or unexpected incident results in harm, the first priority should be to attend to the care of the patient. Immediate emergencies must be dealt with at the earliest and the safety risk should be addressed and reduced if possible. Disclosure should be made at a time when the patient is physically and emotionally stable, and has recovered sufficiently to be able to understand the information.

Stages of Disclosure

Disclosure is often an ongoing process in which multiple disclosure conversations may occur over time, depending on the patient's condition and the concerns that arise. Disclosure generally occurs in two broad stages.

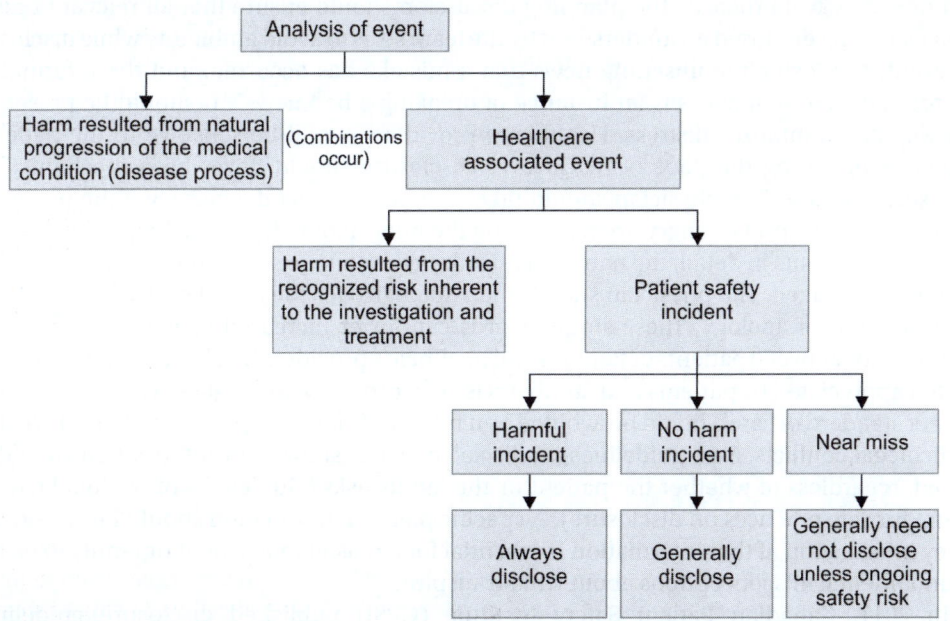

FLOWCHART 1: Circumstances when disclosure should take place.
Source: Disclosure Working Group. Canadian Disclosure Guidelines: Being open with patients and families. Edmonton, AB: Canadian Patient Safety Institute; 2011. Reproduced with permission.

First Stage of Disclosure (Initial Disclosure)

It is the initial discussion with the patient that should take place as soon as reasonably possible after an event. This stage of disclosure should focus on the medical condition as it now exists, and the probability of any further investigations or treatments. At this stage, all the contributors to the patient safety incident might not be clearly known or understood. Only the agreed upon facts that are known should be communicated during this stage. Other important components of this stage includes:
- An apology for what has happened.
- Avoidance of blame and speculation.

Second Stage of Disclosure (Postanalysis Disclosure)

During this stage, the reasons for the event are better understood. Patient should be informed about the additional facts known after the analysis, action taken to prevent similar events, if such improvements are possible. In postanalysis stage of disclosure, leadership and management representatives may take an active role, and the healthcare providers should be updated about the results of the analysis and encouraged to participate in the discussions.

Figure 1 summarize the disclosure process that starts with detection of patient safety incident and passes through various stages depending upon the nature of incident. The Canadian Patient Safety Institute has provided a detailed checklist for disclosure process, as a part of a published document: "Canadian Disclosure Guidelines-Being Open with Patients and Families" (**Box 2**).[21]

What to Say?

Before disclosing the error, healthcare providers involved in the disclosure process should plan how they will proceed. The planning discussion should ensure that all relevant agreed upon facts to be disclosed are understood by the team so as to avoid ambiguity while disclosing the event. Disclosing the upsetting news that a mistake has occurred, and the information regarding the consequences is an instance of breaking a bad news.[19] It should be presented in a way that minimizes distress. Healthcare providers should be sensitive to the patient's responses in setting the pace of disclosure. Disclosure should never be a mechanical or insensitive process. The physician should take care, not to react defensively if the patient or families become upset or angry upon receiving the information. It may be helpful to describe the course of events in detail, the nature of mistake, consequences, and remedial action taken or to be undertaken. The physician should then apologize for the mistake. Use the words *I'm sorry* as a part of apology. These simple words can foster increased respect and improved relationships between patients or families and healthcare providers involved. Genuine concern is often appreciated by patients and families. Use of words such as 'negligence', 'fault', 'failing to meet standard of care' should be avoided as it may imply legal assertions capable of creating medicolegal conflicts. New guidelines on disclosure suggest that, key information should be shared, regardless of whether the patient or the family asks (Guidelines of National Quality Forum for safe practices on disclosure). A specific piece of information should be considered as key information, if that information is essential for a reasonable patient or family to be free of fundamental misconceptions about what transpired.[20]

In 2011, Canadian Patient Safety Institute (CPSI) published disclosure guidelines, which evoke CPSI's main guiding theme *Ask-Listen-Talk – Good healthcare starts with good*

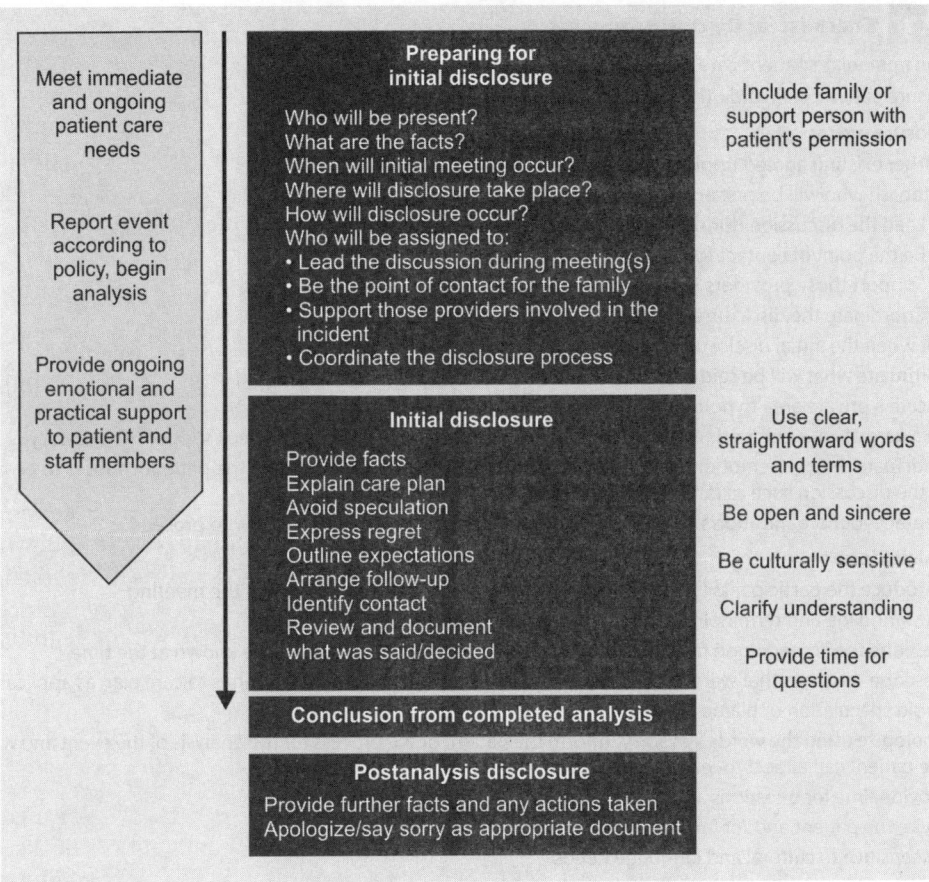

FIG. 1: The Disclosure process.
Source: Disclosure Working Group. Canadian Disclosure Guidelines: Being open with patients and families. Edmonton, AB: Canadian Patient Safety Institute; 2011. Reproduced with permission.

communication.[21] These guidelines support and encourage individuals and organizations to develop their own disclosure policies. For detailed information, this publication is available as a free download at *www.patientsafetyinstitute.ca*

Disclosure must occur if there has been harm related to a patient safety incident, or if there is a risk of potential future harm. In the case of a near miss, disclosure is discretionary based on whether it is felt the patient would benefit from knowing, e.g., if there is a residual safety risk. A discussion with the patient should take place regardless of the origin of the harm. Although the term 'disclosure' is used to describe the communications after the patient safety incident, any harm resulting from the disease process or healthcare should be discussed with the patient. Harm that has resulted from the inherent risks of an investigation or treatment should always be communicated to the patient. Such harm should not prematurely be attributed to simply a complication of the investigation or procedure. Incidents should be appropriately examined to understand all of the contributors involved. An analysis may indicate a combination of reasons actually resulted in the harm.

> **BOX 2** **Checklist for Disclosure process.**
>
> - The immediate patient care need are met
> - Ensure patient, staff and other patients are protected from immediate harm
>
> **Disclosure process plan**
> - Gather existing agreed upon facts
> - Establish who will be present at the meeting (s), and who will:
>   - Lead the discussion during the meeting(s)
>   - Be the point of contact for the family
>   - Support those providers involved in the incident
>   - Coordinate the disclosure process
> - Set when the initial disclosure will occur
> - Formulate what will be said and how effective disclosure will be accomplished
> - Locate a private area to hold disclosure meetings, free of interruptions
> - Be aware of your emotions and those providers involved in the process and seek support if necessary
> - Anticipate patient's emotions and ensure support is available, including who the patient chooses to be part of the discussion such as family, friends or spiritual representatives
> - Contact your organization's support services for disclosure if uncertain on how to proceed
>
> **Initial disclosure**
> - Introduce the participants to the patient, functions and reasons for attending the meeting
> - Use language and terminology that is appropriate for the patient
> - Describe the agreed upon facts of the patient safety incident and its outcome known at the time
> - Describe the steps that were and will be taken in the care of the patient (changes to care plan as applicable)
> - Avoid speculation or blame
> - Apologize using the words "I'm sorry." Inform the patient of the process for the analysis of the event and what the patient can expect to learn from the analysis, with appropriate timeliness
> - Provide time for questions and clarify whether the information is understood
> - Invite the patient and /or family to discuss the event from their point of view
> - Be sensitive to cultural and language needs
> - Review what was discussed and document what was said and decided, giving the patient an opportunity to read and review the documentation about the disclosure in the medical record
> - Offer to arrange subsequent meetings along with sharing key contact information
> - Offer practical emotional support such as spiritual care services, counseling and social work, as needed
> - Reimburse expenses related to the disclosure process, as appropriate
> - Facilitate further investigation and treatment if required
>
> **Susbequent and postanalysis disclosure**
> - Continued practical and emotional support as required, for the patient, family and providers
> - Reinforcement or correction of information provided in previous meetings
> - Further factual information as it becomes available
> - A further apology which might include an acknowledgment of responsibility for what has happened as appropriate
> - Describe any actions taken as a result of internal analyses such as system improvements
>
> **DOCUMENT the disclosure as per organizational policies and practices and include:**
> - The time, place and date of disclosure
> - The names and relationships of attendees
> - The facts presented
> - Offers of assistance and the response
> - Questions raised and the answers given
> - Plans for follow-up with key contact information for the organization
>
> *Source*: Disclosure Working Group. Canadian Disclosure Guidelines: Being open with patients and families. Edmonton, AB: Canadian Patient Safety Institute; 2011. Reproduced with permission.

CONCLUSION

Disclosing medical errors and near misses has a key role in patient safety. Although most clinicians believe that medical errors should be disclosed to the patients, in real situations they do not disclose under the guise of protecting the physician-patient relationship, and because of professional repercussions, guilt and fear of malpractice lawsuits. Patients and families desire disclosure of medical errors by healthcare providers. Failure to disclose medical errors is likely to be perceived as fraudulent concealment and deception.[15] Clinicians are more at risk of lawsuits if the patient comes to know about the mistake from some other source. Healthcare sector is now accepting the concept of disclosure of medical errors to the patients, and evolving their policies in favor of error disclosure. It is recommended that the clinicians, other healthcare providers, and healthcare institutions should develop and implement specific policies and systems of error disclosure. For a quality healthcare that endorses patient safety, a culture encouraging disclosure of medical errors is indispensable.

REFERENCES

1. www.brainyquote.com/quotes/kcywords/errors.html#tsvZs8vSWHgpjM20.99
2. Gawande A. Complications. New York: Penguin Books. 2002.
3. Kohan LT, Corrigan JM, Donaldson MS, editors. To err is human: building a safer health system. Washington: National Academy Press. 2000.
4. Brenan TA, Leape LL, Laird NM, Hebert L, Localio AR, Lawthers AG, et al. Incidence of adverse events and negligence in hospitalized patients: results of the Harvard medical practice study. NEJM. 1991;324:370-6.
5. Kramann SS, Hamm G. Risk management: extreme honesty may be the best policy. Annals of Internal Medicine. 1999;131(12): 963-7.
6. Institute of Medicine, "To err is human: building a safer health care system" (Linda T. Kohn et al eds., national academics press. 1999).
7. Hobgood C, Peck CR, Gilbert B, Chappell K. Medical errors - what and when: what do patients want to know? Acad Emwrg Med. 2002;9:1156-61.
8. Dr. Neeraj Sardana v. Rashmi Kakkar, Uttarakhand SCDRC, Dehradun. Medical Law Cases - For Doctors. 2008;1(9):19-24.
9. Gerula v. Flores (1995), 126 DLR (4th) 506, 128 (Ont CA).
10. Integrated patient safety/risk management program. Albany (NY): VA Healthcare Network, Upstate New York; 1998 June 1.s 3b. Available: www.va.gov/visns/visn02/vitalsigns/patientsafety.html (accessed 2013 June13).
11. Philip CH, Alex VL, Gerald R. Bioethics for clinicians: Disclosure of medical error. CMAJ. 2001;164(4):509-13.
12. American College of Physician. American College of Physicians Ethics Manual. 6th edn. 2012. Available from: http://www.acponline.org/running_practice/ethics/manual/manual6th.htm#confidentiality.
13. Wu AW, Folkman S, McPhee SJ, Lo B. Do house officers learn from their mistakes? JAMA. 1991;265:2089-94.
14. Victorof M. The right intentions: error and accountability. J Fam Pract. 1997;45:38-9.
15. Robertson G. Fraudulent concealment and the duty to disclose medical mistakes. Alberta Law Rev. 1986;25:215-23.
16. Finkelstein D, Wu AW, Holtzman NA, Smith MK. When a physician harms a patient by a medical error: ethical, legal, and risk-management considerations. J Clin Ethics. 1997;8:330-5.
17. Goldberg RM, Kuhn G, Andrew LB, Thomas HA Jr. Coping with medical mistakes and errors in judgment. Ann Emerg Med. 2002;39: 287-92.
18. Novack DH, Detering BJ, Arnold R, Forrow L, Ladinsky M, Pezzullo JC. Physicians' attitudes toward using deception to resolve difficult ethical problems. JAMA. 1989;261:2980-5.
19. Campbell ML. Breaking bad news to patients. JAMA. 1994;271:1052.
20. Gallagher TH, Bell SK, Smith LK, Mello MM, McDonald TB. Disclosing harmful medical errors to patients. Tackling three tough cases. Chest. 2009;136(3):897-903.
21. Disclosure Working Group. Canadian Disclosure Guidelines: Being open with patients and families. Edmonton, AB: Canadian Patient Safety Institute. 2011.

CHAPTER 4

End of Life Care Decisions: Ethical and Legal Issues

Rashmi Datta, Pradeep Sreevastava, Arvind Kumar Singh

> *"Dying can be a Peaceful Event or a Great Agony when it is inappropriately sustained by Life support."*
>
> —Roger Bone[1]

■ INTRODUCTION

End of life (EOL) care is the care provided for people who are likely to die within the next 12 months (including people with incurable and life-threatening conditions and those who die unexpectedly) and their families and carers. Consideration of EOL issues is an evolving phenomenon in India. Advances in medical technology, diagnostics, therapeutics, and intensive care can prolong the natural course of a critical disease or the aging process. However, a prospective determination about which patients will benefit from aggressive management and life-support is difficult. In a subset of critically ill patients, it may be obvious (as per the existing evidence on the disease's severity and reversibility) that the chances of meaningful survival and/or the return to an economically viable life are limited.[2,3]

Most doctors equate EOL issues as a strategic withholding of cardiopulmonary resuscitation (CPR) in the event of a cardiac arrest. Although thorough understanding of withholding and/or withdrawing treatment is extremely crucial, but it describes only what doctors decide not to do. The EOL issues also include, what should be done? From the patient's point of view, a host of uncontrolled factors (personal beliefs, cultural and religious influences, peer and family pressure) also have effects on EOL issues. Paternalism is still a cultural standard in India, and it is customary for physicians to inform the family of bad news rather than the patient, and decisions have to be made taking the family into consideration. In such circumstances, conflicts may arise regarding continuation of life-support.[3-5]

■ PALLIATIVE CARE AT THE END OF LIFE

In India, about 80% of the total healthcare bills are paid by the patients or their relatives. Currently, the intensive care in India is limited (less than one hospital bed/1,000 people and an even lesser number of ICU beds). Often, terminally ill patients are taken back to their homes either for performing socially pertinent rituals, or due to the exorbitant cost of critical care.[3,6] The concept of Managed or Palliative Care emerged from the notion that intensive care is expensive. The principle is that unnecessary healthcare costs can be reduced through a variety of mechanisms, including economic incentives for physicians and patients to select less costly forms of care; programs for reviewing the medical necessity of specific services and controls on inpatient admissions and lengths of stay.[7]

The World Health Organization defines palliative care as "an approach that improves the quality of life of patients and their families facing the problems associated with life-threatening illness, through the prevention and relief of suffering by means of early identification and impeccable assessment and treatment of pain and other problems, physical, psychosocial and spiritual."[8] Palliative care wards are now established with designed medical plan of the patient focusing not only on EOL issues such as DNR but also on pain management and symptom control including dyspnea, nausea, confusion, delirium, skin problems, and oral care. Psychological issues such as depression, sadness, anxiety, fear, loneliness need to be considered in those patients not on mechanical ventilation.[9]

■ MAGNITUDE OF THE PROBLEM

Data from western countries show that termination of medical treatment is currently the norm. In European countries withholding of therapy is reported in 38% of patients and withdrawal of therapy in 33%, although there were considerable variations amongst the countries. More than 85% of Americans die without CPR, and nearly 90% of decedents in American ICUs have withholding or withdrawal of medical treatments.[10,11]

There is a paucity of data on EOL decisions in India. Few studies[4,12] have been performed in Indian ICUs. A unicentric survey on the practices of EOL decision-making in North India noted that 78% patients received full resuscitation; in the 22% who were classified as receiving limitation of care, 18.8% were transferred out of the ICU terminally (left against medical advice) for financial or other reasons. Only 1.6% of ICU deaths had do-not-resuscitate (DNR) orders and life-support was withheld in another 1.6%.[4] In another Indian study, it was revealed that 34% of deaths in Mumbai had terminal limitation of therapy. Nearly 25% of these patients were not intubated; 67% were initially intubated and ventilated but failed to recover and, subsequently, had no further escalation of therapy and 8% had withdrawal of therapy.[12]

In India, medical practitioners are often reluctant to reveal individual EOL practices due to fear of punitive action. Life-support systems are rarely withdrawn; though not starting therapies tends to be more acceptable. These decisions, if made, are usually based on institutional policies for want of a uniform Governmental policy as in the West.[5,6,13,14]

■ MEDICAL FUTILITY

Medical futility is a professional judgment that permits doctors to withhold or withdraw care deemed to be inappropriate without subjecting such a decision to patient approval. Treatment should be defined as futile only when the intended goal will, in all probabilities, not be accomplished.[15,16] Medical futility was first defined by Schneiderman and colleagues as "quantitatively futile when it is shown to be useless in the last 100 cases in which it has been tried and qualitatively futile when it would result in nothing better than permanent unconsciousness or persistent dependence on intensive care."[17] Jecker's modification described futility as, "a treatment which cannot provide a minimum likelihood or quality of benefit and is not owed to the patient as a matter of moral duty."[18]

The Ethics Committee of the Society of Critical Care Medicine issued consensus statement regarding futile and other possibly inadvisable treatments. The consensus statement specified that:[19]

- Treatments should be defined as futile only when they will not accomplish their intended goal.
- Treatments that are extremely unlikely to be beneficial, are extremely costly, or are of uncertain benefit may be considered inappropriate and hence inadvisable, but should not be labeled futile.
- *Policies to limit inadvisable treatment should have the following characteristics*:
  - Be disclosed in the public record.
  - Moral values acceptable to the community.
  - Not be based exclusively on prognostic scoring systems.
  - Articulate appellate mechanisms
  - Be recognized by the courts.

In February 2005, the Indian Society of Critical Care Medicine (ISCCM) published guidelines for limiting the life prolonging interventions and providing palliative care toward the EOL (**Box 1**).[20]

BOX 1 | **Guidelines for limiting life-prolonging interventions and providing palliative care toward the end of life in Indian ICUs**

- The physician has a moral obligation to inform the capable patient/family, with honesty and clarity, the poor prognostic status of the patient when further aggressive support appears nonbeneficial. The physician is expected to initiate discussions on the treatment options available including the option of no specific treatment
- When the fully informed capable patient/family desires to consider comfort care, the physician should explicitly communicate the available modalities of limiting life-prolonging interventions. If the patient or family do not desire the continuation of life-supporting interventions the available options for limiting the supports should be identified as follows:
  - Withdrawal of life-support
  - Withholding of life-support
  - Do-not-resuscitate status
- The physician must discuss the implications of forgoing aggressive interventions through formal counseling sessions with the capable patient/family, and work toward a shared decision-making process. Thus, he accepts patient's autonomy in making an informed choice of therapy, while he fulfils his obligation of providing beneficent care
- Pending consensus decisions or in the event of conflicts between the physician's approach and the family's wishes, all existing supportive interventions should continue. The physician however, is not morally obliged to institute new therapies against his better clinical judgment
- The proceedings of the counseling sessions, the decision-making process, and the final decision should be clearly documented in the case records, to ensure transparency and to avoid future misunderstandings
- The overall responsibility for the decision rests with the attending physician/intensivist of the patient, who must ensure that all members of the caregiver team including the medical and nursing staff represent the same approach to the care of the patient
- If the capable patient/family consistently desires that life support be withdrawn, in situations in which the physician considers aggressive treatment nonbeneficial, the treating team is ethically bound to consider withdrawal within the limits of existing laws
- In the event of withdrawal or withholding of support, it is the physician's obligation to provide compassionate and effective palliative care to the patient as well as attend to the emotional needs of the family

■ WITHHOLDING OR WITHDRAWAL OF LIFE SUPPORT

As terminally ill patient progresses toward death it may be difficult to decide, when the medical treatment becomes futile? Once it is decided that the treatment is futile, the question arises as to withdraw or withhold life-sustaining treatment. Withdrawal of therapy means removal of a therapy which was started in an attempt to sustain life but has now become futile and is now just prolonging the process of death. Withholding of life support means that a treatment or procedure which may keep the patient alive who without such treatment would die is not given or performed. It refers to the concept of no therapeutic escalation by DNR.

There are two situations in the ICUs when the decision regarding withholding or withdrawal of life-sustaining treatments may be considered: When the prognosis for survival is poor, with or without treatment or when the potential benefits of treatment, in terms of quantity and quality of life, are not worth the financial and emotional burden (in the judgment of the patient or the surrogate decision-maker).[21] Doctors usually experience more difficulty in withdrawing rather than withholding life-sustaining measures. Therapies typically withheld/withdrawn include CPR, life-saving surgery, intrusive palliative procedures, balloon pumps, ventilators, dialysis, pacemakers, vasopressors, blood, antibiotics, and insulin. Parenteral and enteral fluids or nutrition are usually not withheld/withdrawn.

All ethical codes including the International Code of Medical Ethics and the Hippocratic Oath are based on humanist philosophy. According to the principles of beneficence, a medical practitioner is expected to alleviate pain and suffering of patients on one hand, and to protect and prolong their lives on the other.[22] Although the bioethical principle of justice, which forms the basis for triage, does lay down guidelines for allocation of healthcare resources, but conventional thinking does not accept termination of life sustaining care, merely on the plea that the resources could be better employed elsewhere.

There are no specific legal directives which accept termination of life sustaining care in situations where financial implications to the patient or family become unbearable. The consensus statement provided by the American College of Chest Physicians/Society of Critical Care Medicine Consensus Panel on Ethical and Moral Guidelines specifies that:

> *"A patient's productivity or economic value must play no role in the decision whether to undertake or withdraw intensive care. All patients must be treated equally."*[23]

If a competent, informed patient asks that support be withdrawn because it is economically burdensome, patient's autonomy should take precedence over the physician's perception of best interest for his patient. The situation is more difficult when the patient is incompetent and a surrogate expresses financial concerns. The physician's obligation in this instance is to ensure that there is no conflict of interest between the surrogate's economic concerns and patient's benefit before withdrawing support. The medical practitioner must try to ameliorate the patient's financial concerns by all means possible, including waiving of fees and involving other members of the healthcare team to help resolve the perceived problem.[2,3,6,24]

■ ADVANCED DIRECTIVES AND DO-NOT-RESUSCITATE ORDERS

Bioethical principle of autonomy is respected in the practice of medicine by following the doctrine of informed consent. Autonomy also implies allowing a competent individual to give advance consent as well as advance refusal to treatment of any nature for a subsequent period of decisional incapacity. Certain countries have accepted that the principle of autonomy entitles a person to even choose self-destruction. This principle has legal status in the United

States by the Patient Self Determination Act 1990 and the Uniform Rights of the Terminally Ill Act 1985. The patient can specify refusal of life-support if terminally ill or in coma (living will) or can nominate the spouse, relative or other person entrusted to make medical decisions when he/she would be unable to do so (durable power of attorney for healthcare). Such documents signed by the patient are called advance directives (ADs).[2,13,15,25]

In practice, a clinician is legally bound to respect the expressed or written ADs of an incapacitated or unconscious patient, irrespective of the outcome. Doctors can and have been penalized for institution of life-saving treatment as it amounts to interference with the patient's bodily integrity.

Do-not-resuscitate directive is a specialized and documented AD which is a well-accepted concept in many developed countries. In 1993, the guidelines by American Society of Anesthesiologists were restricted to the care of patients with DNR directives for cardiac arrest under anesthesia in the operating room where the chance of survival in 'witnessed arrests' is high. These evolved into the 2003 limited aggressive therapy order (LATO) in the US which offered patients the option of giving consent for CPR, for other "higher-success" situations in addition, including a witnessed cardiopulmonary arrest in which the initial cardiac rhythm is ventricular tachycardia or fibrillation and cardiac arrest resulting from a readily identifiable iatrogenic cause.[13,26]

Advance directives including DNR and LATO have not received legal sanction in India.[3,6,13] Therefore, doctors may be held liable to have violated the Law should they issue unwritten, verbal DNR recommendations to the patient's caregiver or relative for terminally ill or patients with poor prognosis. Many hospitals are now adopting futility policies based upon ISCCM guidelines. However, similar guidelines are lacking in an operating room set-up.[3,5,11,20]

EUTHANASIA

Euthanasia (Greek; *Eu* means Good, *thanatos* means Death), by definition, is an intentional killing of a person whose life is perceived to be not worth living by an act of commission or omission. Euthanasia may be categorized as follows.

Active Euthanasia

Active euthanasia is an act of commission when termination of life is done at the patient's request. It entails the use of lethal substances or forces to kill a person such as with lethal injection given to a person with terminal disease in terrible agony.

Passive Euthanasia

Passive euthanasia entails withholding of medical treatment for continuance of life, such as removing ventilator machine, from a patient in coma.[27] It is an act of omission under directives of a doctor and should be termed "Medical futility" implying pointlessness of continued care.

Voluntary Euthanasia

In voluntary euthanasia the consent is taken from the patient.

Nonvoluntary Euthanasia

In nonvoluntary euthanasia the consent is unavailable, e.g., when the patient is in coma, or is otherwise unable to give consent.

A distinction is sometimes drawn between euthanasia and physician assisted suicide (PAS), the difference being in who administers the lethal medication. In euthanasia, a physician or third party administers it, while in PAS, it is the patient himself who does it, though on the advice of the doctor. In Switzerland, euthanasia is illegal but PAS even by nonphysicians is legally condoned since 1918 under Article 115 of the Swiss Penal Code (SPC).[28,29] An important idea behind this distinction is that in "passive euthanasia" the doctors are not actively killing anyone; they are simply not saving him.

The general legal position all over the world seems to be that while active euthanasia is illegal unless there is legislation permitting it; passive euthanasia is legal provided certain conditions and safeguards are maintained. In India active euthanasia is illegal and a crime under section 302 or at least section 304 IPC. Physician assisted suicide is a crime under section 306 IPC (abetment to suicide).

In India, debate on euthanasia kick-started after a plea for euthanasia by Kolavennu Venkatesh, a young chess player who fought a bitter legal battle to end his life before a debilitating muscular degeneration killed him. Unfortunately, he died 2 days after the Andhra Pradesh HC rejected his plea for euthanasia Apart from his eyes, Venkatesh left behind a debate on the ethical and legal aspects of euthanasia.[30,31]

■ IMPLICATIONS TO HUMAN ORGAN TRANSPLANTATION ACT

Under the Human Organ Transplantation Act, 1994, human organs can be legally removed from the body of a person pronounced brain-dead by a board of medical experts constituted in accordance with the provisions of the Act, and a valid consent for removal of the organs had been given by the person during his lifetime or by the next-of-kin if the person is <18 years of age. It may be pertinent to note that the concept of Brainstem Death is accepted only where Organ Transplantation is to be undertaken. It is not accepted as the basis for declaring clinical death for purposes of the Registration of Births and Deaths Act.

Human Organ Transplantation Act is silent on stopping life-support treatment in a certified brain-dead individual if consent for organ harvesting is not forthcoming. It would account for euthanasia and is punishable (see below). Additionally 'non heart-beat donors' (NHBD) do not fall under the purview of the act. In these donors, a person is declared dead by cardiopulmonary criteria after establishing that circulation and respiration have ceased and their function will not resume. Consensus is also lacking on the time before any intervention geared toward organ retrieval is attempted (heparin to prevent intravascular clotting and phentolamine to maintain vascular perfusion) as these cannot be considered as beneficial to the patient. As such, would their use not seem to violate the ethical responsibility to the still alive patient?[3,6,32]

Legal Aspects of End of Life Issues in India

In India, the law regarding End of Life issues is predominantly silent and relatively archaic at places, with a lack of specific legislation on this subject. The Constitution of India not only guarantees the right to live but also provides directives to the State to provide healthcare to all citizens. This is illustrated in the following provisions of the constitution of India:
- *Article 21—Protection of life and personal liberty*: No person shall be deprived of his life or personal liberty except according to procedure established by law.

- *Article 14—Equality before law*: The state shall not deny to any person equality before the law or equal protection of the laws within the territory of India.
- *Articles 39 and 47* of the Directive Principles of State Policy.

In Gian Kaur vs. State of Punjab (1996 2 SCC 648), Constitution bench of Supreme Court of India stated that, "*Article 21 only guarantees right to life and personal liberty and in no case can the right to die be included in it.*" This clearly means that Article 21 does not allow termination of life in a dying person or in a vegetative state.

A physician who practices euthanasia would be charged under Sec 299 or Sec 304 A, IPC, depending on the method used. Relatives who participated or were aware of such intention of the physician could be charged under Sec 107 and 202 IPC. In cases where the entire process is undertaken at the behest of relatives, they could be charged under Sec 299 or 304 IPC as well. A physician might cite the provisions of Sec 87, Sec 88 and Sec 92, IPC to defend himself in cases where he is alleged to have used terminal sedation for an act of mercy killing. Intent will become a material consideration in such a case.[2,4,5,21,33]

In Naresh Marotrao Sakhre vs. Union of India (1995 Cri LJ 96), Bombay High Court held that, euthanasia or mercy killing is nothing but homicide whatever the circumstances in which it is effected.

In a landmark case of Aruna Ramchandra Shanbaug vs. Union of India and others, the Supreme Court legalised passive euthanasia by means of the withdrawal of life support to patients in a permanent vegetative state (PVS) subject to the safeguards laid down in the judgment. The court laid out guidelines for passive euthanasia. The Court stated that, the decision for withdrawal of life support of a patient in permanent vegetative state can be taken only by the 'next of kin' (parents or the spouse or other close relatives, or in the absence of any of them, a person or a body of persons acting as a next friend) or the attending doctor with the caveat that the decision should be taken bonafide in the best interest of the patient. The decision then requires to be ratified by the High Court concerned. An application is to be filed to the Chief Justice of the High Court who will constitute a bench of at least two judges to decide on the issue. Before doing so they will consult a panel of at least three experts, consisting of a neurologist, psychiatrist, and a physician as recommended by the State, who will examine the patient and submit their report to the Court. Simultaneously, notice will be issued to the State, near relations or in their absence, close friends. The views of the near relatives and committee of doctors would be given due weight by the High Court before pronouncing a final verdict which shall not be summary in nature. At paragraph 135, it was declared: The above procedure should be followed all over India until Parliament makes legislation on this subject. It means that, these guidelines will be the law until Parliament enacts legislation on the subject.[34]

■ CONCLUSION

Medical practitioners and healthcare administrators have unending apprehensions while dealing with EOL decisions particularly termination of life support. There is a felt need to have specific legislation on EOL care issues. An acceptable definition of medical futility will be prerequisite to any change in the law and medical fraternity need to come to a consensus on this issue. Until legal sanction is given to medical futility, effective communication with the patient's relatives remains the key. Patients approaching EOL and their families must be communicated in a sensitive and supportive manner by the healthcare providers and take EOL decisions with the knowledge, skills and attitude needed to provide quality care.

There must be clear documentation of efforts to achieve resolution with the patient and family, emphasizing that limiting the use of life-sustaining treatments will not lead to abandonment. In case there is a doubt whether, the EOL care decisions are legally appropriate or not, the matter should be referred to the institutional Ethics Advisory Committee.

■ REFERENCES

1. Bone RC. Reflections; a guide to end of life issues for you and your family. Evanston IL: National Kidney Cancer Association. You and I are dying. 1997.pp.4-7.
2. Yeolekar ME, Mehta S, Yeolekar A. End of life care: issues and challenges. J Postgrad Med. 2008;54(3):173-5.
3. Datta R, Chaturvedi R, Rudra A, Jaideep CN. End of life issues in the intensive care units. Med J Armed Forces India. 2013;69(1):48-53.
4. Mani RK. Limitation of life support in the ICU: ethical issues relating to end of life care. Indian J Crit Care Med. 2003;7:112–7.
5. Sharma H, Jagdish V, Anusha P, Bharti S. End-of-life care: Indian perspective. Indian J Psychiatry. 2013;55(Suppl 2):S293-8.
6. Chakravarty A, Kapoor P. Concepts and debates in end-of-life care. Indian Journal of Medical Ethics. 2012;9(3):202-6.
7. WHO, 2002. Palliative care for older people: better practices. ISBN 978 92 890 0224 0.
8. Cooper CC, Gottlieb MC. Ethical Issues with Managed Care: Challenges Facing Counselling Psychology. The Counselling Psychologist. 2000;28:179-236.
9. Bowen L. The multidisciplinary team in palliative care: a case reflection. Indian J Palliat Care. 2014;20(2):142-5.
10. Prendergast TJ, Claessens MT, Luce JM. A national survey of end-of-life care for critically ill patients. Am J Respir Crit Care Med. 1998;158:1163-7.
11. Sprung CL, Cohen SL, Sjokvist P, Baras M, Bulow HH, Hovilehto S, et al. End-of-life practices in European intensive care units: the Ethicus Study. JAMA. 2003;290:790-7.
12. Kapadia F, Singh M, Divatia J, et al. Limitation and withdrawal of intensive therapy at the end of life: practices in intensive care units in Mumbai, India. Crit Care Med. 2005;33:1272-5.
13. Puri VK. End-of-life issues for a modern India-Lessons learnt in the West. Indian J Crit Care Med. 2005;9:81-5.
14. Barnett VT, Aurora VK. Physician beliefs and practice regarding end-of-life care in India. Indian J Crit Care Med. 2008;121(3):109-15.
15. Sridhar P, Renuka PK, Bonanthaya R. End of Life and Life After Death - Issues to be Addressed. Indian J Palliat Care. 2012;18(3): 226-9.
16. Mohindera RK. Medical futility: a conceptual model. J Med Ethics. 2007;33:71-5.
17. Helft PR, Siegler M, Lantos J. The rise and fall of the futility movement. N Engl J Med. 2000;343:293-6.
18. Schneiderman LJ, Jecker NS, Jonsen AR. Medical futility: its meaning and ethical implications. Ann Intern Med. 1990;112: 949-54.
19. Consensus statement of the Society of Critical Care Medicine's Ethics Committee regarding futile and other possibly inadvisable treatments. Crit Care Med. 1997;25(5):887-91.
20. Mani RK, Amin P, Chawla R, Divatia JV, Kapadia F, Khilnani P, Myatra SN, Prayag S, Rajagopalan R, Todi SK, Uttam R, Balakrishnan S, Dalmia R, Kuthiala A. ISCCM position statement: limiting life-prolonging interventions and providing palliative care towards the end of life in Indian intensive care units. Indian J Crit Care Med. 2005;9:96-107.
21. Mani RK, Mandal AK, Bal S, Javeri Y, Kumar R, et al. End-of-life decisions in an Indian intensive care unit. Intensive Care Med. 2009;35(10):1713-9.
22. International Code of Medical Ethics of the World Medical Association. World Medical Association Bulletin. 1949;1(3): 109-11.
23. Ethical and Moral Guidelines for the Initiation, Continuation, and Withdrawal of Intensive Care: American College of Chest Physicians/Society of Critical Care Medicine Consensus Panel. Chest. 1990;97(4):949-58.
24. Bansal RK, Das S, Dayal P. Death Wish. JK Science Journal of Medical Education and Research. 2005;7(3):169-71.
25. Jeong SY, Higgins I, McMillan M. The essentials of Advance Care Planning for end-of-life care for older people. J Clin Nurs. 2010;19(3-4):389-97.
26. Choudhry NK, Choudary S, Singer PA. CPR for Patients Labeled DNR: The Role of the Limited Aggressive Therapy Order. Ann Intern Med. 2003;138(1):65-8.
27. Bernat JL. Medical futility: definition, determination, and disputes in critical care. Neurocrit Care. 2005;2(2):198-205.

28. Hurst SA, Mauron A. Assisted suicide and euthanasia in Switzerland: allowing a role for non-physicians. BMJ. 2003;326:271-73.
29. Keiser O, Spoerri A, Brinkhof MWG, Hasse B, Gayet-Ageron, A, Tissot F, Christen A, Battegay M, Schmid P, Bernasconi E, Egger M for the Swiss HIV Cohort Study and the Swiss Nation. Suicide in HIV-Infected Individuals and the General Population in Switzerland, 1988-2008. Am J Psychiatry. 2010;167:143-50.
30. Venkatesh is gone, but his struggle lives. The Times of India. 2004;18.
31. Ministry of External Affairs, Government of India. Healthcare. Available: http://meaindia.nic.in/indiapublication/healthcare.htm.
32. Bardale R. Issues related with non-heart-beating organ donation. Indian J Med Ethics. 2010;7(2):104-6.
33. Dogra TD, Rudra A. Lyons Medical Jurisprudence and Toxicology, 11th Edn, Delhi Law House. 2005.
34. Katju M, Mishra S. Judgment in the Supreme Court of India on Criminal Original Jurisdiction Writ Petition (Criminal) No 115 of 2009 by Aruna Ramchandra Shanbaug (Petitioner) versus Union of India and others. 2011. Source: http://judis.nic.in/supremecourt/chejudis.asp.

CHAPTER 5

Medicolegal Aspects of Discharge Against Medical Advice

Krishnadutt H Chavali, Swapnil S Agarwal, VP Singh

> *"Your most unhappy customers are your greatest source of learning."*
> —**Bill Gates, Microsoft**

■ INTRODUCTION

Discharge against medical advice (DAMA) is a problematic situation in which a patient leaves the healthcare establishment before the healthcare provider recommends discharge.[1] It is also known by other names, leave against medical advice (LAMA), or at-own-risk (AOR) discharge. An AOR discharge, LAMA, or DAMA is understood to occur whereby a patient leaves the hospital without informing or leaves after consultation with a medical team but before assessment and/or treatment have been completed.

Studies have empirically demonstrated that patients who leave against medical advice (AMA) have higher risks of adverse medical outcome.[2,3] This can in turn be a potential area of "negligence suit" against the medical practitioner and/or the healthcare provider. A properly executed DAMA can thus provide significant legal safeguard against the risk of medical negligence liability. In addition to the legal implications, such discharges are often associated with adverse medical outcomes for the patient.

When the patient leaves the hospital before completion of medical treatment and against medical advice, there occurs breakdown in therapeutic relationship between patient and physician. Dissolution of patient-physician relationship terminates the physician's duty of care and professional liability with respect to care of the patient. However, professional obligations of the medical practitioner do not end abruptly. Although, acceptance of DAMA by the medical practitioner can be seen as respecting patient autonomy, it not only raises clinical, ethical, and legal issues for the treating physician but also leads to adverse health outcomes thereby burdening the health system even more.[4,5] To effectively manage a case of DAMA as per the clinical, ethical, and legal requirements, a thorough understanding of the associated medicolegal aspects cannot be overemphasized.

■ HOW PREVALENT IS DAMA?

Discharge against medical advice is a universal problem in healthcare sector, plaguing both developing and developed countries. The rate of DAMA varies among different hospitals, institutes, and countries due to multiple reasons. Furthermore, there are studies that have documented a higher rate in developed as compared to developing countries. In prospective study, from India the incidence of DAMA was 3.84% in the emergency department (ED) of a private hospital over 3 months.[6] As per another Indian study at a tertiary care hospital with attached medical college for neonates in ICU, conducted setting, prevalence was 25.4%.[7] In another retrospective study, it was found that, about 3.3% of patients left hospital of DAMA against medical advice. Most of them were from ward followed by ICU.[8] In yet another study it has been documented that there is considerable variation in prevalence rates of DAMA ranging from 0.002 to >35%.[9] In the US, each year 1–2% of all hospital discharges (approximately 500,000 patients) are designated as DAMA.[10]

■ CAUSES AND PREDICTORS OF DAMA[4,11]

Why Patients Leave Against Medical Advice?

A patient can have multiple reasons for leaving a treatment against medical advice. Reasons such as partial recovery, lack of trust in service quality, feeling uncomfortable, and even financial constraints are given by patients. Low literacy levels and rural background have also been found as reasons for DAMA.[12] DAMA has a multifactorial etiology, and patients leave the hospital against medical advice due to various reasons (**Box 1**). Thorough understanding of the reasons why patients leave against medical advice can help to identify those at higher risk and thus intervene earlier to prevent the occurrence of DAMA.

Who is at Risk of DAMA?

Early identification of patients at risk may help in designing the preventive strategies, thereby decreasing the occurrence of DAMA. A study suggested that early identification of "at-risk of DAMA" patients and improved modalities to prevent DAMA among these patients may reduce the negative outcomes associated with DAMA patients.[13] Various predictors like the male, substance abuse, mental and emotional problems, lack of health insurance, younger age, race/ethnicity, income, primary diagnosis, severity of illness, and hospital location/type and size have all been suggested.[14] Various factors suggestive of an impending DAMA may be categorized as shown in **Table 1**.[4]

BOX 1	Causes of discharge against medical advice.

- Dissatisfaction with the quality of care
- Patient expected a shorter stay
- Patient's condition is not improving
- Preference for another hospital
- Believes that the condition terminal
- Disliking of the hospital environment
- Financial difficulties
- Insensitive behavior and poor communication
- Not understanding the need for further testing or treatment

TABLE 1: Predictors of impending DAMA.

Patient related factors	Hospital related factors
• Previous medical history • Behavior while in the hospital • Younger age • Male gender • No health insurance • Low socioeconomic status • Alcohol and drug abuse • Psychiatric disease • Persons with less social support (single) • Past history of DAMA	• Failure to orient the patient to treatment on admission • Inefficient admission and discharge procedure • Inadequate staffing patterns • Punitive or threatening atmosphere in the hospital • Poor doctor-patient relationship • Failure to establish a supportive provider-patient relationship

(DAMA: discharge against medical advice)

■ LEGAL STATUS OF DAMA

Dissolution of the Therapeutic Relationship

Approval of DAMA by the clinician is seen as respecting patient autonomy. DAMA evidences an irretrievable breakdown in the patient-physician relationship, when patient leave the hospital before completion of medical treatment and against medical advice. Dissolution of the therapeutic relationship terminates the physician's duty of care and professional liability with respect to care of the patient. It is commonly assumed that the execution of DAMA provides protection from future liability for both the doctors and the hospital.

Is there any Protection Against Future Litigation?

The protection afforded against medical negligence lawsuits in cases of DAMA emanates only when the following is established:[15]
- Termination of legal duty to treat the patient. Establishing that no further obligation to care exists to treat the patient who is competent, fully aware of, and assumes responsibility for the repercussions of severing their therapeutic relationship with the doctor.
- Creation of affirmative defense of "assumption of risk." The patient's ability to competently assume the risks of his actions (leaving against medical advice) is determined by the patient's competence to make a competent decision. To make a competent decision, an individual must be able to:
  ○ Understand the information relevant to the decision;
  ○ Retain that information;
  ○ Use or weigh that information as part of the process of making the decision; or
  ○ Communicate his decision (by talking, sign language, or any other means).
- Documentary evidence of patient's refusal of care and execution of all necessary steps of discharge process.
- Reasonable care (consistent with the prevailing standards of care) was provided up to the point in which the relationship was terminated.

Validity of DAMA

The validity of DAMA pivots on the assumptions that in such requests the patient is fully informed and competent to invoke an AOR discharge, and that care up to the point of the AOR discharge meets prevailing clinical standards. Legally, considering and respecting patient autonomy, no patient can be forced to undertake a treatment that he or she does not want to, at a place that he or she is not interested to avail of the service. It is well within their right to decide whether to continue with a treatment at the particular place or leave it irrespective of the stage up to which the treatment may have progressed.

Duty of Doctor in DAMA

In case there is a request for DAMA, doctors must appropriately discharge their legal responsibilities as follows:[4]
- Assessing the patient's decision-making capacity, trying to comfort the patient, and resolving the issues related to DAMA so as to prevent the DAMA.
- Providing appropriate information to the patient about his or her condition, treatment options, and the potential risks as well as the risk of noncompliance with medical advice and alternative treatment options.
- Establishing that the information provided has been understood and duly considered and any misunderstandings and/or gaps in comprehension clarified.
- Documenting all the necessary aspects of discharge process as per hospital policy and applicable laws.
- Getting the patient's acknowledgement that he or she received the necessary information and the assumption of risks by signing the DAMA form.

■ CONSEQUENCES OF DAMA

Discharge against medical advice is associated with higher risk of adverse medical outcomes. Such discharges can in turn be a potential area of "negligence suit" against the medical practitioner and/or hospital. Often, the consequences of discharges against medical advice are unwelcome. It is important to understand the consequences so as to resolve them at the earliest opportunity.

Risk to the Patient

Poor Outcomes

Most of the studies have shown that patients have had poor outcomes in cases of DAMA. Patients with chest pain who left against medical advice had a higher risk of myocardial infarction than other patients with similar characteristics who stayed in the ED to complete their workup.[13] Similarly, asthma patients who left against medical advice had an increased risk of both relapse and subsequent ICU admissions.[16]

High Healthcare Costs

Despite being a small percentage of total discharges, these patients have disproportionately high healthcare costs. One study reported that healthcare costs among these patients were 56% higher than expected.[17]

High Morbidity, Mortality, and Hospital Readmissions

Patients with DAMA suffer higher than expected rates of morbidity, mortality, and hospital readmission. Case-control study in an urban teaching hospital, patients discharged AMA from the general medicine service had a higher (21% vs. 3%) 15-day readmission rate as compared to patients with age, gender, and diagnosis-matched controls.[10,16,18] As per a study with California State Inpatient Database, as compared to patients who were discharged home, patients discharged AMA had significantly higher 30-day readmission rates, higher rates of multiple readmissions and likelihood of being readmitted at different hospitals.[19]

Poor Insurance Claim Settlement

The potential risk, other than medical, is of nonsettlement of claims from the insurer. It is still unclear whether insurance companies, who offer reimbursement of medical costs, would proceed with settlement of claims for patients who get discharged against medical advice. But there is always a risk of nonsettlement.

Risk to the Doctor/Hospital

Risk of Litigation

All patients who leave against medical advice are at potentially high-risk for initiating a "suit of medical negligence." Estimates show that 1 in 300 DAMA cases results in a medical negligence lawsuit compared to 1 in 30,000 standard ED visits.[20]

Factors Related to Impending Litigation

Whether a case of DAMA would later end up as malpractice lawsuit depends on many factors. Important factors predicting high chances of future litigation are:

- *Reason for DAMA:* Early detection and timely rectification of risk factors related to impending DAMA may help in designing the preventive strategies, thereby decreasing the occurrence of DAMA. If financial constraint is the cause of the DAMA, the healthcare provider should consider of providing feasible alternatives so that the patient can continue with the treatment. This should be provided at right time because sudden financial burden and withdrawal from treatment leading to an unfavorable outcome can have serious medicolegal implications with the provider liable to be sued for deficiency in services.

   Failure to regularly attend to the patient and rude behavior of the medical practitioner or the supportive staff can also be reasons for seeking DAMA and also a lawsuit for deficiency of services. There have been instances where support staff has been rude and callous with the patient/relatives resulting in heated arguments. With an unfavorable outcome in such cases, the doctor or the hospital can be accused of deliberate inaction and can be sued for damages.

- *Improper counseling*: Improper counseling, especially in cases with expected poor prognosis is one of the factors for taking DAMA. If the patient seeks DAMA due to a poor prognosis being advised casually and his health improves at the new medical facility, he or she may accuse the previous healthcare provider for providing misleading information or deficiency in service.

   Counseling should also include the expected outcomes associated with DAMA. If the patient or attendant is not clearly acquainted with inherent risk of morbidity and/or mortality associated with DAMA, then if any complication occurs after the DAMA, provider

can be accused of providing incomplete information, and absence of "shared and informed decision making" is deemed as deficiency in service.
- *Incomplete/incorrect documentation*: It is a well-known maxim that "what is not documented, in not done." Healthcare providers must ensure that everything that is shared with patient or relative is not only clearly documented but also duly acknowledged by the patient or attendant by affixing their signature. This would avoid the allegation of not sharing the risks of DAMA in a prospective legal dispute. With the technology available, healthcare establishments may also consider video recording of the communication between the patient and the doctor in order to keep a record. Of course, this should be done with the knowledge and consent of the patient or legal guardian.

■ MANAGING DAMA: A PRACTICAL APPROACH

A practical approach toward managing patients, who intend to leave the hospital against medical advice, requires an understanding of ethical and legal obligations. Patients, who have decision-making capacity, have a legal right to refuse the treatment, even if doing so is apparently harmful to the patient. Honoring patient autonomy in decision making sometimes can conflict with doctor's ethical obligation to beneficence. DAMA does not obviate a doctor's responsibility to advocate for patient's well-being, and therefore, reasonable efforts should be made to protect these patients from impending harm that may occur due to their decision of refusing the medical advice. Ideally, in such cases, the healthcare provider and patient should work together as a team to select the best course of action for the particular individual.[21] Shared decision making between patient and doctor has a vital role in optimizing medical care and minimizing the harm, and may even obviate the need to DAMA.

Assess Decision-making Capacity

When a patient refuses medical advice, it is most important to assess the patient's decision-making capacity and document clearly that the patient can understand their condition, available treatment options, and consequences of not accepting the proposed treatment.[22] Decision-making capacity can be determined by assessing the following elements:[23]
- *Understanding*: Patient's ability to understand the meaning of information provided by the physician.
- *Appreciation*: Patient's ability to determine how facts are relevant to his or her condition.
- *Reasoning*: Patient's ability to use the information to make decisions regarding his or her care.
- *Ability to express a choice*: Patient's ability to clearly communicate the choice of treatment.

If Patient Lacks Capacity

A patient, who lacks decision-making capacity, is unable to refuse or give consent for treatment. In case a patient is found to lack capacity, healthcare providers are required to take decision of continuing with the treatment or discontinuing it (as per advance directives if available), and/or consider the choice of the surrogate decision-maker (as per hospital policy based on applicable law). In circumstances, when a patient (who lacks capacity) has a life-threatening medical condition, then under the "emergency consent principle" the provider may treat even without consent to prevent serious and irreversible harm or death. The circumstances of the situation should invariably be noted down in the case notes at the earliest possible time for the record and possible future use.

Adequate Information and Disclosure of Risks

The patients should be provided all information relevant to an AMA decision, including their diagnosis, treatment options available, and the risks and benefits of accepting or refusing treatment. It is important that patients confirm their understanding of this information and demonstrate reasons for deciding to leave against medical advice. A patient's signature on an AMA form, by itself, does not indicate informed consent. It is important to thoroughly discuss with the patients about the risks and consequences of leaving AMA. The elements noted in **Box 2** should be discussed in detail.[24]

BOX 2 | **AIMED approach for DAMA patients.**[24]

A (Assess)
- Severity of illness (How sick is the patient?)
- Degree of risk to patient's health (What is at stake?)
- Decision making capacity (Is capacity intact or impaired?)

I (Investigate)
- *Patient's reason for leaving:* Talk to the patient to understand why the patient is acting against his/her best interest. Talk empathetically to the patient, "I am worried about you. Why do you want to leave before your care is complete?"
- *Try resolve the concerns:*
  - Comfort the patient by symptom management
  - Sometimes, the medical condition itself needs proper management
  - Ensure that opioid, alcohol, or nicotine withdrawal (if present) are managed adequately
  - Discuss care plan with the patient
  - Sometimes patient has pressing responsibilities like child and elder. Such concerns can be addressed with a call to a relative or friend

M (Mitigate)
- *Mitigate harm:* If all attempts to convince the patient to continue treatment are exhausted and patient is determined to leave, then, try to mitigate the harm by offering the best possible alternate care plan that the patient will accept after DAMA.
  - Offer maximal necessary treatment acceptable to patient
  - Provide optimal follow-up plan and discharge instructions

E (Explain)
- *Explain risks and benefits:*
  - Explain original plan of care, along with benefits and risks of following or refusing to follow the plan
  - Explain alternate treatment plan along with associated risks and benefits
  - Explain the discharge instructions including reasons to return
  - Explain the patient that he/she is welcome to return any time if circumstances change

D (Document)
- Assessment of decision-making capacity
- Discussion on original treatment plan offered
- Risks and benefits of accepting or refusing treatment, explained to the patient
- Discussion on patient's reasons for refusing investigation or treatment, and the decision to leave against medical advice
- Efforts to address the concerns and resolve the issue
- Recommendations for alternate care plan including risks and benefits
- Discharge instructions and when to return
- If patient refuses to take part in discharge discussion or refuses to sign DAMA form, this should also be documented, and get signature of two witnesses in presence of whom the patient denied

(DAMA: discharge against medical advice)

Adequate Documentation and DAMA Forms

The importance of appropriate documentation of the process of DAMA cannot be overemphasized. There is a requirement that the patient should be provided with the appropriate information, determined to be competent, and allowed to ponder on the information before arriving at a decision to refuse further treatment (against medical advice). The documentation should include all these necessary requirements before acquiescence to DAMA is deemed acceptable. Medical records of the patient should include:

- Assessment of decision-making capacity.
- Information provided to the patient pertaining to diagnosis, treatment options available.
- Risks and benefits of accepting or refusing treatment.
- The patient's reasons for refusing investigation or treatment.
- The decisions made by patient to leave against medical advice.
- Efforts to address the concerns and resolve the issue.
- Recommendations for alternate treatment plan along with associated risks and benefits.
- Discharge instructions and when to return for follow-up.
- Getting signatures of the patient, treating doctor, and two witnesses.
- If the patient refuses to sign the DAMA form, reading it aloud, documenting the refusal to sign, and noting that the patient was made aware of the risks of LAMA.
- Getting signature of two witnesses who witnessed the fact of patient's refusal to sign.

Although, simple signing of a DAMA form does not confer absolute medicolegal protection, a signed DAMA form is acknowledgment that a discussion with the patient of the risks of discharge has occurred. It is the right of the patient to be given a summary of the treatment provided to the patient even if he or she seeks DAMA. Failure to give a discharge summary or referral note to the patient can be deemed as deficiency of service by courts of law.

It is common practice to document that the patient left the hospital despite an explicit medical recommendation to the contrary. Typically, the consent for DAMA is similar to the one shown in **Table 2**. In practice, these documents do not confer legal protection.[23,25,26] In fact, it is not possible to have a document that absolves the healthcare team from responsibility for adverse events. The Canadian Medical Protective Association acknowledges that physicians can be held responsible for adverse outcomes when patients leave against medical advice, but nonetheless recommends trying to obtain a signed DAMA form documenting that a discussion outlining the risks of discharge has occurred.[27] Whenever a patient leaves hospital under circumstances that do not seem ideal, the focus should be on establishing the patient's capacity and arranging the safest modality for follow-up, rather than creating conflict. For example, in a study, a high proportion of medical staff reported informing patients erroneously that they would not have insurance coverage for their hospital visit if they left against medical advice.[23] This would initiate distrust and can be a risk for future litigation.

The DAMA forms must be designed and executed in medicolegally effective manner so as to avoid culpability, in case a lawsuit claim arises as a consequence of associated poor outcome. A practical approach with the acronym AIMED has been proposed (**Box 2**) to ensure that essential ethical, legal, and medical elements are included and documented in each case where patients desire to decline medical care and leave against medical advice.[24]

TABLE 2: Informed consent for discharge against medical advice.

Name of the Patient: .... Age/Sex: ....

Name of the Guardian: .... Relation to the Patient: ....

Hospital No. of Patient: .... Department: ....

Ward: .... Name and No. of Unit under Treatment: ....

Diagnosis: ....

Admission Date: .... Time: ....

I/We have been informed by the treating doctor about my/our relative's critical condition and that I/he/she needs continuing hospitalization for monitoring and further treatment which, if not provided, may be detrimental to my/our relative's health.

In spite of being made aware that discontinuation of further monitoring and treatment under hospitalization can have serious adverse effects to my/our relative's condition, I/we wish to discharge myself/our relative from hospital against medical advice. I am informed that ambulance facility shall be made available on demand even if I/we take discharge against medical advice either to my/our home or another medical facility.

Patient's Name: .... Sign: .... Date and Time: ....

Name of LAR*/NOK**: .... Relationship: ....

(Sign: ....) Date and Time: ....

(* Legally Authorized Representative / ** Next of Kin)

This consent has been explained to the patient/representative in my presence.

Name of Witness: .... Address: ....

(Sign: ....) Date and Time: ....

Name of Doctor: .... Sign: .... Date and Time: ....

CONCLUSION

Despite the advances in documentation and communication, DAMA continues to be a bitter experience both for patients and their doctors, and is associated with adverse outcomes including higher readmission rates. Autonomy of the patient must be respected and the doctor should not consider it an insult to his ego that the patient wishes to leave his care to avail of the services of another doctor or establishment. Rather, on receipt of a request of a patient seeking DAMA, it is the duty of the healthcare facility or doctor to ensure that the patient understands the implications of his decision and also that the patient is provided all the support so as to reach the next hospital or home safely. Health of the individual should be the prime concern for any doctor. In fact, if this aspect is taken care of for every patient, the number of DAMAs can be minimized to a large extent. Modifiable patient characteristics that serve as predictors for DAMAs should be identified and addressed, and strategies should be developed to reduce the adverse outcomes associated with DAMA.

REFERENCES

1. Ding R, Jung J, Kirsch TD, et al. Uncompleted emergency department care: patients who leave against medical advice. Acad Emerg Med. 2007;14(10):870-6.
2. PSNet. (2005). Case and Commentary: Discharge against Medical Advice. Agency for Healthcare Research and Quality. [online] Available from: https://psnet.ahrq.gov/webmm/case/96/Discharge-Against-Medical-Advice. [Last Accessed on August, 2019].
3. Stern TW, Silverman BC, Smith FA, et al. Prior discharges against medical advice and withdrawal of consent: what they can teach us about patient management. Prim Care Companion CNS Disord. 2011;13(1). pii: PCC.10f01047.
4. Al Ayed I. What makes patients leave against medical advice? J Taibah Univ Med Sci. 2009;4(1):16-22.
5. Choi M, Kim H, Qian H, et al. Readmission rates of patients discharged against medical advice: a matched cohort study. PLoS One. 2011;6(9):e24459.
6. Naderi S, Acerra JR, Bailey K, et al. Patients in a private hospital in India leave the emergency department against medical advice for financial reasons. Int J Emerg Med. 2014;7(1):13.
7. Devpura B, Bhadesia P, Nimbalkar S, et al. Discharge against medical advice at neonatal intensive care unit in Gujarat, India. Int J Pediatr. 2016;2016:1897039.
8. Gautam N, Sharma JP, Sharma A, et al. Retrospective evaluation of patients who leave against medical advice in a tertiary teaching care institute. Indian J Crit Care Med. 2018;22(8):591-96.
9. Eze B, Agu K, Nwosu J. Discharge against medical advice at a tertiary centre in South Eastern Nigeria. Sociodemographic and clinical dimensions. Patient Intell. 2010;2:27-31.
10. Glasgow JM, Vaughn-Sarrazin M, Kaboli PJ. Leaving against medical advice (AMA): risk of 30-day mortality and hospital readmission. J Gen Intern Med. 2010;25(9):926-9.
11. Franks P, Meldrum S, Fiscella K. Discharges against medical advice: Are race/ethnicity predictors? J Gen Intern Med. 2006;21(9):955-60.
12. Awasthi S, Pandey N. Rural background and low parental literacy associated with discharge against medical advice from a tertiary care government hospital in India. Clin Epidemiol Glob Health. 2015;3(1):24-8.
13. Lee TH, Short LW, Brand DA, et al. Patients with acute chest pain who leave emergency departments against medical advice: prevalence, clinical characteristics, and natural history. J Gen Intern Med. 1988;3(1):21-4.
14. Spooner KK, Salemi JL, Salihu HM, et al. Discharge against medical advice in the United States, 2002-2011. Mayo Clin Proc. 2017;92(4):525-35.
15. Levy F, Mareiniss DP, Iacovelli C. The importance of proper against-medical-advice (AMA) discharge: how signing out AMA may create significant liability protection for providers. J Emerg Med. 2012;43(3):516-20.
16. Baptist AP, Warrier I, Arora R, et al. Hospitalized patients with asthma who leave against medical advice: characteristics, reasons, and outcomes. J Allergy Clin Immunol. 2007;119(4):924-9.
17. Kahle CH, Rubio ML, Santos RA. Discharges against medical advice: considerations for the hospitalist and the patient. Hosp Med Clin. 2015;4(3):421-9.

18. Hwang SW, Li J, Gupta R, et al. What happens to patients who leave hospital against medical advice? CMAJ. 2003;168(4):417-20.
19. Olufajo OA, Metcalfe D, Yorkgitis BK, et al. Whatever happens to trauma patients who leave against medical advice? Am J Surg. 2016;211(4):677-83.
20. Bitterman RA. Against Medical Advice: When should you take "no" for an Answer? Lecture Presented at ACEP Scientific Assembly. Chicago, IL: 2008.
21. Gillick MR. Re-engineering shared decision-making. J Med Ethics. 2015;41(9):785-8.
22. Searight HR. Assessing patient competence for medical decision-making. Am Fam Physician. 1992;45(2):751-9.
23. Alfandre D, Schumann JH. What is wrong with discharges against medical advice (and how to fix them). JAMA. 2013;310(22):2393-4.
24. Clark MA, Abbott JT, Adyanthaya T. Ethics seminars. a best-practice approach to navigating the against-medical-advice discharge. Acad Emerg Med. 2014;21(9):1050-7.
25. Schmidt MJ, Dostal KU. Optimizing outcomes when patients leave against medical advice. JCOM. 2007;14(12):645-53.
26. Devitt PJ, Devitt AC, Dewan M. Does identifying a discharge as "against medical advice" confer legal protection? J Fam Pract. 2000;49(3):224-7.
27. CMPA Good Practices Guide. Leaving Against Medical Advice (AMA). [online] Available from: https://www.cmpaacpm.ca/serve/docs/ela/goodpracticesguide/pages/communication/Informed_Discharge/leaving_against_medical_advice-e.html. [Last Accessed on August, 2019].

CHAPTER 6

Violence Against Doctors: Causes, Effects, and Solutions

Sundeep Mishra

> *"Violence can never be justified, least of all against someone who is ostensibly attempting to save a person's life."*
> —**Sumanth Raman**[1]

■ INTRODUCTION

Sacrifice is part of the great tradition of medicine, a tradition that compels doctors into one of the most hazardous occupations. The list of dangers is actually quite long: Risk for communicable illnesses—both common and rare, stresses that lead to extremely high rates of burnout, depression, substance abuse, and suicide that outpace other professions (of similar level of education, gender, and generation), and serious occupational hazards like workplace violence both physical and verbal. Each and every practicing doctor has been touched by these issues, either directly or as witness. As per an Indian Medical Association study, more than three-fourths of physicians have witnessed some form of violence at workplace. On the other hand, individuals entering the profession are either completely unaware or have only limited understanding of the potential long-term consequences that are often understated or ignored.[2] Some occupational hazards have indeed been studied, but there is no comprehensive analysis of workplace risk for physicians like those that have been done for other professions especially those related to workplace violence.

Violence directed against the physician and the healthcare workers seems to be a common phenomenon worldwide. However, this phenomenon has been given a scarce consideration and minimal lip service not only in lay public, media, and law administrators but also in medical community. As a matter of fact, the subject of aggression and violence against physicians and its remedies does not figure anywhere either in medical curriculum or continuing medical education.[3] Multiple anecdotal reports suggest that the problem is increasing globally but systematic data is lacking.[4-10] However, it is likely to be more prevalent in those healthcare settings like India, which were traditionally socialistic but have recently turned to capitalistic model of healthcare.[11]

Although violence is common in many workplace settings especially those dealing with social and financial sectors, it can under no circumstance be condoned in hospitals. Although in reality in-hospital violence is just a superficial symptom of a deeper malady afflicting overall healthcare system, the hospitals cannot be allowed to become battlegrounds for the simple reason that sick people need a peaceful environment where they can get sympathy, empathy, support, etc. At the same time, the healthcare professionals also need a stable and peaceful environment if they are to provide selfless care (rather than worry about their personal safety). On a long-term basis, the threats and violence could have a bad impact on the physician's psychology leading to post-traumatic stress syndrome (PTSD) in majority of the physicians, something which is akin to a problem faced by war veterans.[12] This manifests as a physician feeling helpless, becoming irritable, introverted, and having thoughts of abandoning medicine or even contemplating suicide.[13] Even more stable personalities might be forced to practice defensive medicine and intent on saving their own skin rather than considering for the patient.

■ DEFINITION

Many people think of violence as a physical assault. However, violence in healthcare setup is a much broader problem. It is any act, in which a person is abused, threatened, intimidated, or assaulted in his/her employment. Generally speaking, workplace violence includes:
- Threatening behavior (shaking fists, throwing objects, or destroying property).
- Verbal or written threats (expression of an intention to inflict harm).
- Harassment (any behavior that demeans, embarrasses, humiliates, annoys a person. This includes inappropriate words, gestures, intimidation, bullying, or other such activities).
- Verbal abuse (insults, offensive language, or disdainful language).
- Physical attacks (hitting, pushing, or kicking).

Violence against doctors is any act of aggression, physical assault, or threatening behavior that occurs in a healthcare setting and causes physical or emotional harm to a health worker.[14] The violence can range from telephonic threats, intimidation, actual verbal abuse, physical but noninjurious assault, sexual harassment, physical assault causing injury; simple or grievous, weaponry attacks, and homicide to vandalism and/or arson. Verbal abuse is the most common type of violence encountered, but there seems to be some gender bias as well, sexual abuse being nearly exclusive in female workers.

■ FACTORS PREDISPOSING TO VIOLENCE

The root cause of the problem is the growing distrust between healthcare sector and lay community compounded by poor patient–doctor communication. The whole society is getting materialistic and healthcare sector is no exception to this. With private capital being infused into healthcare sector, corporate hospitals, pharmaceutical and device industry, and business professionals in the hospital administrator seat, the mentality of physicians has also changed from a charitable to a profit making. Instead of quality of patient care, the focus has shifted to numbers and "targets being achieved" in terms of patients seen in OPD, investigations and therapeutic procedures done and often the doctor's reimbursement is based on these numbers.[15] However, healthcare is unlike any other capitalistic profession due to several factors:
- It is a highly technical branch, not easily understood by lay people.
- Although science, it is not a very exact (linear) and structured branch like computer science, for example often the disease is poorly understood, its causation not that well established, its diagnosis unclear, despite best attempts, the response to treatment is uncertain and dependant on so many ifs and buts. Thus, it is really a journey into unknown for most patients, and it is the "unknown" which mankind fears the most.
- Disease is in a negative domain for the patients and their loved ones and, very few individuals can face a negative situation cheerfully.

- Most people, at least in developing countries, do not budget for unforeseen medical calamity, and thus do not set aside sufficient reserves for any such eventuality, and therefore when it portends a financial disaster and in the emotional confusion, the patients and their relatives may transfer the blame on hospital and their staff. Statistically highest number of violent incidents occur in the setting of emergency departments, intensive care units (ICU) and surgical/interventional theaters, where the first news of bad luck is broken.[16]
- Often therapeutic options are limited and not readily acceptable, and thus recipients of bad information (disease) often bear a grudge against the person who breaks the bad news, almost invariably the doctor, so it is a kind of "shoot the messenger."
- The doctors and healthcare staff are trained in their own technical profession but often, they lack training in communication skills or empathy skills.

SITUATION UNIQUE TO INDIA

- The primary healthcare infrastructure in the country is eroding perhaps due to general lack of awareness, low priority accorded to it, and low investment in this area. Additionally a peculiar tendency to directly consult the specialists/super-specialists has led to the fact that patients who could have been diagnosed in the earliest stages of their disease often slip through the primary care centers to present at some superspecialist/tertiary hospitals with advanced and even incurable disease.
- Low coverage of population with health insurance.
- Lack of communication skills in physicians which contributes to very tenuous patient–doctor relationship which is especially prone to breaking down into violence.
- Rudimentary health insurance structure.

WHAT LEADS TO VIOLENCE BY ATTENDANTS/RELATIVES?

Physician Related Factors

- *Misunderstandings:* Miscommunication at any level from explanation of etiology, disease course, prognosis, need for investigations and treatment options.
- *Mishappenings:* When the disease course and prognosis is not properly communicated to the patient, if a mishap occurs, the treating doctor and staff may be perceived as callous or inconsiderate.
- Dissatisfaction with the course of treatment.
- Disagreement with physician on modalities, option, and course of treatment.
- Malpractice
- *Conflict of interest:* Inability to obviate the feeling that many doctors prescribe unnecessary investigations and medicines to obtain undue benefits from medical industry.
- Perceived lack of communication (collaboration) or inability to share information between doctor and patient.
- *Casual opinion:* Criticism by other/second opinion doctor.

Patient Related Factors

The second problem is that the patient and their attendants are in most vulnerable phase of their existence, i.e., faced with temporary or permanent disability and even death. In this state they are fearful, anxious and in doubt. At this moment they require empathy and humane behavior and not challenge by the doctor or staff.

- In many government hospitals there is overcrowding, long waiting time to meet doctors, absence of a congenial environment, multiple visits to get investigations done and then subsequently to consult doctors, concept of bed sharing by two and sometimes three patients, floor beds and poor hygiene and sanitation.
- Even in private hospitals there could be prolonged waiting times—delay in attention or admission of sick patient or perceived delay in investigation and treatment.
- *Perceived (and real) lack of availability of doctor (senior doctor)*: Currently, there is a shortage of trained specialists. Furthermore, even in the available specialists there is a skew in distribution in favor of urban areas. As a consequence, very few experts are available in low resource setting which has even led to quacks occupying this medical space.[17]
- *Perceived lack of caring by physician or staff*: Many physicians, especially in governmental sector, are overburdened by the clinical load due to twin reasons of paucity of staff and inability of private sector to cater for really poor and low middle-class. Hugely overburdened OPDs, casualty, and wards in governmental hospitals are a common sight which contributes to overstretching not only infrastructure but also medical manpower, contributing to a perception of a lack of caring by the hospital staff.
- *Altered states of attendants*—intoxication, mental illness, severe anxiety or stress.
- *Problems of public hospitals*—dysfunctional equipment, poor quantity and quality of paramedical and supportive staff (and doctors being at apex have to take blame for it).
- Low insurance cover of the general population is also a big contributing factor, being one of the most common causes of leading a previously middle-class family into poor class.[18] It is a common knowledge that most incidents of violence occur at the time of preparation and payment of the medical bill.[19]
- *Low health related literacy*: While overall literacy has improved in the country, healthcare literacy still remains very low. Many caregivers fail to understand the disease process and even more importantly the available therapeutic options.

Hospital Related Factors

Hospitals are a home to medical equipments and facilities but often do not pay much attention to security. At least most government hospitals in India are deficient in security.
- Lack of security personnel in casualty, ICU and other risk prone areas; lack of police post nearby.
- Lack of security equipment, metal detectors, scanning devices, etc.
- Lack of security protocols, e.g., who will respond and when?
- Percentage of expenditure in healthcare is amongst the lowest all over world. This has led to very few government hospitals in India and it has been estimated that <20% of health needs are catered to by government hospitals. Furthermore, even these government hospitals are at present plagued by poor infrastructure and lack of adequate manpower undertaking healthcare. Thus, majority of lay public is forced to go to private sector for health needs. Bulk of healthcare service is provided by small and medium private healthcare establishments which is isolated and disorganized, and woefully lack in security arrangements.[20]

Role of Community

Weak and Ineffective Laws

There are no effective laws for the protection and safety of the medical personnel in private arena. In government sector while it is a non-bailable offense to assault a uniformed public servant like government doctors, the rules are hardly ever strictly enforced and lay public being aware of this weak implementation has no qualms in "exacting revenge" from the doctor and the hospital staff in any eventuality of mishap with their patient. Rather, since these acts go regularly unpunished it provokes mob violence, one incident after another. The Medicare Service Persons and Medicare Service Institutions (Prevention of Violence or Damage or Loss of Property) Act has been notified in 19 states in the past 10 years, but has failed to address this core issue. As a matter of fact, very few cases have even reached courts after filling of a *challan* and till date no person accused of assault on a medicare establishment has ever been penalized under this Act at least in the States of Punjab and Haryana from 2010 to 2015.

Community Leaders

Another problem could be small time community leaders/troublemakers. This is more of a problem in government hospitals or employee insurance hospitals who cater to a significant population of working class (unlike corporate hospitals which deal nearly exclusively with intellectual or elite class). These individuals might consider the health crisis as an opportunity to "show off" their leadership skills or they may grudge the perceived power enjoyed by the physicians (at that point of time) and feel that their own power is in jeopardy and may feel slighted. They may react by organizing others from patients, relatives and friends, inciting violence against so-called established power, i.e., the healthcare professionals including doctors.

Lack of Faith in Judicial Process

In India, lay public do not have adequate faith in the legal process of the country. Society, in general, believes that the doctors are often "well connected" and will get away with anything, forcing a common man to take law into his/her own hand.[21]

Role of Media

The media is forever in search of a good story. The story of an underdog fighting a huge establishment is ever popular. In this whole scheme the poor and defenseless patients become an underdog fighting against the huge and established but corrupt medical system led by highly intellectual and "powerful" physicians. This is a good recipe for any successful journalistic endeavor but gives a very poor image to an average doctor. Thus, press indulges in the sensationalization of every related news item, often completely ignoring the real facts.

■ HOW TO ANTICIPATE VIOLENCE IN HEALTHCARE SETTING?

The key remedy is to remain alert for such incidents of violence. There are certain tell-tale signs which can be looked for to anticipate any violence, easily identified as an acronym STAMP (**Table 1**):[22,23]

- Undue staring is an important early indicator of possible violence. This is generally deployed on mid-level health workers like nurses to intimidate them into improper action, but if they refuse, can culminate into violence.
- Lack of eye contact/shifty gaze is another important cue which is reflective of anger and passive resistance although there could be some cultural reasons to avoid eye contact.
- Tone and volume of voice is a very important clue to impending outburst but caustic and sarcastic replies with a normal tone are also important.

TABLE 1: Signs to anticipate violence—STAMP.

S	Staring/lack of eye contact
T	Tone and volume of voice
A	Anxiety
M	Mumbling
P	Pacing

- Signs of anxiousness, frequently rubbing hands, tapping hands or feet, nonseasonal perspiration should be accounted for before they reach a dangerous level.
- Signs or substance abuse or drug intoxications should be kept in mind and appropriate steps taken.
- Mumbling, using slurred/incoherent speech or repeatedly asking the same question or making the same statements are important signs to be recognized. Mumbling can be interpretive of mounting frustration and a cue for violence.
- Pacing is another indication of mounting agitation as well as staggering, waving arms or pulling away from healthcare personnel attempting to treat them.

■ MANAGING VIOLENCE IN HEALTHCARE SETTING

At the Time of Violence[23]

If violence is impending or actually occurring:
- Remain calm in the face of provocation and do not raise your voice but try to let things blow over.
- Obtain all the documentary evidence of violence. It is a good idea to earmark some hospital staff who will take photographs, audio/video records of the violence.
- All medical record of the patient should be photocopied immediately because there is a huge possibility that interested person/mob could carry away the original record.
- Inform the legal counsel/lawyer immediately.
- Inform the police immediately by phone, sending someone to police post, and SMS but importantly keep a record of such attempts to contact law enforcing agency.
- Identify the troublemakers/community leader(s) inciting violence.
- Get written, signed statements from all individuals present (physicians, nurses and other paramedical staff, patients, relatives, and other bystanders) in context of the violence.
- Lodge a First Information Report with the police.
- While registering a complaint make sure that it is registered under the relevant Act, i.e., Protection of Medical Personnel.
- It is very important not to try to "settle" the issue by paying hush money which seems more as an admission of guilt than otherwise.

■ PREVENTING VIOLENCE IN HEALTHCARE SETTING

Preventive Tips for the Physicians

- *Better communication:* This is the most workable strategy with the intellectual class—
  - The physicians have to understand that patients and relatives are going through extraordinary fear, anxiety, and doubt and thus may not behave rationally. Further the

doctors have to understand that patients come from different backgrounds, educational and economic classes.
- Patient and their caregivers should always be kept in loop at each and every medical step, e.g., investigation, diagnosis or treatment.
- Although doctor has to provide services to so many patients in limited time, never act in hurry while interacting with the patient. The problem of time constraints can probably be overcome by having more supportive staff.
- Give sufficient opportunity to the patient and family to speak. Listen to them patiently. Patients feel satisfied if they are being heard and understood.
- In case complications appear during hospital stay, a senior doctor should counsel the patient/relatives. This will give them assurance that best possible care is being provided.
- Incorporate philosophy of medicine, ethics, and empathy training in medical curriculum. Medical education system needs to be reorganized. The importance of teaching morals, ethics, and empathy to budding doctors cannot be overstressed. Good empathy training could lead to good doctors. It is particularly important to show empathy for suffering and sympathy in financial dealings. The patient should be treated as a fellow human and not some abstract problem or worse made fun of or treated with ridicule.
- Proper and written consent in word and spirit in the patients' own dialect and language with witnesses must be obtained before undertaking major investigations or treatments especially of surgical procedures. The consent should delve upon the purpose of investigation/intervention, its possible outcome, clearly detailing commonly occurring life-threatening/non-life-threatening complications, the available alternatives, advantages/disadvantages of each one of them. In case the patient refuses, the consequences of refusal must be discussed and mentioned explicitly in the consent form. While performing an intervention only those procedures be done for which consent has been obtained unless it is life-saving.
- Second opinion should be given very carefully, with careful choice of words. At the same time patient may be encouraged to seek a second opinion as a strategy to build confidence. If second opinion is different from your own opinion, the reasons for difference must be discussed and the final choice strictly left to the patients/caregivers.
- It is important never to overreach in attempts to treat a patient. One should realize the limits of what medicine can do as well as limit of available infrastructure and most importantly of self. Never do any procedure beyond the scope of one's training and facilities. The dictum "do no harm" holds true for entire medical specialty.
- Proper documentation is the key to all successful modern medical practice. Accurate and proper documentation may not directly prevent violence but after violence records may be seized by police. Unfortunately, in very sick patients the focus is entirely on saving life and documents are not in order but it, documentation is still important. Try to keep photocopies of important documents because they might be lost in the chaos of ensuing violence. It may be a good idea to employ a staff or at least delegate the work of record keeping to one of the medical staff, so that this aspect is not overlooked.
- *Certain safety habits can be suggested:*
    - Pay a close attention to surroundings when you come out of office; avoid looking at your phone as you walk in hospital area.
    - Pay close attention to the cars parked around when coming and leaving the hospital premises.
    - Lock the car door immediately after entering.

Preventive Tips for the Hospital Administrators

- *Strengthening the security:*
  - Security personnel (preferably army background) should be posted at the entrance of every hospital, ICU, and operation theaters and should not let anyone through without checking for appropriate identification.
  - Weapons/weapon-like objects should be confiscated before allowing passage to anyone.
  - All attendants must register at the front desk and be given a visitor badge to be worn at all times.
  - Restrict entry of attendants to clinical workplace. No more than two attendants should be allowed with the patient.
- Establish a Hospital Committee (PRO) specializing in effective communication which can satisfy the patients/attendants.
  - Trained psychologists (counselors) should be available to cater for emotional needs of patients and their caregivers when required.
  - Since India is a diverse country with several official languages and also medical tourism is showing a huge growth, language translators should be available who can prevent incidences of miscommunication.
- Hospital workplaces should establish a policy for assessing and reporting threats, which would allow employers to track them to see whether prevention strategies are working.
- Reduce the waiting times for everything and if they cannot be done at least explain why these times are there in the first place.
- Every hospital should have an emergency algorithm including an evacuation plan in case of a major act of violence.
- At the time of designing a hospital, attention should be directed to workplace's landscaping, parking lot, and outdoor lighting keeping in mind security aspects.
- *Displaying information and also the laws governing the safety of doctors up-front:*
  - To satisfy the intellectual class
  - To make them aware of consequences of violence against doctors
- Involving media in their activities.
- Healthcare personnel must have some training in martial arts, which might save their life in some instances.

■ STRONG AND EFFECTIVE LAWS: ESSENTIAL IN FIGHT AGAINST VIOLENCE

Strengthening the Law Against Violence

It is very important to make "violence against doctors", a non-bailable offense for all medical areas; private or public. There is indeed a need to modify the Indian Penal Code to allow for tougher penalty against the perpetrators of such violence. On January 7th, 2018 "Prevention of Violence Against Doctors, Medical Professionals and Medical Institutions Bill, 2018" was tabled in Lok Sabha, demanding strict action against those who create violence in hospitals against doctors. The bill shall come into force on such date, as the Central Government may, by notification in the Official Gazette, appoint.

Key Features of the Bill

- *Prohibition of Violence:* Any act of violence against a doctor, medical professional or medical institution shall be prohibited and mitigated at all levels.
- *Cognizance of offence:* Any offence committed under this Act shall be cognizable and non-bailable and triable by the Court of Judicial Magistrate of the First Class.
- *Penalty and compensation:* Whoever commits or attempts to commit or abets or incites the commission of any act of violence in infringement of the provisions of section 3, shall be punished with imprisonment which shall not be <6 months but which may extend up to 5 years and with fine which shall not be < ₹5,000 but which may extend up to ₹500,000 in addendum to recovery of the entire damage to the property or belonging of all concerned including the witnesses if any; in actual. If the accused does not pay or is financially incompetent to pay the penalty at that time it shall be recovered as if it were an arrear of land revenue and any property belonging to his immediate relatives may be attached in recovery of the said penalty.
- *Explanatory Note:* It shall be the responsibility of every doctor, medical professional or medical institutions, as the case may be, before start of any treatment or procedure to make an explanatory note containing:
  - the present medical condition of the patient
  - expected procedures and treatment
  - possible outcome
  - expected time to be taken for recovery
  - chances of failure of the prescribed procedures
  - expected expense per unit of medication, procedure, treatment and service pertaining details as applicable, to be provided with, and categorically explained to the patient in person or his nearest kin, attendant or escort, as the case may be and a confirmation of understanding either in writing or a verbatim ascent in front of minimum two attesters shall also be obtained.
- *Cases of medical negligence:*
  - The Central Government shall, by notification in the Official Gazette, in order to provide able and timely assistance to the victims of medical negligence or mismanagement, establish a District Wise Committee or for the area as may be specified in such notification to hear appeals and grievances of the victims of medical negligence or mismanagement and to aid and advice such victims for taking recourse to an appropriate forum for a suitable relief and at its own cost.
  - The Committee established under sub-section (1) shall consist of experts one each from the field of medicine, law, consumer movement, health management and human rights and shall be chaired by the Member of Parliament of the respective constituency.
- *Central Government to provide funds:* The Central Government shall, after due appropriation made by Parliament by law in this behalf, provide, from time-to-time, adequate funds for carrying out the purpose of this Act.
- *Act to have overriding effect:* The provisions of this Act and rules made there under shall have effect notwithstanding anything inconsistent therewith contained in any other law for the time being in force.
- *Act to supplement other laws:* The provisions of this Act shall be in addition to and not in derogation of any other law for the time being in force.
- *Power to make rules:* The Central Government may, by notification in the Official Gazette, make rules for carrying out the purposes of this Act.

Implementation of Effective Laws

Often, the real challenge faced in preventing violence against doctors is poor implementation of existing laws. A lack of implementation of existing laws has obstructed efforts to protect doctors from the menace of violence. Law meant for protection of doctors against violence needs to be stricter and should be implemented promptly and effectively. Law enforcing authorities should be particularly sensitized to this aspect and must realize that their mandate is to maintain law and order. The rule of law must be respected and adhered to by the society at large.

Role of Media in Preventing Violence

Media has a very important role to play. They should also write positive things about the profession or at least both sides of the issue in situations like this; they should avoid journalism of sensationalism and avoid provocative headlines. While in short-term these kinds of reports get a few eyeballs but in the long run might prove counterproductive for the society.

Health Related Literacy

There is a need to educate not only lay public but also first-contact physicians in some cases, for example myocardial infarction. There is a need of clear guidelines and management algorithms forlay the public and even physicians.[24]

Insurance Schemes

Mass insurance schemes should be offered to cover the whole population. Several states have their own schemes but national schemes like the currently launched Pradhan Mantri Jan Arogya Yojana (PMJAY) scheme and older Rashtriya Arogya Nidhi for BPL patients are revolutionary steps in this direction.

■ CONCLUSION

In a predominantly capitalistic society, healthcare and primary education are perhaps the only remaining professions in India, which lay public expect to function on socialistic model. This would ensure a cost-effective, high-class healthcare delivery to practically the entire population. However, in reality medicine (as also education) is no longer treated as a welfare activity but rather a profit-making venture, at least by the corporate sector. This difference in perception between the society in general and the healthcare providers has led to serious gap between what is expected and what is delivered on health front. One of the outcomes of this mismatch is violence against doctors (among other problems) which is seriously threatening the status quo in this profession. On the other hand, while violence on road (road rage), public places, even schools is common (though not condonable), it can under no circumstance be acceptable in hospitals. The hospitals simply cannot be allowed to become battlegrounds for the simple reason that sick people need a peaceful environment where they can get sympathy, empathy, support, etc. Even healthcare professionals need a stable and peaceful environment so as to to give selfless care rather than worry about their personal safety. Thus, if the hospital environment is exposed to violence, its practitioners might start practicing defensive medicine, and focusing on saving their own skin rather than treating a patient. One of the major factors contributing to violence is not only monetary considerations but also a lack of communication and a failing doctor-patient bonding. Solution lies in not only changing attitudes and practices of physicians and hospitals but also regulators, media and even lay public.

REFERENCES

1. Raman S. Why the Threat of Violence against Doctors though Unacceptable may be getting us Better Healthcare. [online] Available from: https://www.thenewsminute.com/article/why-threat-violence-against-doctors-though-unacceptable-may-be-getting-us-better-healthcare. [Last Accessed on August, 2019].
2. Dey S. Over 75% of Doctors have Faced Violence at Work, Study Finds. Times of India; 2015. [online] Available from: https://timesofindia.indiatimes.com/india/Over-75-of-doctors-have-faced-violence-at-work-study-finds/articleshow/47143806.cms. [Last Accessed on August, 2019].
3. Mishra S. Do we need to change the medical curriculum: regarding the pain of others. Indian Heart J. 2015;67(3):187-91.
4. Mäulen B. An ever increasing incidence of violence against physicians. MMW Fortschr Med. 2013;155(5):14-6, 18, 20.
5. Püschel K, Cordes O. Tödliche Bedrohung als Berufsrisiko. Dtsch Arztebl. 2001;98:A153-7.
6. Tolhurst H, Baker L, Murray G, et al. Rural general practitioner experience of work-related violence in Australia. Aust J Rural Health. 2003;11(5):231-6.
7. Alexander C, Fraser J. Occupational violence in an Australian healthcare setting: implications for managers. J Health Manag. 2004;49(6):377-92.
8. Magin PJ, Adams J, Sibbritt DW, et al. Experiences of occupational violence in Australian urban general practice: a cross-sectional study of GPs. Med J Aust. 2005;183(7):352-6.
9. Koritsas S, Coles J, Boyle M, et al. Prevalence and predictors of occupational violence and aggression towards GPs: a cross-sectional study. Br J Gen Pract. 2007;57(545):967-70.
10. Miedema BB, Hamilton R, Tatemichi SR, et al. Monthly incidence rates of abusive encounters for Canadian family physicians by patients and their families. Int J Family Med. 2010;2010:387202.
11. Mishra S. Violence against doctors: the class wars. Indian Heart J. 2015;67(4):289-92.
12. Kowalczuk K, Jankowiak B, Krajewska-Kułak E, et al. Aggression as the cause of stress among physicians. Ann Acad Med Stetin. 2009;55(3):70-5.
13. Hinsenkamp M. Violence against healthcare workers. Int Orthop. 2013;37(12):2321-2.
14. Workplace Violence: Law and Legal Definition. [online] Available from: http://definitions.uslegal.com/w/workplace-violence/. [Last Accessed on August, 2019].
15. Mishra S. What ails the practice of medicine: the Atlas has shrugged. Indian Heart J. 2015;67(1):1-7.
16. Kuhn W. Violence in the emergency department: Managing aggressive patients in a high-stress environment. Postgrad Med. 1999;105(1):143-8, 154.
17. Mishra S. Who is a cardiologist: usurpers spawn? Indian Heart J. 2015;67(6):509-11.
18. Ramakrishnan S, Mishra S, Chakraborty R, et al. The report on the Indian coronary intervention data for the year 2011–National Interventional Council. Indian Heart J. 2013;65(5):518-21.
19. Kalra A. Govt to Cut Health Budget by nearly 20 percent for 2014-15. Business Today 23; 2014.
20. Healthcare Indicators. [online] Available from: http://www.ita. doc.gov/td/health/india_indicators05.pdf. [Last Accessed on August, 2019].
21. Madhok P. Violence against doctors. Bombay Hosp J. 2009;51(2):301-2.
22. STAMP System can Help Professionals to Identify Potentially Violent Individuals. Eurek Alert! The Global Source for Science News. Washington, DC: Black Lack Publishing; 2007. [online] Available from: http://www.eurekalert.org/pub_releases/2007-06/bpl-ssc062007.php. [Last Accessed on August, 2019].
23. Nagpal N. Incidents of violence against doctors in India: Can these be prevented? Natl Med J India. 2017;30(2):97-100.
24. Aggarwal K, Mishra S. Heart attack guidance for physicians: When to suspect, how to diagnose, what to do? Indian Heart J. 2017;69(Suppl 1):S6-7.

SECTION 3
Patient Safety Initiatives: A Key to Medicolegal Safety

Chapter 7   Patient Safety and Risk Management
Chapter 8   Healthcare-associated Infections: A Threat to Patient Safety
Chapter 9   Communication Skills in Healthcare: A Tool to ensure Patient Satisfaction

CHAPTER 7

Patient Safety and Risk Management

Sameer Mehta

> "A culture of safety is a journey, not a destination.
> It requires our continuing diligence."
>
> — **Terry J Moulton**

■ INTRODUCTION

The concept of patient safety may be traced back in the medical writings as early as 5th century BC, when the ancient Greek Hippocratic oath was written, which does contain language propounding that the physician and his assistants should not cause physical or moral harm to a patient. The first known published version of Primum non nocere, a Latin phrase that means "first, do no harm," dates to the medical texts from the mid-19th century, and is attributed to the 17th century English physician Thomas Sydenham.[2] From those olden times to now, medicine and its practice has come a long way, and healthcare outcomes have significantly improved with the scientific discoveries of modern medicine.

However, many studies have shown that hospitalized patients are at risk of suffering variety of harms, some of which may be preventable.[3] In 1999 the report "To Err Is Human", published by the Institute of Medicine drew global attention toward the problem of preventable harm in medicine.[4] A major consequence of this knowledge has been the development of patient safety as a specialized discipline. Patient safety has acquired greater significance with organizations developing and adopting strategies to manage the risks. Modern medicine has acquired far more structured approach toward the concept of patient safety and risk management. Healthcare standards too have evolved with times to make healthcare organizations a safer place. While the level of healthcare is certainly improving in India, there is certainly a long way to go in the field of patient safety and risk management. This chapter attempts to cover certain basic guidelines, drawing from standards that make for a safer environment and in complying with which the hospital is better equipped to defend itself in case of an exigency. This, by no means, purports to be an exhaustive compendium on the subject—but seeks to cover some common and not so common aspects of safety that would be of interest to the reader.

■ STRATEGIES FOR SAFETY IN HEALTHCARE

Emergency Care and Patient Safety[5]

Emergency departments (ED) have inherent risks for errors due to the urgency of care needs and intricacy of communication that can result in patient harm. The ED environment is fast-paced, busy and tiring, and it requires quick thinking, a broad depth of knowledge about many medical conditions, and a broad range of skills to provide emergency care. Often, patients reach the ED for the first time, with incomplete medical records, unaware of their medical condition or medications, or not in a position to communicate this information. Such a situation can significantly increase the risk for harm. Various factors related to safety issues in the ED can be deconstructed as: (i) patient related, (ii) provider related, and (iii) environment/system related (**Table 1**).[5-7]

Possible Solutions

Developing and maintaining a "culture of safety" can minimize the risks and actual occurrence of harm to the patients. In the emergency care setup, a culture of safety encourages teamwork, event reporting, communication openness, transparency with feedback and learning from errors, and administrator collaboration for safety.[8] The reporting of errors, adverse event and near misses should be encouraged, without fear of blame or loss of employment. By creating an environment that promotes reporting of adverse events and near misses, the true safety problems are identified and can be targeted for improvement.

In the ED, doctors may be simultaneously treating multiple patients with similar conditions or with similar names. In cases of critically ill patients, verbal orders may be used for medication, followed by written/computer orders, when the doctor is able to leave the bedside. In addition, wide range of medications with different doses and different routes (intravenous, intramuscular, subcutaneous, or oral) are administered based on various patient-specific factors (age, gender, body weight, medical condition, etc.). Considering all of these factors, it is not surprising that in a prospective observational study it was reported that up to 60% of ED patients experienced medication errors. The study concluded that medication errors in the ED are common, and most errors occur in the prescribing and administering phases.[9] To reduce the medication errors in EDs, addition of clinical pharmacist (CPs) can greatly improve medication safety. CPs can intercept prescribing errors in the ordering system before they are administered and before they result in patient harm. Pharmacists can recommend appropriate antibiotic dose and timely administration of medications for emergent conditions. They can prevent errors with formulation confusion, look-alike/sound-alike (LASA) medication confusion, weight-based dose errors, and dosing frequency errors.

TABLE 1: Safety factors in the emergency department.[5-7]

Patient related issues	Provider related issues	Environment/System related issues
• Age extremes	• Experience	• Inadequate staff
• Communication barriers	• Fatigue	• Inexperienced staff
• Vague/atypical complaints	• Cognitive errors	• Communication problems
• Cognitive impairment	• Missed test results	• Overcrowding
• Complex medical conditions	• Procedural errors	• Boarding of admitted patients
• Lack of knowledge of medical problems and medications	• Transitions of care	• Lack of equipment/equipment breakdown
		• Inadequate consultation services
		• Lack of previous medical records

Overcrowding in the ED has detrimental effects on patient safety, as crowding is associated with higher morbidity and mortality, delayed pain control, and inferior healthcare.[10] The practice of keeping admitted patients on stretchers in hospital ED after they have been admitted to the hospital because no inpatient or observation beds are available called boarding, causes crowding in the ED, and can be harmful to patients. Boarding increases patient's morbidity, lengths of hospital stay, and mortality. Strategies that optimize bed management reduce boarding by improving the efficiency of hospital patient flow, but these strategies are grossly underused.

There is no specific law governing emergency care in India. As per the principle of "right to life and dignity" as enshrined in Article 21 of the Constitution, it is imperative to not turn away any patient who lands up in the hospital in need of the emergency care. In *Parmanand Katara judgment*, the Supreme Court emphasized the need for making it obligatory for hospitals and medical practitioners to provide emergency medical care.[11] Hospitals and medical practitioners have to initially screen the patient to decide if he requires emergency medical treatment. The hospital has to provide definitive emergency care when it is equipped with infrastructure, diagnostics and clinical skill sets to attend to the patient. However, the hospital may provide basic care to stabilize the patient and refer onward to another hospital or to a medical practitioner having facilities, if it is not equipped adequately to provide definitive emergency care.

■ RADIOLOGY AND IMAGING

The radiology and imaging services largely cover diagnostics and certain therapeutic modalities. Functional elements include radiation emitting modalities such as X-ray, computerized axial tomography (CT scanners), positron emission tomography (PET scanners), single photon emission computer tomography (Gamma scanners), linear accelerators, mammography, orthopantomography, etc., nonradiating imaging techniques include ultrasound sonography, magnetic resonance imaging (MRI), echocardiography, etc. All the ionizing-radiation-emitting and the nuclear medicine modalities are governed by the Atomic Energy Regulatory Board (AERB). AERB has laid down very specific guidelines for installation and monitoring of these modalities, and compliance is mandatory.

Often, trained staff and radiologists working in the radiology department are aware of the dangers posed by radiation exposure, and follow all safety procedures. The increased usage of radiology devices by other departments in the hospital has emerged as a serious safety issue. The workers handling radiology equipment in other departments like OT, endoscopy room, and orthopedics may not have adequate personal protective equipment like lead aprons, dosimeters, etc. Other hospital staff including ward boys, nurses, anesthesiologists, etc., are also vulnerable as they may not be aware of the radiation risk from the equipment placed within their surroundings. Hospitals should provide dosimeters to their workers, and ensure that the exposure to radiations to the healthcare workers is within the safe limit. In India, there is a shortage of radiologists and trained workers, resulting in wide gap between demand and supply. Hospital should assure appropriate credentials and training on safety issues for healthcare providers and other workers handling imaging equipment.

There are potential risks in the MRI environment, not only for the patients, accompanying family members, attending healthcare professionals, and others who are exposed to magnetic fields of MR scanners, such as security or housekeeping personnel, firefighters, etc. Many cases of magnetic resonance imaging (MRI) of adverse incidents involve patients, equipment, and personnel. American College of Radiology has laid down guidelines for MRI

TABLE 2: Four zone model for MRI safety.[12]

Zone I	Zone II	Zone III	Zone IV
This region includes the all areas freely accessible publicly, basically everything outside the MRI itself.	It is the interface between the zone 1 and the other zones. Here patients are met and transforms into candidates for MRI examination. The history and other questioning are done here.	• This is any area (beyond the MRI scanner room) where there is a potential magnetic field danger to persons, or any area from which there is access to the MRI scanner room. Zone III is to be physically restricted from Zone II, and persons in Zone III are to be under the continuous supervision of MRI personnel. • Patients are accepted and prepared to enter the scanner. Restrict access to zone three controlled by the MR personnel.	This is the MRI scanner room itself. This zone is highly hazardous due to the strong magnetic field and hence the restricted area and should be under direct visual observation.

safety in its Guidance Document for Safe MR Practices.[12] It describes a process by which patients, personnel, and equipment are required to pass clinical/physical screenings prior to being granted access to the areas immediately around the MRI scanner room. It essentially propounds a four-zone layout that allows checking of ferrous ingress before one reaches the magnet room. Hospitals that institute such zoning with installation of ferrous detectors create a safer environment for both the patient and the staff (**Table 2**).

Another less known stipulation is the mandate to maintain the waiting area for radiology at negative pressure—implying that air being circulated in the space does not flow into adjacent spaces. This is based on the premise that there could be patients with active Koch's in the waiting area for X-ray and hence the measure of containing the potential spread. The containment, however, is possible when the architectural layout allows so.

■ COUNSELING ROOMS—INFORMED CONSENT

Informed consent is a written permission secured by the treating doctor from the patient/patient kin to proceed with the treatment/intervention, having explained the risks and benefits thereof, including the possible consequences. Certain medical imaging examinations require significant radiation dose. While obtaining consent the issue of radiation risk must be addressed for these examinations. While the ethical and the legal implications are covered elsewhere in this compendium, it is important to plan for such rooms in the hospital judiciously. The Code of Ethics protects patient privacy. In keeping with the code, it is important that the discussion around the health condition and the future course of action with its implications is done in a setting that allows confidentiality and privacy. Legally, the doctor and the hospital are obliged to establish that the patient is adequately briefed as to the pros and cons of the course of action. The common practice, therefore, is to institute what may be termed a counseling room where such interaction takes place. It is advisable to video-record the preconsent counseling session, especially in high risk cases. Ensure that the CCTV signage is present in the counseling room and the patient is specifically informed of this fact. The room is often equipped with an audio-visual recording facility to capture the interaction. The location of a room, depending on the clinical facility it serves, may be preferred juxtaposed between the restricted and the nonrestricted zones such that the doctor in greens need not step out into the nonrestricted zone in order to maintain clean practices. A counseling room thus serves to secure the rights and obligations of both the clinician and the patient in a safe setting without compromising on patient privacy.

■ ISOLATION ROOMS

Isolation rooms are designed to isolate patients for better airborne infection control. An airborne infectious isolation room is intended for an infectious patient that could potentially expose others to the infective organism. A protective environment room is designed to accommodate an immune-compromised patient who is at a greater risk of contracting infection from others. A combined isolation room accommodates a patient that is both infectious and immune-compromised. The design metrics are beyond the purview of the present context. However, it is important that the hospital's infection control risk assessment team determines the type and the numbers at the outset as these rooms have atypical and intricate engineering requirements. These present challenges in retro-fits to be undertaken in an operational facility. A hospital that receives and admits patients with such clinical indications without commensurate provisions would risk exposing the patients to infection.

Although patient isolation is an established aspect of infection control, it may also negatively influence direct patient care and patient satisfaction. Studies have found that time spent by healthcare professionals in direct patient care is either less frequent or shorter with patients in isolation, than with patients not in isolation.[13] In a study that assessed patient safety, it was found that isolated patients had more errors in processes of care, and had increased likelihood for adverse events as compared with patients not in isolation.[14] For example, isolated patients were more likely to have either incomplete recordings of vital signs, or to have days with no vital sign recordings at all. In addition, they had more days with either no nursing narrative notes, or physician progress notes recorded in the chart. Isolated patients were twice as likely as control patients to experience adverse events per 1,000 days. Patients in isolation were as much as eight times more likely to experience supportive care failures such as falls, ulcers, and fluid and electrolyte abnormalities. Not surprisingly, patients in isolation expressed greater dissatisfaction regarding their care.[13]

It is very important to inform the patient about the isolation procedures, rather than just putting them in place with no explanation. While the isolation procedures may be familiar to the hospital staff, most patients do not have the same perspective. Take time to educate the patients why isolation is a must with their illness. Patient education at the time of isolation is a critical component of the process to reduce anxiety and distress. As the problem of antibiotic-resistant bacteria in hospitals continues to grow, the role of isolation as an infection control intervention will further increase in future. Attention must be paid to the patient safety issues related to isolation, and adverse effects should be monitored and managed appropriately.

■ MEDICAL RECORDS

Medical records are the documents that collate the patient care, in which sufficient data is recorded in the sequence of events to justify the diagnosis and warrant the treatment and the end results. These are important for ongoing patient management as much as they are for posterity. Hospitals are increasingly shifting to electronic medical records (EMR) wherein the patient data is available on the computer network. It is important that the record is maintained safely by way of duplicating/mirroring the same on another server/cloud so that in case of any loss of data in the primary server, records can yet be accessed through the alternative storage. In 2013, Ministry of Health and Family Welfare, Government of India has provided a guideline for the implementation of electronic health record in India. The guideline was further revised in the year 2016 to provide better direction to the Indian healthcare institutions in implementing electronic health record. These guidelines stress on ethical, legal, and social issues associated with the use of electronic health record.

Where records are maintained physically, the practice in certain countries is to house these in a fire-safe enclosure. This underscores the critical need for safekeeping of records for continuity of treatment without a break in access. Patient privacy is another important metric when it comes to patient information, especially with data now being disseminated and relayed over the electronic medium. India does not as yet have a law as elaborate as Health Insurance Portability and Accountability Act (HIPAA) in the United States that provides data privacy and security provisions for safeguarding medical information. However, any local entity that officially collaborates with a healthcare establishment covered under HIPAA will be, by dint of the laws applicable to them, also required to comply. Thereby, measures to prevent physical theft and loss of devices containing electronic data and measures to protect networks and devices from data breaches and unauthorized access assume significance.

A well-designed and properly implemented EMR system has a potential to enhance patient safety by effectively addressing various areas of concern, particularly those related to medication safety, diagnostic errors, and communication issues.[15] Computerized physician order entry (CPOE) has been shown to reduce medication-related errors. Proper implementation of interoperable health information technology (HIT) system is very useful in establishing effective communication methods in healthcare.[15] EMR can improve patient safety by detecting missed diagnoses, producing diagnostic error alerts to prevent misdiagnosis and assisting the practitioner in gathering and synthesizing patient information.[16]

Despite the well-established benefits of various EMR functionalities, some studies have identified potential disadvantages associated with this technology. These include financial issues, changes in workflow, temporary loss of productivity associated with EMR adoption, privacy and security concerns, and several unintended consequences which may include dosing errors, failure to detect fatal illnesses, and delays in treatment, increased medical errors, negative emotions, changes in power structure, and overdependence on technology.[15] The risk of harm related to using EMRs can be reduced by identifying and addressing the unintended consequences, effectively and at the earliest.

■ PATIENT ACCESSIBILITY

Access to health services means, "the timely use of personal health services to achieve the best health outcomes."[17] It requires: (i) Gaining entry into the hospital, accessing a location where needed health care services are provided (geographic availability), and (ii) Finding a health care provider whom the patient trusts and can communicate with. Accessibility barriers are obstacles that make it difficult for patients and individuals with disabilities to access the healthcare system. There are several barriers, both visible and invisible. Patients waiting for or not receiving proper care is one of the major problems associated with patient access. Patient safety is at risk when a hospital's access system is vulnerable. To assure patient safety, it is very important to improve the hospital accessibility system.

The Government of India enacted the Persons with Disabilities (PWD) Act, 1995 and signed and ratified the UN Convention on the Rights of Persons with Disabilities (CRPD) in 2008. Design guidelines and standards established by different authorities such as Central Public Works Department, National Building Code and Ministry of Social Justice and Empowerment were compiled into a comprehensive document under the aegis of Ministry of Urban Development, titled "Harmonised Guidelines and Space Standards on Barrier Free Built Environment for Persons with Disability and Elderly Persons, 2015."[18] Hospital and healthcare facilities are classified as category 4 and the applicable guidelines and standards appear in Chapter 5 of the document. Despite the government initiating awareness campaigns, this is yet not adequately reflected in healthcare buildings. Seemingly elementary provisions such as handrails, grab bars, leveled and nonslippery surfaces, etc., are only the few among the various safety parameters covered in the document. Adoption of these standards and guidelines essentially make the healthcare facility a safer place. Accreditation norms such as JCI call for compliance for infrastructure that enables a differently abled person to negotiate and transact independently insofar as feasible to make the facility inclusive and safe.

■ PATIENT HANDLING AND MOVEMENT ASSESSMENT

The practice of manual patient handling (lifting, transferring, positioning, and sliding patients without assistive technology) is a risky activity that increases the risk of injury, pain, and negative health outcomes to patients, and puts caregivers at considerable risk for musculoskeletal injury. It is an unsafe practice for both patients and caregivers. The solution to the safety issues associated with manual patient handling lies in safe patient handling (SPH) with assistive patient handling and movement (PHAM) technology. PHAMA is a process, focused on SPH and movement along with mobility equipment to facilitate the transfers. Safe patient handling activities can significantly reduce overexertion injuries by replacing manual patient handling with safer methods guided by the principles of ergonomics. Ergonomics is the process of designing or arranging workplaces, products and systems to best suit the capabilities of workers. The ergonomic approach to patient handling seeks to maximize the safety and comfort of patients during handling.

It is expected and known that some patients are infirm to a point where they need assistance in moving in and out of the bed. Hospitals are also seeing an increasing incidence of obese patients that the caregivers may find difficult to maneuver without a risk to both the patient and themselves. Lifts and hoists are now available to enable safer management of such patients. From a design perspective, structural considerations, space for maneuvers and movement, space for storage of mobility equipment, door openings, choice of water closets, etc., are a few instances that merit attention. A PHAMA must analyze both the physical characteristics of patient handling as well as the procedural aspects in order to minimize safety risks to both patients and staff.

■ INFECTION CONTROL

People get to a hospital to be treated and cured and the last thing one expects is to actually acquire infection. The World Health Organization states, "Of every 100 hospitalized patients at any given time, 7 in developed and 10 in developing countries will acquire at least one healthcare-associated infection."[19] Infection prevention and control (IPC) is a practical solution to the problem of morbidity and mortality caused by infection to the patients.

It becomes imperative then that one adopts the standards and the best practices that help fight the scourge of nosocomial infection. An infection occurs if there is completion of infection chain which is made up of six different links (**Fig. 1**):
1. Pathogen (infectious agent)
2. Reservoir
3. Portal of exit
4. Means of transmission
5. Portal of entry, and
6. The new host.

To prevent the infection, each link can be interrupted, or broken, through various means. One of the main sources of these agents, in the hospital, is the diseased patients. The pathogens use body fluid secretions, blood, feces, and droplets expelled by the respiratory track, among others, as a portal of exit. The main routes for the spread of infections are—contact, droplet, and airborne transmission. The modes of transmission include direct contact during patient handling, indirect contact with contaminated surfaces (fomites) and airborne propagation (also a mode of indirect contact). Infection prevention and control has a key role in the field of patient safety. It aims to prevent pathogens from coming into contact with a person in the first place.

The WHO has provided detailed information about the infection control program in its publication: Practical Guidelines for Infection Control in Health Care Facilities.[20] The infection control program should be designed and strictly implemented in order to reduce the infection risk. For instance, administrative controls based on the stringent protocols require, among others, that universal precautions (hand hygiene, gloves when touching blood and secretions, etc.) must be used on all patient's manipulation.

Engineering design plays a significant role in the infection control for hospitals. Building design of the hospital must incorporate the systems that gears up the infection control program. Layout design must be planned in stringent relationship with the infection control measures to provide adequate patient, staff, materials, and waste flows in order to prevent cross contamination. Basic knowledge on dynamics of droplet infection is a useful plan of the infection control measures that are used to size the gap between patient beds to reduce the risk of cross infection by droplet direct contact. Infection control program generally demands that patients with airborne communicable diseases (e.g., tuberculosis, measles, etc.) must be isolated in an airborne infection isolation (AII) room. A protective

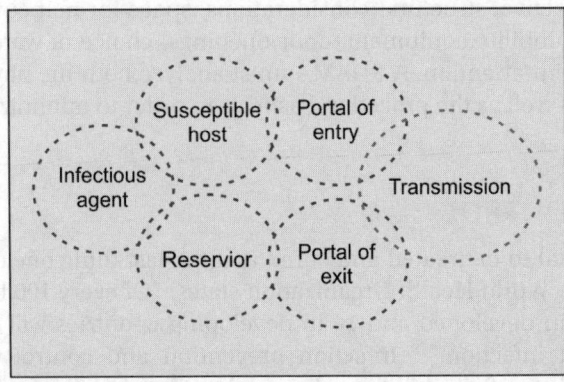

FIG. 1: The infection chain.

environment room is required for isolation of immunocompromised patients (e.g., bone marrow transplant, oncology, etc.). Studies have shown that there is a definitive association between the transmission of airborne infections and the ventilation of the building, and that insufficient ventilation increases the risk of disease transmission.[21] The sufficient evidence of the association between ventilation, the control of airflow direction in buildings, and the transmission and spread of infectious diseases supports the use of negatively pressurized isolation rooms for patients with the infectious diseases such as measles, tuberculosis, influenza, and severe acute respiratory syndrome (SARS) in hospitals.[22] Source isolation or elimination is more effective than the use of increased ventilation rates, for the prevention of airborne communicable diseases in the hospital setting. The WHO has provided guidelines on natural ventilation for infection control in healthcare settings, and this approach can be a feasible solution for many design settings for the low-income developing countries.[23] Contact infection is best countered by clean hands and clean surfaces. One cannot overemphasize the need for providing hand wash fixtures in adequate numbers and at all locations such that the caregiver is encouraged to wash hands between seeing two patients. Surfaces are expected to be free of crevices and shall be seamless insofar as possible, to ease cleaning. Else, contact infection control is a matter of universal precautions.

Airborne infection control is a function of heating, ventilation, and air conditioning (HVAC) design. ASHRAE 170[24] standards prepared by a Project Committee of the American Society of Heating, Refrigerating and Air-conditioning Engineers (ASHRAE) is a design standard specifically meant for ventilation of healthcare facilities. This covers the design parameters of temperature, humidity, pressure gradient, air changes, filtration, etc. It recognizes the need to inhibit *Aspergillus* and is by far the best known and recognized guideline toward implementing an airborne infection control program. Some standards have sought to define the size of the air diffusion plenum at a minimum of 6' × 8'. It requires a certain study to draw appropriate inferences from ASHRAE 170 to understand that the clean and aseptic zone emerges as nearly 10' × 10', which also tends to align with Health Technical Memorandum 03-01, the corresponding UK standard. This assumes significance as the unidirectional airflow that is intended to entrain particulate matter out of the aseptic zone must cover not merely the patients and the surgical team, but also the instrumentation tray that must not be subject to turbulence.

In times of increasing consumer activism, it is important to not merely comply with the standards and the best practices, but document and demonstrate these too. A healthcare facility would do well to constitute an Infection Control and Risk Assessment team configured to review, address, and recommend matters pertaining to HVAC and plumbing systems along with materials/surfaces in interiors.

Monitoring Differential Pressure

A healthcare facility has certain rooms that are mandated to be maintained at differential air pressure in a bid to control infection. Operating rooms, isolation rooms, soiled utility rooms, laboratories, etc., are a few instances. It is important that these rooms are not merely designed for differential pressure but are also equipped for monitoring to check that the differential pressure is maintained on an on-going basis. This puts the healthcare facility on a sounder footing in case of an outbreak. It merits mention that Centre for Diseases Control, Atlanta, a bellwether institution where it comes to infection control, mandates the monitoring as a critical requirement in healthcare facilities too.

■ MEDICAL GASES

Medical gases constitute essential services. Medical gas supply systems in hospitals are utilized to supply specialized gases and gas mixtures to various parts of the facility. The gases commonly handled by such systems include—oxygen, medical air, nitrous oxide, nitrogen, carbon dioxide, and medical vacuum. The gases used in anesthesia are generally supplied under high pressure, either in cylinders or via pipeline with cylinders on anesthesia machines for emergency backup. Oxygen, nitrous oxide, and medical air are usually supplied from pipeline. The services may be stand-alone or centralized. A centralized system allows averting movement of heavy cylinders within the facility and allows ease of monitoring.

In exercise of the powers conferred by sections 5 and 7 of the Explosives Act, 1884 (4 of 1884) and in supersession of the Gas Cylinders Rules, 2004 (except as respects things done or omitted to be done before such supersession), the Central Government made the Gas Cylinders Rules, 2016.[25] The objective of these rules is to ensure safety of the general population occupied with the activity of filling, ownership, transport, and import of such gases. Regulatory authorities emphasize the practice of various safety procedures to facilitate easy identification and to avoid mixing of the containers. They also insist that the handling of these gases should be done only by a trained professional. Although regulatory measures are in place to ensure safety in the manufacture and distribution of medical gases, intermittent accidents do occur which have the potential to cause injury to patients and healthcare providers. Therefore, safety should be the highest priority and all necessary precautions must be taken and backup plans must be instituted to minimize the risk of any unfortunate incident.

Safety Measures Related to Medical Gases

- To ensure safety, it is very important to establish a monitoring system to maintain a stable supply of medical gases.
- The system should trace the flow of gases from the source, through the pipeline, and to the various outlets from where these gases are used in the hospital.
- The systems should indicate: (i) The amount of gas remaining in the different tanks, (ii) The operating condition of the supply station, and (iii) The gas pressure applied to each area where the gas is in use.
- The medical gas outlet should have such a design that it is impossible to allow a cross-connection to a different medical gas. For example, connecting a hypoxic patient to a carbondioxide supply. Use pin patterns that will only fit into the correct female connector. The use of Diameter Indexed Safety Systems (DISS) compliant terminal outlets that will ensure one does not plug a probe for one system into another, unintended system. In other words, a probe for oxygen will not fit into an outlet for suction or medical air or nitrous oxide.
- *Color coding:* Bright colors respectively designed to the particular kind of gas.
- There must be a provision of back-up or stand-by that allows for uninterrupted service. Where manifolds are the primary source, two banks of cylinders should be maintained—one duty and the other stand-by. As the primary source depletes, the stand-by takes over by way of solenoid valve operation without having to resort to any electrical intervention. Where compressors and pumps are concerned, similar provision of duty and stand-by that may alternate, are made, to allow a degree of safety in supply.
- Provision of audio-visual alarms at plant room and/or on the building management system console as also in the clinical departments close to the nurse stations allows for safeguards in case of deviation in the flow and/or pressure beyond the accepted range.

- A periodic check of the constituents of each gas would be in order to ensure that the parameters specified by the applicable pharmacopeia are met.

Storage of Cylinders[26]
- The storage area should be cool, dry, ventilated, and clean area constructed of fire resistant material. Cylinders should not be exposed to dampness, corrosive chemicals, and fumes as they may damage the cylinders and valve protection caps.
- It should have good access for deliveries and a reasonable level floor surface.
- It should have segregation of "Full" and "Empty cylinders."
- Cylinders with an oldest fill date should be used first.
- Prominent signs of no smoking, no open flames or sparks, etc., should be displayed over the storage area.
- Cylinders should always be kept in place with chain or any other restraining device.
- The suitable trolley/cart should be used to transport and support the cylinders.

■ SMART HOSPITALS

Medical science and technology, both are changing the way healthcare is being delivered. There are real and practical applications of artificial intelligence that encompass early detection and diagnosis, treatment and predictive analysis including prognosis. This is set to grow as the database expands and algorithms get calibrated and recalibrated. However, simpler networking tools that allow interfacing of equipment to servers and thereby allow staff to access data on the move, go a long way in facilitating better patient management. A nurse is constantly working among beeps and there is a very human possibility that such an alarm-alert would go unnoticed, training notwithstanding. Technology now allows handheld devices akin to mobile phones that alert the nurse to medication time, action checklists and alarms; allows charting and internal communication on the go; and importantly, allows seamless handover on change of shift. This makes for a smart hospital focused on patient safety, easing the recording and traceability.

■ RISK MANAGEMENT

Risk may be defined as a probability or threat of damage, injury, liability, loss, or any other negative occurrence that is caused by external or internal vulnerabilities, and that may be avoided through preemptive action.[27] Risk management is a planned and a structured process to identify, classify, and evaluate the risks and then to manage and control them. The aim is to ensure the best value for the project in terms of cost, time, and quality by balancing the input to manage the risks with the benefits from such act. Risk management in healthcare is a continuous and proactive process of developing and implementing the strategies to optimize patient well-being and to prevent harm or to limit patient injury. Risk management should be a common thread throughout the entire organization.

The Process of Risk Management[28]
Risk management is a process that may be divided into following five basic steps (Dickson, 1995):
1. Risk identification
2. Risk assessment

3. Development of risk management strategies
4. Implementation of risk management strategy
5. Evaluation of risk management activities

Risk Identification

The first step of risk management is to identify the risks that may threaten and/or jeopardize the patient, healthcare provider, and healthcare organization. It is challenging to recognize all the threats a healthcare organization faces. Healthcare risk managers can uncover threats by engaging everyone—patients, healthcare providers, administrators, and all other personnel involved with the healthcare organization.

Sources of Risk Identification

- Brainstorming with clinicians, staff and administrators, and quality managers
- Tracing the journey of a patient from admission till discharge
- Retrospective screening of patient records
- Root cause analysis of incident reports, sentinel event reports, quality committee reports, reports of accreditation bodies
- Facility management and safety committee report
- Patient complaints and satisfaction survey results
- Specialized committee reports (such as morbidity and mortality committee, medication management and use, infection control, blood utilization, facility management and safety committee).

Risk Assessment

After identifying the risks, specific analysis is done to determine potential risks. It is an evaluation of the risk to determine:

- What could possibly happen?
- What is the likelihood of occurrence of the event (measuring risk)?
- How severe will be the outcome if something did happen?
- How can the likelihood of occurrence be mitigated and to what degree?
- What can be done to reduce the impact?

Development of Risk Management Strategies

- *Avoidance of risk:* If the risk is high and the benefit is low in carrying out any particular procedure/activity, then avoidance of such procedure/activity will be appropriate.
- *Prevention of risk:* Hospitals and health-care providers can take steps to prevent the possibility of mistakes. Prevention is developing the programs that will prevent occurrence of events that could lead to adverse outcomes. For example, clinical practice guidelines may reduce medical errors.
- *Transfer of risk:* A high-risk case can be transferred to a higher level of expertise for appropriate care.
- *Reduction of risk*: Reduction is the strategy that begins immediately after the harmful event has occurred. One of the most important risk reduction strategies is the immediate care of and attention to the persons threatened or injured. Impact of harmful event can be reduced by many ways:
  - Early investigation and care to the patient can reduce the medical risk.

- Thorough documentation of the steps taken to mitigate the effect of harmful event can reduce the risk of legal liability.
- Honest disclosure can be helpful in reducing the loss associated with harmful event.

Implementation of Risk Management Programs

A risk management program is to be implemented based on the best risk management strategies compatible with the prime objective of patient safety. An important strategy that aims to manage or reduce the risk of bad outcomes is the implementation of activities on the basis of analysis of morbidity or mortality audits. The audit process should enable healthcare providers to learn from harm events in an objective and nonpunitive environment. This audit process should address potential causes or circumstances surrounding the bad outcome (mortality/morbidity), not only those attributable to individual human error but also to those that may be attributed to system-based failure. Implementation of risk management plan should be oriented toward learning, sharing, and implementing interventions that are known to be efficient for avoiding another similar situation. A no-blame approach contributes to improve the safety culture and will also improve the implementation of risk management programs.

Evaluation of Risk Management Activities

Evaluation refers to reviewing the risk management activities and of the whole experience with the risk management strategy. A committee may be appointed to evaluate general or specific activities. Risk management is a continuous process that starts with identification and analysis of risk, followed by development and implementation of risk management strategies, and continues with frequent evaluation of risk management activities and their results; the process is then repeated.

■ CONCLUSION

Recent advancement in medical science and technology and better understanding of the disease mechanism have created an efficient but immensely complex healthcare system. This complexity brings many challenges for healthcare professionals in continuing to keep the patients safe. Every day, more than a million people are treated safely in the hospitals, but there are times when things go wrong. Safety has become a prominent topic in the medical field since the Institute of Medicine in 1999 released its landmark report "To Err Is Human." The patients who come to the hospitals, seeking care, do so with the hope that they will get cured, all the while assuming that, they do not expose themselves to any new danger. Creating the system where this assumption is justified is the real challenge for healthcare system. Safety in healthcare has often been compared with safety in aviation. In the first instance the concept of safety in medical field is a relative term, since life itself is a high risk phenomenon which permits no absolute safety. While healthcare has much to learn from aviation, the transfer of lessons from aviation to healthcare needs to be modulation, considering the specific characteristics of healthcare system. There are many opportunities for safety concepts in aviation that can be considered for adoption in healthcare. A focus on systems rather than individuals, need for actions to be proactive, rather than solely reactive to harmful events and an evaluation of latent risk factors that may end up as a harmful event, are some of the important lessons that we can learn from aviation. If a culture of safety is to be achieved, we must rethink and rebuild the processes through which healthcare is delivered.

REFERENCES

1. Moulton TJ. A culture of safety is a journey, not a destination. It requires our continuing diligence. [online] Available from: https://www.twitter.com/navymedicine/status/. [Last accessed Aug., 2019].
2. Sokol DK. "First do no harm" revisited. BMJ. 2013;347:f6426.
3. WHO Patient Safety Curriculum Guide for Medical Schools. [online] Available from: https://www.who.int/patientsafety/education/curriculum/who_mc_teachers-guide.pdf. [Last accessed Aug., 2019].
4. Kohn LT, Corrigan JM, Donaldson MS, et al. To Err Is Human: Building a Safer Health System. Institute of Medicine, Washington (DC): National Academy Press (US); 2000.
5. Farmer BM. Patient safety in the emergency department. Emerg Med. 2016;48:396-404.
6. Jepson ZK, Darling CE, Kotkowski KA, et al. Emergency department patient safety incident characterization: an observational analysis of the findings of a standardized peer review process. BMC Emerg Med. 2014;14:20.
7. Sklar DP, Crandall C. What do we know about Emergency Department Safety? Perspectives on Safety. Patient Safety Network. [online] Available from: https://psnet.ahrq.gov/perspectives/perspective/88/what-do-we-knowabout-emergency-department-safety. [Last accessed Aug., 2019].
8. Verbeek-VanNoord I, Wagner C, Van Dyck C, et al. Is culture associated with patient safety in the emergency department? A study of staff perspectives. Int J Qual Health Care. 2014;26(1):64-70.
9. Patanwala AE, Warholak TL, Sanders AB, et al. A prospective observational study of medication errors in a tertiary care emergency department. Ann Emerg Med. 2010;55(6):522-6.
10. Bernstein SL, Aronsky D, Duseja R, et al. The effect of emergency department crowding on clinically oriented outcomes. Acad Emerg Med. 2009;16(1):1-10.
11. Parmanand Katara v. Union of India AIR 1989 SC 2039.
12. Kanal E, Barkovich AJ, Bell C, et al. ACR guidance document on MR safe practices: 2013. J Magn Reson Imaging. 2013;37(3):501-30.
13. Abad C, Fearday A, Safdar N. Adverse effects of isolation in hospitalised patients: a systematic review. J Hosp Infect. 2010;76(2):97-102.
14. Stelfox HT, Bates DW, Redelmeier DA. Safety of patients isolated for infection control. JAMA. 2003;290(14):1899-905.
15. Tanner C, Gans D, White J, et al. Electronic health records and patient safety: co-occurrence of early EHR Implementation with patient safety practices in primary care settings. Appl Clin Inform. 2015;6(1):136-47.
16. Singh H, Giardina TD, Meyer AN, et al. Types and origins of diagnostic errors in primary care settings. JAMA Intern Med. 2013;173(6):418-25.
17. Millman M; Institute of Medicine (US) Committee on Monitoring Access to Personal Health Care Services. Access to Health Care in America. Washington (DC): National Academies Press; 1993.
18. Harmonised Guidelines and Space Standards for Barrier-Free Built Environment for Persons with Disability and Elderly Persons. Government of India. Ministry of Urban Development. [online] Available from: https://cpwd.gov.in/publication/harmonisedguidelinesdreleasedon23rdmarch2016.pdf. [Last accessed Aug., 2019].
19. Health Care-Associated Infections Fact Sheet. [online] Available from: https://u.osu.edu/korzen.1/2016/09/23/health-care-associated-infections-fact-sheet/. [Last accessed Aug., 2019].
20. WHO. Practical Guidelines for Infection Control in Health Care Facilities. [online] Available from: http://www.wpro.who.int/publications/docs/practical_guidelines_infection_control.pdf. [Last accessed Aug., 2019].
21. Barbosa BP. The role of engineering design in the infection control for hospitals. Tr Civil Eng Arch. 2018;1(2):39-42.
22. Li Y, Leung GM, Tang JW, et al. Role of ventilation in airborne transmission of infectious agents in the built environment—a multidisciplinary systematic review. Indoor Air. 2007;17(1):2-18.
23. WHO. Natural Ventilation for Infection Control in Health Care Settings. 2009. [online] Available from: https://www.who.int/water_sanitation_health/publications/natural_ventilation.pdf. [Last accessed Aug., 2019].
24. ANSI/ASHRAE/ASHE Standard 170-2008. American Society of Heating, Refrigerating and Air-Conditioning Engineers, Inc.; [online] Available from: http://www.saludcapital.gov.co/DSP/Infecciones%20Asociadas%20a%20Atencin%20en%20Salud/Comites/2016/Abril/ASHRAE-Standard-170-2008qq.pdf. [Last accessed Aug., 2019].
25. The Gas Cylinder Rules. New Delhi: The Gazette of India, Ministry of Commerce and Industry; 2016.
26. Guidance for the Storage of Gas Cylinders in the Workplace. BCGA Guidance Note GN2—Revision 5. British Compressed Gases Association; 2012. [online] Available from: https://www.agaseurope.com/media/2444/guidance-for-the-storage-of-gas-cylinders-in-the-workplace.pdf. [Last accessed Aug., 2019].
27. businessdictionary. Risk (Definition). [online] Available from: http://www.businessdictionary.com/definition/risk.html. [Last accessed Aug., 2019].
28. Alam AY. Steps in the process of risk management in healthcare. J Epid Prev Med. 2016;2(2):118.

CHAPTER 8

Healthcare-associated Infections: A Threat to Patient Safety

Rahul S Kamble

> *"Bacteria often find their way into patient's bodies through the lines and tubes that doctors use to deliver drugs and nutrition."*
> — **Consumer Reports.**
> **America's Antibiotic Crisis**[1]

■ INTRODUCTION

Healthcare-associated infection (HAI) is a serious patient safety issue, as it continues to occur, and leads to morbidity, mortality, and escalating healthcare expenditure. Originally HAI was referred to the infections associated with admission in an acute-care hospital (formerly called, nosocomial infection), but now the term applies to infections acquired in the continuum of settings where patient receives healthcare (e.g., long-term care, home care, and ambulatory care). These unanticipated infections develop during the course of treatment, and may result in increased morbidity and mortality; prolong the duration of hospital stay; and necessitate additional diagnostic and therapeutic interventions, thus generating added financial burden to the patients. HAIs are considered an undesirable outcome, and being preventable in some cases, these are often considered an indicator of the quality of patient care, an adverse event, and a major patient safety issue.

Multiple factors like, recent advances in quality healthcare, patient preferences, and financial incentives have shifted more medical procedures to outpatient settings; thus, fewer patients are admitted to hospitals. Medical procedures are shifting into outpatient facilities, mainly due to technological advances such as, minimally invasive surgical procedures. The disturbing fact is that the average duration of inpatient admissions has decreased while the frequency of HAIs has increased.[2,3] The true incidence of HAIs is likely to be underestimated as hospital stays may be shorter than the incubation period of the infecting microorganism (a developing infection), and symptoms may not manifest until days after patient discharge. Studies have found that between 12% and 84% of surgical site infections (SSIs) are detected after the patients have been discharged from the hospital, and most become evident within 21 days after the surgical operation.[4,5] In high-income countries, for every 100 hospitalized patients, 7 develop at least one HAI and the frequency of HAIs in intensive care units (ICUs) is at least 3-fold higher (approximately 30%).[6] The data available indicate that the burden of HAIs in low- and middle-income countries like India is high, with an estimated pooled prevalence of 15.5 per 100 patients, and is more than double the prevalence in Europe and the US.[7]

These data demonstrate the critical link between infection prevention and control, and improving patient safety.

■ WHAT IS HEALTHCARE-ASSOCIATED INFECTION?[8,9]

According to World Health Organization (WHO), HAI, also referred to as "nosocomial" or "hospital" infection, is an infection occurring in a patient during the process of care in a hospital or other healthcare facility which was not present or incubating at the time of admission. They are unrelated to the original illness that brings patients to the hospital and are neither present nor incubating as at the time of admission. HAI can also appear after discharge. A particular infection should be considered healthcare associated, only if:
- It was not present or incubating when the patient was admitted to the hospital.
- The infection does not represent a complication or extension of an infectious process that was present at the time of admission.
- The infection occurred >48–72 hours after admission, and within 10 days following discharge or longer if it is related to a surgical procedure, a *Clostridioides difficile* infection or an antibiotic-resistant organism.

For the purposes of National Healthcare Safety Network (NHSN) surveillance in the acute care setting, the Center for Disease Control (CDC) has defined HAI as a localized or systemic condition resulting from an adverse reaction to the presence of infectious agent(s) or its toxin(s). There must be no evidence that the infection was present or incubating at the time of admission to the acute care setting.

What are the Sources of Healthcare-associated Infections?

Healthcare-associated infections may be caused by infectious agents from endogenous or exogenous sources.
- Healthcare-associated infections are endogenous when the patient's own germs infect the patient or when the infection sets in because of the patient's particular vulnerability. Endogenous sources of infectious agents can be body sites such as the skin, nose, mouth, gastrointestinal (GI) tract, or vagina that are normally inhabited by microorganisms.
- Exogenous infections are those, whose source is found outside the patient's body. They include infections transmitted through patient care personnel, visitors, medical equipment, medical devices, or by a contaminated hospital environment (air, water, and food).

The distinction between endogenous and exogenous infections is important since some decisions reveal judicial reluctance to impose medical liability for endogenous infections.[8]

Important Facts Related to Healthcare-associated Infection

- Direct observation of the infection site or the patient chart or the other clinical records help in forming the clinical evidence.
- For certain infections, diagnosis by the physician or surgeon based on direct observation or during medical examination or surgical procedure or diagnostic procedure, is an acceptable criterion for HAI, unless there is contradictory evidence. For example, one of the criteria for SSI is "surgeon or attending physician diagnosis." Unless stated clearly, diagnosis by physician alone is not an acceptable criterion for any specific type of HAI.
- Infections among infants due to passage through the birth canal are also considered HAIs.

Which Infections are NOT Healthcare-associated

The following infections are not considered to be associated with healthcare:
- Those infections which are associated with complications or extensions of infections already present at the time of admission; unless a change in pathogen or presenting symptoms strongly suggests that the infection has been acquired after hospital admission.
- Infections like herpes simplex, toxoplasmosis, rubella, *Cytomegalovirus*, or syphilis among infants which are acquired transplacentally and manifest in <48 hours after birth; and
- Reactivation of a latent infection [e.g., herpes zoster (shingles), herpes simplex, syphilis, or tuberculosis].

The following conditions are not infections:
- Colonization, i.e., presence of microorganisms on skin, on mucous membranes, in open wounds, or in excretions or secretions but there are no clinical signs or symptoms; and
- Inflammation as a tissue response to injury or stimulation by noninfectious agents, e.g., chemicals.

Common Healthcare-associated Infections

Surgical Site Infections

Surgical site infection is a type of HAI involving the surgical site within 30 days of the procedure, or within 90 days if an implant is in place and the infection is related to the operative procedure. SSIs are categorized into following three types:

1. Superficial Incisional Infection

Superficial incisional infection occurs within 30 days of procedure and involves only skin and subcutaneous tissue of incision. Patient has at least one of the following:
- Purulent drainage from superficial incision.
- Organisms isolated from aseptically obtained culture of fluid or tissue from superficial incision.
- Superficial incision that is deliberately opened by a surgeon and is culture-positive or not cultured and patient has at least one of the following clinical findings: Pain or tenderness, localized swelling, redness, or heat.
- Diagnosis of SSI by surgeon.

2. Deep Incisional Infection

Deep incisional infection occurs within 30 days or 90 days of surgery and has implant if after the 30 days and involves deep soft tissues of incision. Patient has at least one of the following:
- Purulent drainage from deep incision.
- Deep incision that spontaneously dehisces or deliberately opened by surgeon and is culture-positive or not cultured and patient has at least one of the following signs and symptoms: Fever (>38°C), localized pain, or tenderness.
- Abscess or other evidence of infection involving deep incision found on direct examination, during invasive procedure, or by histopathologic examination or imaging test.
- Diagnosis of SSI by surgeon.

3. Organ/space Surgical Site Infection

Organ or space infection occurs within 30–90 days of the surgery, and if implant has been put, after the 30 days and involves any part of the body except the skin incision, fascia or muscle

layers, opened or manipulated during the operative procedure. At least one of the following conditions is present:
- Purulent drainage appears from the drain put into the organ or the space.
- Organism is isolated from the culture of fluid or tissue taken from organ or the space.
- Abscess or other evidence of infection in the organ or the space is detected by direct examination, or by histopathological examination or by imaging test.
- Surgical site infection is diagnosis clinically by the surgeon.

Ventilator-associated Pneumonia

In ventilator-associated pneumonia (VAP), both possible and probable VAPs are included. The patient is on a ventilator for ≥3 days and >14 days since last ventilator-associated condition (VAC).

Ventilator-associated Condition

For the diagnosis of VAC, after a period of stability or improvement of 2 or more days, at least one of the following conditions should be present:
1. Increase in FIO_2 of ≥20 points for 2 days or more
2. Increase in PEEP ≥3 cm for 2 days or more

Within window period [2 days before + 2 days after the VAC date (total 5 days)] meets both criteria:
- The patient has a temperature >38°C or <36°C or white blood cell count ≥12.0 × 10^9/l or 4.0 × 10^9/l and
- New antimicrobial agent(s) is started and continued for ≥4 days to the patient.
- Within window period meets at least one of the criteria mentioned below:
  - Purulent respiratory secretions (one or more specimens) defined as Gram stain of 4+ white blood cell (WBC) and 1–2+ epithelial cells
  - Positive culture of sputum endotracheal aspirate, BAL, lung tissue or protected specimen brushing.

AND

The organism is NOT excluded: "Normal respiratory flora," "normal oral flora," mixed respiratory flora," "mixed oral flora," "altered oral flora" or other commensal flora of the oral cavity or upper respiratory tract: *Candida* species or yeast not otherwise specified; coagulase-negative *Staphylococcus* species; and *Enterococcus* species, when isolated from cultures of sputum, endotracheal aspirates, bronchoalveolar lavage, or protected specimen brushings

OR

Excluded organisms isolated from cultures of lung tissue or pleural fluid including *Candida* species or yeast not otherwise specified, coagulase-negative *Staphylococcus* species or *Enterococcus* species

OR

Test result meets one of the following criteria:
- Positive pleural fluid culture (from thoracentesis or initial placement of chest tube) or
- Positive lung histopathology or
- Positive diagnostic test for *Legionella species* or
- Positive diagnostic test for respiratory viruses.

Central Line-associated Bloodstream Infection

Criteria: The surveillance is restricted to ICU patients who:
- Have a central line in place for >2 days or central line has been discontinued for <3 days.
- There is a pathogen in one or more blood cultures and infection is not suspected at another site and all elements of laboratory findings confirmed blood stream infection (BSI) first present together on or after the 3rd hospital day.
- The patient has at least one of the following: Fever (>38°C) or chills or hypotension (systolic <90 mm Hg) and positive laboratory results that are not related to an infection at another site and common commensal organism is cultured from two or more blood cultures, drawn on separate occasions and criteria elements occurred within a time frame that does not exceed a gap of 1 day and all elements of laboratory results confirmed BSI first present together on or after the 3rd hospital day.

Catheter-Associated Urinary Tract Infection (CAUTI) in Residential Care

Criteria: Resident must have indwelling urinary catheter and at least **ONE** of the following:
- Fevers, rigors **OR** new onset hypotension with NO alternate sign of infection
- Acute change in mental status **OR** functional decline with no alternate diagnosis **AND** leukocytosis (WBC > 14,000)
- New onset suprapubic pain or costoverterbral angle pain or tenderness
- Purulent discharge around catheter or acute pain, swelling of testes, epididymis or prostate

AND
- Urine culture (> 10^6 CFU/ml) correlates with symptoms

OR
- Positive blood culture & urine culture with same organism with no alternate site of infection
- Fever (>38C) or chills, new flank or supra-pubic pain or tenderness, change in character of infection

■ TRANSMISSION OF INFECTION

Transmission of infection in a hospital may occur if the following three elements are present: (1) A source of infecting microorganisms, (2) A susceptible host, and (3) A means of transmission of the microorganism to the host.

Source of Microorganisms

A study[10] reviewed 1,022 outbreak investigations and reported that the most common sources of infectious agents causing HAI are: The patient, medical equipment, environment of the hospital, healthcare personnel, contaminated food, and contaminated equipment.

Susceptible Host

Patient factors are important predisposing factors for HAIs. Immunocompromised patients, may be due to age, underlying diseases, use of drugs, or surgical treatments are at a higher risk of acquiring HAIs. Extrinsic risk factors for the susceptible host include surgical or other invasive procedures, diagnostic or therapeutic interventions (e.g., invasive devices, implanted foreign bodies, organ transplantations, and immunosuppressive medications), and personnel exposures.

Means of Transmission

The spread of microorganisms may occur through four common routes: Contact (direct and indirect), respiratory droplets, airborne spread, and common vehicle.

■ THE BURDEN OF HOSPITAL-ACQUIRED INFECTION

World Health Organization estimates HAIs to occur among 7–12% of the hospitalized patients globally, with >1.4 million people suffering from infectious complications acquired in the hospital at any time.[11] A survey amongst 55 hospitals of 14 countries representing the four WHO regions (Europe, Eastern Mediterranean, South-East Asia, and Western Pacific) showed that 8.7% of hospital patients had HAIs. The estimated prevalence of HAIs in the United States (US) is 4.5% corresponding to 9.3 infections per 1000 patient days; while that in Europe is reported to be 7.1% corresponding to a cumulative incidence of 17.0 episodes per 1000 patient days.[12] A multicenter and prospective cohort surveillance of device-associated infection by the International Healthcare Associated Infection Control Consortium (INICC) in 55 ICUs of 8 developing countries including India revealed an overall rate of 14.7% HAI corresponding to 22.5 infections per 1000 ICU days.[13] Various studies have reflected an increasing trend in HAI incidence across India over the last decade as mentioned in **Table 1**.[14-20]

■ PREVENTING HOSPITAL-ACQUIRED INFECTION

"If you know how to prevent infections, you know how to protect patients from most adverse events."

Many preventive measures have been recommended as mentioned in **Table 2**.[21-23] These measures are applied to reduce morbidity, length of hospital stay, mortality, and hospital costs. Among the published guidelines three main approaches are as follows:
1. Elimination of endogenous healthcare-associated pathogens to reduce oropharyngeal, intestinal, and skin colonization.
2. Use of methods to prevent cross contamination and to control various sources of healthcare-associated pathogens that can be transmitted from patient-to-patient or from

TABLE 1: Trend in HAI incidence across India.

Studies	HAI rate (%)	HAI per 1000 patient days
Ramana (2012)[14]	41.0	–
Sood (2011)[15]	04.3	6.16
Datta (2010)[16]	29.1	–
Shalini (2010)[17]	27.4	–
Kamat (2008)[18]	34.0	40.66
Habibi (2008)[19]	52.2	28.6
Mehta (2007)[20]	04.4	9.06

(HAI: healthcare-associated infection)

TABLE 2: Strategies for prevention of HAIs.[21-23]

	General measures	Healthcare-associated pneumonia	Bloodstream infections	Surgical site infections
Personnel	Educational programs: Hand-washing, gloves, gowns, etc., control of infections at risk for healthcare workers; immunization	Maintenance, disinfection of respiratory equipment (endotracheal tubes, suctioning devices, ventilators etc.); careful use of invasive exploratory endoscopies	Careful manipulation of catheters: Aseptic technique for insertion; search for source of bacteremia (infection foci)	Preparation of operative team (surgical gloves, gowns, masks, etc.)
Patient	Patient isolation: Single room for high-risk patients; antibiotic prophylaxis; specific conditions (neutropenic, burn patients), SDD; topical treatments for colonized sites	Oropharyngeal decontamination: Treatment of healthcare associated sinusitis; local antibiotics (aerosols); gastric alkalinization; semi-recumbent position; care of enteral nutrition	Duration of catheterization, changed at appropriate intervals; adjusting for severity of underlying disease; blood cultures with best techniques (automated) for rapid identification of pathogens; SDD limits translocation and endotoxin release	Wound classification (clean, clean-contaminated, dirty); minimize preoperation stay; suitable skin preparation, hair removal; antibiotic prophylaxis
Treatment	Optimal use of antibiotics, control of antibiotic use (antimicrobial use audits)			
Environmental measures	HAIs surveillance: Close cooperation with microbiology; computerized systems in surveillance and fast transmission of data; proper elimination of medical waste	Surveillance of air conditioning humidities, hot water nebulisers (*Legionella*); isolation precautions; isolation guidelines	Hospital and intensive care unit surveillance (epidemiology); disposable catheters, close cooperation with microbiology	Limiting source of exogenous contamination; excellent surgical technique, limiting dead space exposing wound; proper wound dressing
Administrative measures	Infection Control Committee: Restriction policies (hospital formulary); guidelines for prevention; consensus conferences; application of guidelines	–	–	Sterilization and suitable disinfection measures for reusable equipment; disposable instruments whenever possible; disposal regulations
Miscellaneous	<ul><li>Hospital design engineers for suitable structure of wards, rooms, specific isolation units, and healthcare facilities</li><li>Close cooperation between authorities, microbiologists, and infectious diseases consultants</li></ul>			

(HAIs: healthcare-associated infections)

personnel to patient, i.e., proper disinfection and care of catheters, respiratory equipment, humidifiers, endotracheal tube, and dialysis systems.
3. Use of antibiotic prophylaxis in postoperative and high-risk patients (burn patients, patients in ICUs, etc.). Aerosolized polymyxin-B and/or endotracheal aminoglycosides can be given to prevent *Pseudomonas* and/or *Acinetobacter* pneumonia which have the highest mortality rates.

■ INFECTION PREVENTION INITIATIVES

Several organizations have analyzed the effectiveness of guidelines, standards of care, and preventive measures in order to recommend evidence-based measures for improving patient safety.

Recommendations by Agency for Healthcare Research and Quality

All healthcare organizations focus on the following infection prevention initiatives:
- Improving hand hygiene.
- Utilizing barrier precautions to prevent transmission of infection.
- Prudent antibiotic use to reduce *C. difficile* and vancomycin-resistant *Enterococcus* (VRE).
- Preventing urinary tract infections.
- Preventing central venous catheter (CVC)-related BSIs.
- Preventing VAP.
- Preventing SSIs.

Initiative by the World Health Organization

The WHO World Alliance for Patient Safety has chosen the prevention of HAI as the first Global Patient Safety Challenge. The WHO launched the first Global Patient Safety Challenge in 2005 and introduced the "5 moments of hand hygiene" in 2009 as an attempt to reduce the problem of HAIs. In order to prevent HAIs, a high level of hygiene is essential, which includes practicing 5Cs in patient care as depicted in **Figure 1**.

The Joint Commission's National Patient Safety Goals

The Joint Commission established the National Patient Safety Goals (NPSGs) in 2002 to address specific areas of concern in regards to patient safety as mentioned in **Table 3**.[24] The Joint Commission determines the highest priority patient safety issues, including NPSGs, from input from practitioners, provider organizations, purchasers, consumer groups, and other stakeholders. Goal 7 was created to address healthcare personnel education and compliance with hand hygiene and the inclusion of healthcare-associated deaths and disability as sentinel events, requiring root cause analysis and follow-up. This NPSG was substantively expanded upon in 2009 to include patient education regarding multidrug-resistant organisms (MDROs) and patient and family engagement in patient safety related to HAIs. Additionally, this goal requires facility implementation of evidence-based practices to prevent device and procedure-associated infections.[24]

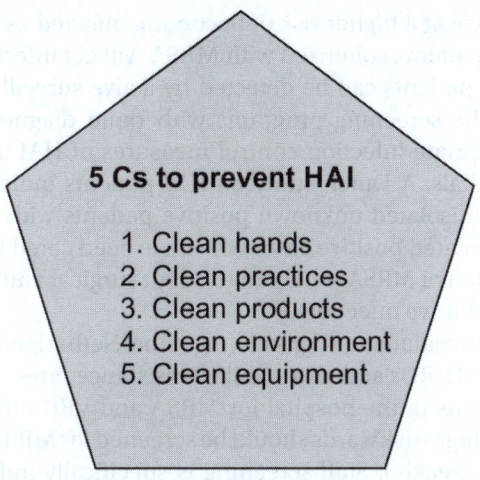

(HAI: healthcare-associated infection)
FIG. 1: The 5 Cs to prevent hospital acquired infections.

TABLE 3: GOAL 7 (reduce the risk of healthcare associated infections).

NPSG.07.01.01	Comply with either the current Centers for Disease Control and Prevention (CDC) hand hygiene guidelines or the current World Health Organization (WHO) hand hygiene guidelines *Applies to:* Ambulatory, behavioral healthcare, critical access hospital, home care, hospital, laboratory, nursing care center, office-based surgery
NPSG.07.03.01	Implement evidence-based practices to prevent healthcare-associated infections due to multidrug-resistant organisms in acute-care hospitals *Applies to:* Critical access hospital, hospital, nursing care center
NPSG.07.04.01	Implement evidence-based practices to prevent central line-associated bloodstream infections *Applies to:* Critical access hospital, hospital, nursing care center
NPSG.07.05.01	Implement evidence-based practices for preventing surgical site infections *Applies to:* Ambulatory, critical access hospital, hospital, office-based surgery
NPSG.07.06.01	Implement evidence-based practices to prevent indwelling catheter-associated urinary tract infections (CAUTI) *Applies to:* Critical access hospital, hospital, nursing care center

(NPSG: National Patient Safety Goals)

Active Surveillance Culture

The most common HAIs are due to the following MDROs: (a) methicillin-resistant *Staphylococcus aureus* (MRSA), (b) Vancomycin-resistant *Enterococci* (VRE), (c) extended spectrum beta lactamases (ESBLs) producing organisms, and (d) *Klebsiella* producing carbapenemases (KPC).

The colonized patients are at a higher risk of becoming infected as compared to the non-colonized one, e.g., 25% of patients colonized with MRSA will get infected. The unrecognized MRSA/VRE/KPC colonized patients can be detected by active surveillance and thus help in preventing transmission. The screening programs with rapid diagnostic tests significantly help in setting up of appropriate infection control measures of HAI and thus can decrease the spread within the hospitals. A Dutch study on ICU patients indicated a 38-fold greater rate of transmission from unisolated unknown positive patients with universal precautions as compared to identified isolated positive cases who have been cared for with gowns, masks, and gloves.[25] Early recognition of MRSA is helpful to adapt surgical antibiotic prophylaxis and prevent surgical site postoperative infections.[26]

Countries with active surveillance programs (e.g., The Netherlands, Denmark, Finland, etc.) control HAI caused by MDROs and also stabilize resistance rates. There should be active screening of incoming patients in the hospital for MRSA and VRE carriage. Additionally, all patients getting admitted to high-risk wards should be screened for MRSA and later they should be screened regularly (e.g., weekly). Staff screening is specifically indicated if transmission continues despite active control measures or if epidemiological aspects of an outbreak are unusual or if there is suspected persistent MRSA carriage by staff.

■ INDICATORS OF HEALTHCARE-ASSOCIATED INFECTIONS

Healthcare-associated infections indicators are a reflection of healthcare quality and patient safety in hospitals. HAI indicators are calculated using surveillance programs and/or systems. **Table 4** provides a list of selected indicators.[27]

TABLE 4: Indicators to control HAIs.

Structure-related indicators (Facility level)	Process-related indicators (Policies and protocols)	Outcome-related indicators (HAIs)
Infection control program approved by top management	Outbreak policy	Catheter-associated urinary tract infections
Annual action plan	Employee infectious diseases screening	Central line-associated bloodstream infections
Annual objectives defined	Staff education	Ventilator associated pneumonia
Infection control budget dedicated	Sterilization and disinfection policy	Ventilator associated event
Hospital infection control committee	Occupational exposure to blood and body fluids policy	Surgical site infections
ICP communication plan	Antimicrobial stewardship	*Clostridioides difficile* associated infections
Human resources for hygiene and cleanliness	Hand hygiene and isolation precautions policy	HAIs due to MDROs
Product purchase committee	• Insertion and maintenance policy for intravascular catheters • Cohort dedicated equipment policy	• Staff exposed to diseases transmissible by blood borne pathogens • Healthcare-associated gastroenteritis

(HAIs: healthcare-associated infections; MDROs: multidrug-resistant organisms)

MANAGEMENT OF HEALTHCARE-ASSOCIATED INFECTIONS

Strategies for Management of Healthcare-Associated Infections

The choice of empiric antibiotic therapy for the treatment of any HAI before microbiology test is available requires:
- Surveillance data of predominant organisms in the hospital on a regular basis.
- Surveillance of the current resistance patterns of these organisms.
- Identification of outbreaks of HAI involving one or more prevalent organisms.

Principles of Empiric Therapy[28]

The conventional empiric therapy should be broad spectrum so as to ensure maximal coverage. Combination therapy with an antipseudomonal penicillin (piperacillin) and aminoglycoside or an antipseudomonal cephalosporin (ceftazidime) and aminoglycoside have been the recommended first-line drugs for long. However, scenarios suggestive of infection due to gram-positive organisms such as MRSA, addition of a glycopeptide should be considered. Rifampicin, fusidic acid, and streptogramins (quinupristin–dalfopristin) also cover most gram-positive organisms. During outbreaks of HAI with high probability of cross contamination of a previously identified endemic MDRO such as *Pseudomonas aeruginosa*, carbapenems (e.g., imipenem or meropenem) in combination with either an aminoglycoside (amikacin) or a fluoroquinolone (ciprofloxacin) are recommended. It is vital that the empirical therapy is reassessed after 2 days or 3 days of initiation. Treatment should be readjusted on the basis of antibiotic sensitivity tests available on day 2 or day 3, and clinical response of the patient.

Specific Empiric Situations

- For suspected anaerobic bacterial infection, e.g., in surgical abdominal polymicrobial infection or in aspiration pneumonia, addition of clindamycin or cefoxitin or metronidazole is recommended. Imipenem can also be a useful alternative for mixed aerobic anaerobic infections.
- In cases of suspected legionellosis infection (atypical pneumonia), erythromycin and rifampicin either alone or in combination are the antibiotics of choice.

Initial Antibiotic Therapy[29]

- *Ceftazidime plus vancomycin*: Vancomycin is the drug of choice for suspected MRSA, penicillin-resistant pneumococci or other gram-positive resistant organisms.
- If vancomycin is not required, then monotherapy with ceftazidime, imipenem, cefepime, or meropenem can be given.
- In case of requirement of combination therapy, ceftazidime plus an antipseudomonal penicillin are the drugs of choice.

Therapeutic Strategies of Documented Healthcare-associated infections

Choice of Antibiotics

Most retrospective studies have shown that combination therapy is superior to monotherapy. However, the drug synergy between the drugs should be known before administration of combination therapy.

Gram-negative Organisms

Monotherapy

Although monotherapy is used less frequently than combination therapy, monotherapy with a third or fourth generation cephalosporin or aztreonam or carbapenems is recommended. Other options include a β-lactam plus a β-lactamase inhibitor such as amoxicillin + clavulanate (co-amoxiclav) or piperacillin + tazobactam or cefoperazone + sulbactam, etc.

Combination Therapy

Beside the conventional combination of a β-lactam antibiotic and an aminoglycoside (offers broad spectrum of antibacterial activity), the combination of ciprofloxacin with ceftazidime in *P. aeruginosa* infection, has also shown efficacy and prevention of emergence of resistance during therapy. It has been confirmed that combination of quinolones and a β-lactam antibiotic reduces the risk of emergence of resistance in *S. pneumoniae, Serratia marcescens, E. cloacae* and *P. aeruginosa*.

Gram-positive Organisms

Multiresistant gram-positive organisms pose specific problems such as MRSA, which are also resistant to rifampicin, aminoglycosides, and fluoroquinolones. The current drugs of choice for the treatment of MRSA infections are vancomycin, teicoplanin, and linezolid.

■ NEWER RESEARCH RELATED TO HEALTHCARE-ASSOCIATED INFECTION

The increased focus on infection prevention has inspired a spurt of invention in the field of environmental disinfection, especially given the growing scientific consensus that the hospital environment plays a significant role in the transmission of antimicrobial-resistant bacteria. The new devices include robots that emit ultraviolet rays and various arrangements that pump cleansing gases into a room. Tests of a Canadian system that releases a vapor composed of ozone and hydrogen peroxide in a sealed room have achieved a 100% microbial kill rate in several hospital rooms contaminated with MRSA.[30]

Now, scientists are exploring the use of the monoclonal antibodies to fight drug-resistant infections, including MRSA and CRE. Some monoclonal antibodies have successfully hindered the growth of *S. aureus*, encouraging the immune system to destroy the bacteria with phagocytes. Molecules necessary to the survival of the drug-resistant bacteria are being attacked by other monoclonal antibodies, a strategy that makes it less likely that the bacteria will be able to mutate to withstand new antibiotics. One group of researchers has developed an antibody vaccine aimed at preventing MRSA from eroding bone around an orthopedic implant; the vaccine targets a protein necessary for bacterial growth.[31] Other drugs are being tested that bypass the bacteria themselves, seeking to lessen the body's response to bacterial infection or deny the bacteria access to the body's resources. Scientists are investigating whether oral doses of probiotics, live microorganisms including some bacteria that may have health benefits, will reduce *S. aureus* nasal and GI colonization. Probiotics are also being looked at as a treatment for CRE. Researchers have developed devices to be inserted in a patient to carry a microchip, which would communicate with the clinicians and nurses with a series of lights alarming any immediate attentions set above every hospital bed.

Scientists are testing faster and more accurate ways to diagnose infections, advances that may help clinicians better judge when and whether to use antibiotics. Instead of relying only on direct clinical symptoms, some researchers are measuring biomarkers released by the body in response to infection. New drug delivery systems that obviate the need for catheters and ventilators may play a key role in the future prevention of infections. Nanomachines, for example, may make it possible to release antibiotics precisely at an infection site deep within the body. Nanomachines have already proven capable of clamping interior arteries and tying sutures in animal studies.

■ MEDICOLEGAL ASPECTS RELATED TO HEALTHCARE-ASSOCIATED INFECTION

Healthcare-associated infection is the infection that occurs in a patient in whom it was not present or incubating at the time of admission to the hospital. The very definition of HAI itself implies a potential for medicolegal problems. Liability for HAIs depends on multiple factors including the following:
- Failure to provide a clean and safe environment during patient care.
- Failure/delay in implementing the infection control measures.
- Failure to carry out routine pre-screening for MRSA or *C. difficile* negative prior to surgical or other admissions.
- Failure/delay in identifying and treating the infection when it has been acquired.

The guidelines on prevention and control of hospital infections provided by various national and international health organizations like WHO may be included as a criterion to determine whether a reasonable care as expected by law has been provided or not. The WHO has recommended the following to reduce HAIs:[32]
- Providing direct patient care using practices that minimize infections.
- Following appropriate practices of hygiene (e.g., hand washing and sterilization of instruments and surfaces).
- Protecting patients from other infected patients and hospital staff who may be infected.
- Complying with the practices approved by the infection control committee.
- Obtaining appropriate microbiological specimens when an infection is present or suspected.
- Notifying the infection control team of cases of HAI, and the admission of infected patients.
- Complying with the recommendations of the antimicrobial use committee regarding antibiotic use.
- Advising patients, visitors, and staff on techniques to prevent the transmission of infection.
- Instituting appropriate treatment for any infections that they have.
- Taking steps to prevent such infections in staff from being transmitted to other persons, especially patients.

In a malpractice lawsuit with allegation of harm suffered as a result of HAI, the complainant may be required to prove that a reasonable healthcare provider/hospital would have foreseen the likelihood of such harm in the absence of certain steps necessary to prevent the infection, and that the healthcare provider/hospital failed to foresee the impending harm, and take the preventive steps.[33] Healthcare providers and hospitals will be held liable for failing to implement adequate infection control measures where such a failure resulted in harm to the patient. The evaluation for negligent conduct in this context is measured against the behavior of a reasonably competent healthcare provider/hospital in a similar position.[34]

An intentional failure to implement adequate infection control measures may indicate that the hospital or hospital managers concerned had either "actual" or "eventual" intention not to implement such measures (e.g., infection control measures are minimized to save costs). In cases where "actual" or "direct" intention is present, the wrongdoers decide not to provide certain infection control measures and know that this is wrong.[35] On the other side, in cases where "eventual" intention is present, the wrongdoers subjectively foresee the likelihood of harm to patients if adequate infection control measures are not implemented and do not care whether or not such harm occurs, i.e., they act with reckless disregard for the consequences of such failure.[36]

All Healthcare-associated Infections are not Preventable!

While fixing the liability for HAIs, it must be recognized that all HAIs are not preventable. There are several predisposing risk factors that may contribute to the occurrence of such infections. It has been observed that certain factors are associated with either an increased risk of colonization or with decreased host defense, which could be divided as risk factors related to: (a) Underlying health condition (e.g., age, smoking habits, and diabetes), (b) The disease process, and (c) Invasive procedure or specific modality used during the treatment.

A study reported that in critically ill patient population, 97% of urinary tract infections are due to catheterization, 87% of cases of BSI of a central line and 83% of cases of pneumonia are associated with mechanical ventilation.[37] The devices have been regarded as important factors in predisposing HAIs. Individuals with weakened immune systems and those expecting a longer stay in any hospital or medical treatment facility are at greater risk of contracting HAI. Hospitals and healthcare providers owe a duty of care to their patients to provide a clean and infection-free environment. Similarly, patients also owe a duty to comply with all medical instructions both during hospital stay and afterwards. In a malpractice lawsuit, a patient may be held responsible for contributory negligence, if the patient did not comply with the medical instructions, resulting in harm related to HAI. For example, if a patient failed to receive recommended follow-up treatment to change wound dressings, or did not take recommended antibiotic medications, a court may determine that the patient is entitled to reduce quantum of compensation or even no compensation at all.

In a case of lawsuit alleging medical negligence on the part of medical practitioner as a result of hospital-acquired infection, following key issues related to the appropriate use of antibiotics may be considered by the court:
- Failure to prescribe the indicated antibiotics.
- Failure to adequately screen for sensitivity or properly monitor antibiotics use.
- Prescribing antibiotics that are clinically contraindicated.
- Inappropriate use of antibiotics for surgical prophylaxis.
- The subtherapeutic use of antibiotics.

To establish a case of negligence against hospital by the patient who acquired an infection during the hospital stay, he/she may be required to prove in a court of law that:
- The hospital breached its duty toward the patient, and did not follow a policy or procedure to prevent the infection.
- The hospital's negligence or deficiency in service caused infection resulting in harm to the patient.

MEDICAL NEGLIGENCE CASES RELATED TO HEALTHCARE-ASSOCIATED INFECTION

Case 1: Patient Suffered Hepatitis C Infection[38]

A recent medical negligence case raised a number of issues related to hospital-acquired infection.

Facts of the Case

The patient was operated for vaginal hysterectomy. After surgery, the patient made an uneventful recovery and was discharged. Though 2 units of blood were reserved for her, no transfusion had been necessary. A month later, the patient developed jaundice. On subsequent investigations, she was tested positive for hepatitis C virus (HCV).

Complainant's Allegation

The patient filed a complaint in the Consumer Forum claiming that, she had acquired the infection during her hospital stay on account of the negligence of the doctors and hospital. Irreparable and grave harm had been caused to her by this negligence resulting in an incurable disease. A sum of ₹ 25 lakhs was claimed as compensation. The following allegations were made by the complainant:
- She was thoroughly investigated preoperatively and had been certified free from HCV.
- Two physicians had clearly told her that HCV could only have been contracted during surgery or in the subsequent hospital stay.
- She had never received any blood transfusion in the past. The only reason, she contracted HCV was due to use of contaminated instruments, syringes, etc., while in hospital.
- All doctors, nurses, assistants and technicians ought to be periodically screened to ensure that they were free of all viruses and infections which they could transmit to the patients whom they dealt with. There is no evidence that the hospital had any such system in place.

Doctor's Defense

The surgeon contended that the surgery had been uneventful, and no blood transfusion had been necessary. Her surgery was done under complete aseptic precautions, and disposable equipment including gloves, syringes, etc., were used. Instruments had been sterilized as per standard hospital protocol and no unsterile instrument was used. The surgeon submitted his own HCV report, which was negative.

Court's Judgment

- The District consumer forum ordered the hospital, five doctors and two pathologists to pay a compensation of around ₹ 6 lakhs after finding them guilty of medical negligence.
- The forum held that the possibility cannot be ignored that there was use of unsterilized equipment, needles or machinery at the time of surgery.
- The forum said, "While conducting blood and urine tests, the doctors ought to have checked if she was suffering from Hepatitis C. But such care and caution was not taken by the opposite parties (hospital and doctors) and she was operated without properly examining and conducting the Hepatitis C test."

Case 2: Patients Lost Vision due to Eye Infection[39]

Facts of the Case
- In two writ petitions under Article 226 of the Constitution, the petitioners alleged that their eyes which were operated upon were damaged due to infection at the Dr BR Ambedkar Memorial Hospital in West Tripura.
- In first civil writ, two petitioners were admitted in the hospital on 17.6.1996 and their left eyes were operated on 18.6.1996 and they were discharged from the hospital on 21.6.1996.
- In second civil writ, the petitioner no. 1 was admitted in the hospital on 18.6.1996 and his left eye was operated on 19.6.1996 and he was discharged on 21.6.1996. Petitioner no. 2 was admitted on 11.6.1996 and her left eye was operated on 12.6.1996 and she was discharged on 24.6.1996. Petitioner no. 3 was admitted on 12.6.1996, her left eye was operated on 13.6.1996 and she was discharged on 26.6.1996.

Patient's Allegation
- The petitioners alleged that their eyes were damaged due to infection at the hospital and the infection in eyes was due to sheer negligence of the Medical Officers of the hospital.
- The petitioners prayed for compensation for the damage caused to their eyes. They claimed compensation of ₹ 2 lakhs each for violation of their fundamental right to life guaranteed under Article 21 of the Constitution of India.

Doctor's Defense
- The patients came to the hospital with their left eyes completely blind and the doctors of the hospital successfully removed the cataract but because of subsequent developments, the petitioners were unable to get back their vision.
- Mr. Saha, senior Govt. Advocate, referred to a publication of the MOHFW, Delhi on hospital-acquired infections and submitted that postoperative infection is worldwide problem. He further submitted that at the time when the petitioners were discharged from the hospital, there was no infection in their eyes and it is quite possible that infection in their eyes took place after they were discharged. Thus, the court cannot record a definite finding that the infection in the eyes of the petitioners was due to negligence on the part of the doctors who conducted the operation.

Inquiry by the Government
- The Government of Tripura constituted a committee and investigated into the causes of infection. The committee visited the hospital on 26.6.1996 and enquired into the matter, examined available records, collected samples and specimen from the O.T. and other steps for microbiological examination and submitted a report dated 3.7.1996. The report issued by the said committee showed that the infection was caused to the eyes of the different patients due to lapse on the part of the authorities.
- The Government constituted another committee which also enquired into the causes of the eye infection of different patients. The committee submitted a report on 25.7.1996, which stated that the infection was a result of contamination in the operation theater. The committee was of the opinion that, "the patients were infected initially around incision and stitch line and the said initial infection progressed to severe intraocular infections. These unfortunate cases were the result of an exogenous infection presumably as a result of some contamination in the operation theatre. The microbiological studies revealed mixed type of infection from bacteria and fungus and the organism were isolated from different

areas of the operation theatre including the floor, overhead lights, walls etc. One of the organisms isolated from the O.T. was also found to be the causative organisms in some patients."

Court's Judgment

- The contention of the State respondents that all the petitioners came to the hospital completely blind cannot be accepted. Cataract in the eyes does not completely blind the eye but only affects the vision of the eye. Further had the cataract operation been successful, the visions in the left eyes could have been restored to a large extent. Instead of the vision of the petitioners being restored in their left eyes, they have lost their left eye completely on account of the infection in the hospital.
- The contention of the State respondents that the infection in the eyes of the petitioners may not have taken place at the hospital has been negatived by the findings of the expert committee constituted by the Government of Tripura. It is clear from the findings recorded by the two expert committees that eyes of the petitioners suffered infection at the Dr BR Ambedkar Hospital where they were operated upon.
- The findings of the two expert committees discussed above clearly indicate that the infection in the eyes suffered by the petitioners were on account of negligence on the face of it.
- The claim of the petitioners to compensation for such damage to their eyes cannot be thrown out by the Court on the ground that such hospital-acquired infection is a worldwide phenomenon and do take place. The petitioners are entitled to compensation for breach of their fundamental right to life under Article 21 of the Constitution from the State Government of Tripura.
- The writ petitions were allowed and respondent nos. 1 and 2 were directed to pay a compensation of ₹60,000 and in addition cost of ₹2000 for the litigation to each of the petitioners in the two writ petitions

■ LEGAL PROVISIONS APPLICABLE TO HEALTHCARE-ASSOCIATED INFECTION

Many countries like UK, US, and Germany have specific legislations and protocols related to HAI which is considered to be in the domain of public health legislation. No such legislation exists in India. Several provisions of The Indian Penal Code which could be applicable in case of HAIs are as given below.[40]

Section 304A IPC (Causing Death by Negligence)

Whoever causes the death of any person by doing any rash or negligent act not amounting to culpable homicide, shall be punished with imprisonment of either description for a term which may extend to 2 years, or with fine, or with both. In case of death due to hospital-acquired infection, Section 304 A IPC could be invoked.

Section 337 IPC (Causing Hurt by Act Endangering Life or Personal Safety of Others)

Whoever causes hurt to any person by doing any act so rashly or negligently as to endanger human life, or the personal safety of others, shall be punished with imprisonment of either description for a term which may extend to 6 months, or with fine which may extend to ₹500, or with both. In case of morbidity due to hospital-acquired infection, the complainant may invoke Section 337 IPC.

Section 338 IPC (Causing Grievous Hurt by Act Endangering Life or Personal Safety of Others)

Whoever causes grievous hurt to any person by doing any act so rashly or negligently as to endanger human life, or the personal safety of others, shall be punished with imprisonment of either description for a term which may extend to 2 years, or with fine which may extend to ₹1,000, or with both. In case of morbidity due to hospital-acquired infection, the complainant may invoke Section 337 IPC.

Section 269 IPC (Negligent Act Likely to Spread Infection of Disease Dangerous to Life)

Whoever unlawfully or negligently does any act which is, and which he knows or has reason to believe to be, likely to spread the infection of any disease dangerous to life, shall be punished with imprisonment of either description for a term which may extend to 6 months, or with fine, or with both.

Section 270 IPC (Malignant Act Likely to Spread Infection of Disease Dangerous to Life)

Whoever malignantly does any act which is, and which he knows or has reason to believe to be, likely to spread the infection of any disease dangerous to life, shall be punished with imprisonment of either description for a term which may extend to 2 years, or with fine, or with both.

■ CONCLUSION

Healthcare providers owe a legal duty of care to their patients. They must exercise the degree of care and skill that could reasonably be expected of a normal and prudent practitioner, and they also have an ethical obligation to act in the best interest of patients. On the similar pattern, the healthcare organizations should also provide a safe environment for the patients so as to prevent them from harm in the course of receiving care. The organizations have a dual duty of setting up of standard protocols for improving patient safety, and then, ensuring that the healthcare staff complies with systems, protocols, policies, and procedures.

The healthcare organizations should have standard updated well-documented protocols for prevention of infection according to the recent evidence of disease virulence, transmission routes, and key control methods. There are many guidelines and recommendations for prevention of infection, and failure to meet those indicates a failure in appropriate standard of care. Even the court of law looks for guidelines and then compares whether those have been followed or not. Proper communication of the lawsuit summaries to the healthcare providers can help the Infection Control Committee in enhancing patient safety and prevention of HAI. If a patient has been harmed or exposed to risk of harm, providers have a duty to disclose that information to the patient or family. When errors have occurred, or when some risk of harm exists, there must be hospital policies available to guide disclosure of patient identifiable health information to regulatory authorities, accrediting bodies, or other government agencies. Greater awareness needs to be created so as to highlight the potential legal implications of HAI.

REFERENCES

1. Consumer Reports. Special Report. America's Antibiotic Crisis. [online] Available from https://www.consumerreports.org/cro/health/hospital-acquired-infections/index.htm. [Last accessed August, 2019].
2. Burke JP. Infection control - a problem for patient safety. N Engl J Med. 2003;348(7):651-6.
3. Stone PW, Larson E, Kawar LN. A systematic audit of economic evidence linking nosocomial infections and infection control interventions: 1990-2000. Am J Infect Control. 2002;30(3):145-52.
4. Weigelt JA, Dryer D, Haley RW. The necessity and efficiency of wound surveillance after discharge. Arch Surg. 1992;127(1):77-82.
5. Sands K, Vineyard G, Platt R. Surgical site infections occurring after hospital discharge. J Infect Dis. 1996;173(4):963-70.
6. World Health Organization. Healthcare-Associated Infections: Fact Sheet. 2014. [online] Available from http://www.who.int/gpsc/country_work/gpsc_ccisc_fact_sheet_en.pdf. [Last accessed August, 2019].
7. Allegranzi B, Pittet D. Healthcare-associated infection in developing countries: simple solutions to meet complex challenges. Infect Control Hosp Epidemiol. 2007;28(12):1323-7.
8. PICNet Surveillance Protocol for Clostridium Difficile Infection (CDI) in BC Acute Care Facilities. 2014. [online] Available from https://www.picnet.ca/wp-content/uploads/PICNet-surveillance-protocol-for-CDI-2014.pdf. [Last accessed August, 2019].
9. CDC/NHSN Surveillance Definition of Healthcare Associated Infection and Criteria for Specific Types of Infections in the Acute Care Setting. 2013. [online] Available from http://www.socinorte.com/wp-content/uploads/2013/03/Criterios-de-IN-2013.pdf. [Last accessed August, 2019].
10. Kohn LT, Corrigan JM, Donaldson MS; Institute of Medicine (US) Committee on Quality of Health Care in America. To Err is Human: Building a Safer Health System. Washington (DC): National Academy Press; 2000.
11. Ducel G, Fabry J, Nicolle L. Prevention of Hospital-acquired Infections: A Practical Guide, 2nd edition. World Health Organization; 2002.
12. Chugh TD. Hospital Infection Control - Are We Serious? Medical Update 2012. [Online] Available from http://www.apiindia.org/pdf/medicine_update_2012/infectious_disease_14.pdf. [Last accessed Aug., 2019].
13. Rosenthal VD, Maki DG, Salomao R, et al. Device-associated nosocomial infections in 55 intensive care units of 8 developing countries. Ann Intern Med. 2006;145(8):582-91.
14. Ramana BV, Chaudhury A. Device associated nosocomial infections and patterns of antimicrobial resistance at a tertiary care hospital. J NTR Univ Health Sci. 2012;1(2):86-9.
15. Sood S, Joad SH, Yaduvanshi D, et al. Device associated nosocomial infections in a medical intensive care unit of a tertiary care hospital in Jaipur, India. BMC Proc. 2011;5(Suppl 6):O16.
16. Datta P, Rani H, Chauhan R, et al. Device-associated nosocomial infection in the intensive care units of a tertiary care hospital in northern India. J Hosp Infect. 2010;76(2):184-5.
17. Shalini S, Kranthi K, Bhat KG. The microbiological profile of nosocomial infections in the intensive care unit. J Clin Diagn Res. 2010;4(5):3109-12.
18. Kamat US, Ferreira AM, Savio R, et al. Antimicrobial resistance among nosocomial isolates in a teaching hospital in Goa. Indian J Community Med. 2008;33(2):89-92.
19. Habibi S, Wig N, Agarwal S, et al. Epidemiology of nosocomial infections in medicine intensive care unit at a tertiary care hospital in northern India. Trop Doct. 2008;38(4):233-5.
20. Mehta A, Rosenthal VD, Mehta Y, et al. Device-associated nosocomial infection rates in intensive care units of seven Indian cities. Findings of the International Nosocomial Infection Control Consortium (INICC). J Hosp Infect. 2007;67(2):168-74.
21. Ostendorf U, Ewig S, Torres A. Nosocomial pneumonia. Curr Opin Infect Dis. 2006;19(4):327-38.
22. Cisneros-Herreros JM, Garnacho-Montero J, Pachón-Ibáñez ME. Nosocomial pneumonia due to Acinetobacter baumannii. Enferm Infecc Microbiol Clin. 2005;23(Suppl 3):46-51.
23. Flanders SA, Collard HR, Saint S. Nosocomial pneumonia: state of the science. Am J Infect Control. 2006;34(2):84-93.
24. The Joint Commission (TJC). National Patient Safety Goals. [online] Available from https://www.jointcommission.org/standards_information/npsgs.aspx. [Last accessed August, 2019].
25. Vriens MR, Fluit AC, Troelstra A, et al. Is methicillin-resistant Staphylococcus aureus more contagious than methicillin-susceptible S. aureus in a surgical intensive care unit? Infect Control Hosp Epidemiol. 2002;23(9):491-4.
26. Gemmell CG, Edwards DI, Fraise AP, et al.; Joint Working Party of the British Society for Joint Working Party of the British Society for Antimicrobial Chemotherapy, Hospital Infection Society and Infection Control Nurses Association. Guidelines for the prophylaxis and treatment of methicillin-resistant Staphylococcus aureus (MRSA) infections in the UK. J Antimicrob Chemother. 2006;57(4):589-608.
27. Blais R, Champagne F, Rousseau L. TOCSIN: A proposed dashboard of indicators to control healthcare-associated infections. Healthc Q. 2009;12:161-7.
28. Chastre J, Fagon JY, Trouillet JL. Diagnosis and treatment of nosocomial pneumonia in patients in intensive care units. Clin Infect Dis. 1995;21(Suppl 3):S226-37.

29. Glauser M, Boogaerts M, Cordonnier C, et al. Empiric therapy of bacterial infections in severe neutropenia. Clin Microbiol Infect. 1997;3(Suppl 1):S77-86.
30. Zoutman D, Shannon M, Mandel A. Effectiveness of a novel ozone-based system for the rapid high-level disinfection of health care spaces and surfaces. Am J Infect Control. 2011;39(10):873-9.
31. Varrone JJ, Li D, Daiss JL, et al. Anti-glucosaminidase monoclonal antibodies as a passive immunization for methicillin-resistant staphylococcus aureus (MRSA) orthopaedic infections. Bonekey Osteovision. 2011;8:187-94.
32. Improving Infection Prevention and Control at the Health Facility. World Health Organization; 2018. [online] Available from https://www.who.int/infection-prevention/tools/core-components/facility-manual.pdf. [Last accessed August, 2019].
33. Carstens P, Pearman D. Foundational Principles of South African Medical Law. Durban: Butterworths Lexis Nexis; 2007. p. 816.
34. McQuoid-Mason D, Mahomed D. A-Z of Medical Law. Cape Town: Juta Legal and Academic Publishers; 2011. pp. 223-4.
35. McQuoid-Mason D, Mahomed D. A-Z of Medical Law. Cape Town: Juta Legal and Academic Publishers; 2011. p. 242.
36. McQuoid-Mason D, Mahomed D. A-Z of Medical Law. Cape Town: Juta Legal and Academic Publishers; 2011. p. 276.
37. Richards MJ, Edwards JR, Culver DH, et al. Nosocomial infections in combined medical-surgical intensive care units in the United States. Infect Control Hosp Epidemiol. 2000;21(8):510-5.
38. South Bombay Hospital, 7 Doctors told to Pay Rs. 6 Lakh to Woman Who got Hepatitis C after Hysterectomy. [online] Available from https://timesofindia.indiatimes.com/city/mumbai/sobo-hosp-7-docs-told-to-pay-rs-6l-to-woman-who-got-hepatitis-c-after-hysterectomy/articleshow/69191871.cms. [Last accessed August, 2019].
39. Haripada Saha and Anr. vs State of Tripura and Ors, 2002 ACJ 1877.
40. Indian Penal Code – Act XLV of 1860.

CHAPTER 9

Communication Skills in Healthcare: A Tool to Ensure Patient Satisfaction

Archana Kumari, Piyush Ranjan

"The most basic of all human needs is the need to understand and be understood. The best way to understand people is to listen to them."
— **Ralph Nichols**

■ INTRODUCTION

Good communication is essential for holistic and effective management of the patients. The patient-centric communication leads to improved compliance and overall patient satisfaction. A good patient-physician relationship has the ability to better understand the patients' perceptions, need, and outcome expectations. It also helps the patients to feel comfortable in sharing relevant personal information which supports the doctors in making appropriate diagnosis and deciding patient-oriented course of treatment. The patients' involvement in the course of treatments further helps in better compliance of the advice, and routine follow-up which in turn, enhances the chances of recovery. These satisfied patients provide job satisfaction for the doctors. Thus, empathetic and effective communication makes the fundamental for successful outcome of the treatment.

In India, medical malpractice litigation against the doctors is increasing, both in number as well as in quantum. Major contributors to the rising claims include increasing awareness of patients toward their rights, patient-centered legal practice, and diminishing professionalism in medical practice. The lawsuit against practicing doctors is majorly on the basis of delayed medical action, negligence with respect to consultation, treatment or drug administration, breached confidentiality and dishonor consent.[1] Often, these situations arise due to miscommunication between doctors and patients or their attendants and the consequences are suffered by both. There are reported acts of violence against doctors, especially in emergency situations. A study from Israel states that 70% doctors and almost 90% supporting staff working in emergency have faced verbal abuse.[2] Post-traumatic stress of these episodes faced by the doctors lead to depression- and anxiety-related work absenteeism, and has a negative impact on physician's family and quality of life.[3] Despite serious emotional and legal repercussions, there is a lack of proper training essential for improving the effective communication skills of healthcare practitioners.

WHAT IS COMMUNICATION

The word communication has been derived from the Latin word *"communis"* which means "to share." Communication may be defined as sharing information and ideas so as to create mutual understanding between the sender and receiver of the information. Communication is a process of sending information via speech, visuals, writing, or any other such method. The communication model includes a sender, who sends the message; encoding of a message; selecting a channel of communication; and the receiver, who receives the message. Decoding is the receiver's interpretation of the sender's message. Here the receiver converts the message into thoughts and tries to analyze and understand it. Sometimes, the receiver will send a message back to the original sender, which is called feedback (**Fig. 1**).

The speech or ideas need to be simple enough to be decoded and understood by the receiver. If the ideas are not presented properly, then decoding is improper and the receiver does not understand. Effective communication is successful delivery of messages from the sender to receiver through a proper communication channel. Communication skill is the competence required for delivery of the message clearly and unambiguously. These skills also involve active listening as an important component to receive the message that others are sending. The content of the messages delivered should be clear, concise, correct, and complete. These messages should be supported with the appropriate body language and tone of message delivery, which depicts the emotional aspect of the communication.[4] Thus, the component channel as well as context of the message is important for effective communication.

Types of Communication

There are three basic types of communication:
1. Verbal Communication
2. Nonverbal Communication, and
3. Paraverbal Communication.

The verbal component constitutes the oral or written communication with appropriate word selection. The nonverbal component includes physical appearance, body language, posture, gesture, and spatial distance. Paraverbal components refer to the tone, pitch,

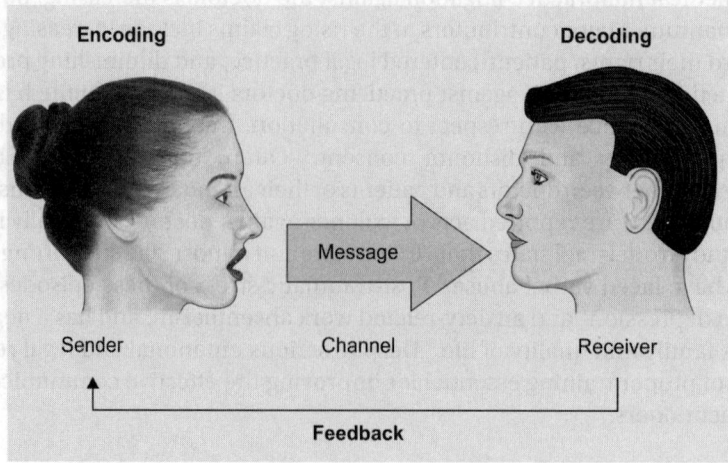

FIG. 1: The basic communication model.

strength, and volume of the voice. During communication, 20% information is communicated through verbal method.[5] The nonverbal and paraverbal components majorly contribute to total message delivery. Despite being important in the delivery and perception of the messages these components are frequently neglected in effective communication.

■ COMMUNICATION IN HEALTHCARE

In healthcare setting, the communication is much more than conveying information. It involves giving and receiving messages which may contain not only facts but opinions, and emotions too. Effective communication in a healthcare setting is one of the most important tools for improving patient satisfaction as well as patient safety. How well a patient understands the information provided by healthcare professionals, have an influence on healthcare decisions that might be taken in future. Effective communication is described to occur when the sender of a message sends the message in such a way that conveys the intent of the message, and the same is understood by the receiver of the message. As a result of the communication from both the sender and the receiver of the message, a shared meaning is created between both the parties.

Importance of Communication Skills for Doctors

A good communication is integral in medical practice to establish a trustworthy patient-doctor relationship, as it enhances the patient's capability to follow recommendations, self-management of chronic conditions, and initiate preventive health behaviors. Effective communication increases the chances of positive treatment outcome and patient satisfaction. A structured communication improves the following aspects of healthcare delivery.

Improvement in Diagnostic Accuracy

While history taking, attentive listening helps the patient to share complete personal information regarding the disease, helping the practitioner to make a better judgment. Studies report that frequent interruption in interview by the doctor may be detrimental to collecting essential information and establishing meaningful relationship.

Compliance with Medical Advice

Low compliance with the treatment has been a major concern for doctors and hospital administration due to increasing healthcare burden, especially in terms of cost. The various reasons for nonadherence to the recommendations are disagreement with doctor due to cost of treatment, personal beliefs, and compliance barriers. The doctors with empathetic attitude, ability to extract and respect patients concerns, and recommending patient-centric treatment are key elements in establishing trustworthy doctor-patient relationships leading to better compliance.

Improved Functional and Emotional Status

Better communication skill while interviewing and discussing the management plan reduces the emotional distress in the patients and leads to better health outcome. Studies characterized physician's interaction styles as person-focused, biopsychosocial, biomedical, and high physician control. Physician's practicing patient focused interactions reported highest quality of care and high physician control was reported the lowest.

Improved Patient Satisfaction

The goal of effective communication is to understand the patient's perception of the disease and treatment related expectations. An effective interaction where the patient is involved in the decision making regarding the course of the treatment and continuity of care enhances patient's satisfaction.

Improved Clinician Satisfaction

The healthcare practitioners with professional life satisfaction are associated with greater patient trust. These doctors may better address patient's concerns establishing a good patient-doctor relationship which in turn increases both patient and clinician's satisfaction. This also helps in reduction of work-related stress.

■ BASIC PRINCIPLES OF GOOD COMMUNICATION

The effective delivery of the message from the sender to receiver is based on three components of communication, i.e., content, process, and context. The content refers to verbal aspects which includes written and oral words. The process refers to nonverbal clues, i.e., body language, tone, eye contact, etc., depicting the way in which the message was delivered, whereas the context refers to situation or environment in which the message was delivered. In consistent messages, the words, tone of voice, and body language all convey the same meaning.

■ TIPS FOR GOOD COMMUNICATION IN OPD SETTING

The medical interview in OPD settings is an opportunity for the doctors to understand the patient's condition and its impact on their functional and mental capacity. This is especially important in cases with chronic illness, where good communication skill is required in allaying anxiety and motivating the patient for good compliance regarding advices. Remember, simply writing a prescription has got no value and is actually wastage of time and energy unless and until adequately honored by patients. The doctor should provide information on what the patient wants to know. A continuous follow-up should be done to check the patient's adherence to the given advice. Detailed discussions should be done regarding nature, course, treatment options, necessity of investigations, and prognosis (both short term and long term) of the disease. Special emphasis should be made on motivating patients regarding sticking to lifestyle modifications. The patient should always be discussed in detail regarding necessity and feasibility of costly investigations and drugs and their effect on main course and outcome of disease.

The Medical Interview with Patient

Prior to the Start of Medical Interview

- Respect the patient's confidentiality and maintain privacy. Do not ask the patient for the reason of his/her visit, if other people are present in the room.
- Be the first one to greet the patient. Do not wait for the patient to start the conversation, as some patients may interpret your silence as indifference. Introduce yourself; shake hands wherever feasible and socially acceptable.
- Address a patient by his/her name whenever required. Do not fumble for name after the patient is in the room.

- Establish eye contact and maintain it at reasonable intervals.
- Try to put the patient at ease. Begin with a general nonmedical conversation in order to develop a comfortable situation for the patient.

Conducting the Medical Interview

Listen Actively

A reliable and complete medical information can be obtained through an active process of listening, observing, and facilitating. During the medical interview with a patient, give full attention to verbal and non-verbal clues from the patient. At the same time, be watchful about your own nonverbal clues like body language, gestures, and eye-contact.

Stay Attuned to Questioning Style

The questions to be asked during the medical interview should evolve from what the patient says, and not just following the predetermined plan. If patient's response is not clear, then restate the question and ask for clarification and this reaffirms to the patient the provider's commitment to understand. Try to comprehend details in simple language. The use of medical jargons and abbreviations can confuse the patient.

Involve the Patient in the Decision Making

Promptly respond to the patient's queries, and provide all necessary information that the patient wants to know. Discuss nature, course, and prognosis of the disease and necessity of investigations. Discuss the treatment options available and effect of the proposed treatment on the main course and outcome of disease.

Offer Empathy

Providing empathy can improve patient satisfaction and compliance to the treatment. The doctor should show empathy by demonstrating a sincere concern toward the patient's pain and distress. An empathic statement would be: "I can see how tough it has been for you to manage with the disease."

■ TIPS FOR GOOD COMMUNICATION IN AN INDOOR AND ICU SETTING

Effective communication between doctors and patients, and their attendants is the key driver for the success of the healthcare system, especially in critical care setting. These are certain tips that will definitely improve one's ability to communicate.

Communicating with the Attendants

Good communication with the attendants assumes great importance especially when patient is critically ill or admitted in ICU. Attendants are apprehensive, and at times have many doubts and queries to be taken care of.
- Never be informal with the attendants. Conduct daily conferences and if possible, twice daily.
- Talk about and appreciate the efforts made by them.
- Most of the attendants have lot of information from unreliable sources. Try to satisfy their queries by giving better references.
- Always explain the dynamic nature of disease. This is especially important in ICU patients.

- Second opinion should be sought proactively. This is important not only in patient management, when one is in doubt, but also helpful in patient's confidence building measure. One will be more convinced and ready to accept bad outcome if the same fact is explained by more than one consultant.
- Never express shock. Always give an impression that situation is under control or will be controlled.
- Never talk low about your colleagues. Be cautious while asking questions with postgraduate medical students on rounds. The absence of senior consultants may make patients feel insecure and creates doubts in their minds regarding the course of the treatment.
- Consent taking is very important part of counseling. Unfortunately, this is neglected, and this important task is delegated to paramedical staff or interns who fail to explain fully and thus doubt sets in mind of attendants while putting signature or give anything in writing. Do not delegate the responsibility to junior staff. Do not downplay procedural risk and never ignore unrealistic expectations. A senior doctor treating the patient must be involved in the final discussion and documentation of the informed consent process. Staff members can provide patient education and can provide the attending doctor with insight into the patient's expectations and level of understanding. However, the ultimate responsibility for verifying informed consent rests with the senior doctor, who is member of the treating team.

Example: A 65-year-old male patient was admitted in ICU. He was a chronic smoker, known case of diabetes mellitus with nephropathy. He was currently admitted for investigation and management of fever and breathlessness. He was diagnosed as a case of pneumonia. The patient did not respond to antibiotic treatment, and subsequently developed ARDS and had to be put on ventilator support. Even after energetic management, the oxygen saturation was not improving. Anticipating the worse outcome, consultant called attendants for communicating the prognosis.

Resident Doctor: "Gentleman, your patient is suffering from very serious condition of lungs. Even in the best setup, the mortality is around 70%. That too when your father smoked a lot, had diabetes with complications and is old enough, there is very little hope and only God knows how long will he be able to survive." (The resident was technically correct).

Son: "I know my father is old and every young man's father must be of same age. He had diabetes and was smoker; that's why we have come to hospital. If only God knows everything then what are you doing?" (The young son showed his emotional outburst).

The resident doctor who has worked really hard all through the night found it hard to accept these words as the reward for his services. The old man died of his illness within 48 hours and the son strongly felt that his father could have been saved if he had taken him to better doctor and abused the doctor in frustration. The doctor was shocked by the attendant's behavior, and it took 1 week for him to get back to normal. The young son developed sense of guilt and still finds it hard to cope with it even after 2 years of the incident.

A better way of explaining the prognosis could have been:
Resident Doctor: "I know and understand........ it is really a tough time for any son whose father is so seriously ill. His chest condition is not responding to the best suitable antibiotics and even after putting him on ventilator we are not getting the desired results."

"You have done a lot for your father and your father is really lucky to get a son like you. Even if the chances are less, we will fight till last breath."

"One who has taken birth has to go some day and every one of us has to meet the same fate sooner or later. God is there and everything is under his control. Pray to him and I can assure you that all of the hospital staffs will keep on putting our best efforts till his last breath."

Son: "Dear Doctor, you are second God. Keep on trying. God will help all of us." Patient's attendant said.

The old man died within 48 hours. His son accepted God's decision as his fate. After the lapse of 2 years, the doctor has forgotten him but the son still remembers that doctor as one who has tried hard to cure his father. They exchange greetings whenever they meet.

■ BARRIERS TO COMMUNICATION

Lack of effective communication has a negative impact on patient-doctor relationship. Both, patient and practitioner can pose barriers to effective communication. Sometimes the clinical set-up might provide challenging conditions for private and confidential exchange of information between patient and practitioner. The key barriers to ineffective conversation are:

- *Lack of training in communication skills:* In India, communication skills as a part of medical curriculum is generally neglected and rarely assessed in medical schools.
- *Non-disclosure of information:* Patients feel neglected in decision-making process, if there is nondisclosure of information regarding different aspects of purpose of treatment, course of treatment, duration, and outcome of treatment. A proper communication might affect patient's choices regarding disease condition and treatment opted.[6]
- *Patient burden:* In India, often, doctors have to treat large number of patients, with more attention to serious patients. Giving less time for building a warm doctor-patient relationship and avoiding to discuss emotional and social impact of patient's situation leads to distress and distrust.
- *Discouragement of collaboration:* Doctor's attitude toward the patients discourages them to voice out their needs, expectations, and confusion regarding the medical condition and course of treatment. Thus, lack of consensus might lead to therapeutic failure.[7]
- *Difficult patients:* Difficult patients are patients with certain behavior issues and can be categorized as argumentative, manipulative, depressed or dependent, etc. Patients of different cultural and ethnic origin or language are also difficult to handle.[5]

■ CONSEQUENCES OF INEFFECTIVE COMMUNICATION

Ineffective communication can have serious consequences in providing optimum care to the patients. Communication is the key to address patient's needs at multiple levels. Clear communication between different healthcare providers in the hospital is essential in successfully treating the patients. Ineffective communications have direct and detrimental impact on various patient related outcomes. The consequences of ineffective communication can be:

- *Medical errors:* Ineffective communication resulting in incorrect or incomplete medical records of patients is one of the most common reasons for medical errors. These errors have potential to cause adverse medical events.
- *Conflict:* The workplace conflict between fellow doctors and other healthcare practitioners can be due to misunderstandings, which originates from lack of communication. The lack of information provided to attendants about their patient's status may also lead to distrust amongst the attendants.

- *Poor decision making:* Lack of patient-doctor communication might lead to poor decision making. Decision making is a process of accurately understanding the problem, searching for possible solutions and determining their impact on outcome. Incomplete information at any stage might lead to wrong medical decisions.
- *Work-related stress:* Ineffective communication increases the work-related stress due to lack of anticipation of outcomes. Poor coordination between various departments, delayed results and tedious paperwork are some of the reasons for work related stress.

■ HOW TO ASSESS THE COMMUNICATION SKILLS OF HEALTHCARE WORKERS?

The doctor-patient communication is integral for the development of patient-doctor relationship. A proper assessment of the doctor's communication skills is essential for enhancing competence leading to better patient satisfaction and health outcome. There are different approaches for assessment of these communication skills. The two broad categories of assessment are survey and observation method with the help of standard clinical observation, audio or video. Questionnaire-based surveys can be easily administered and addressed. The qualitative method through recordings is tedious but helps in providing an insight into the specific nonverbal and paraverbal characteristics of patient and doctor communication.

The Accreditation Council for Graduate Medical Research (ACGME) has identified written examination, global rating, multisource feedback, and procedure case logs for the assessment of communication skills.[8] In a multicenter study in China, multisource feedback was used to assess the professionalism and communication of the residents. The results concluded that MSF is an internally valid and reliable tool for assessing the interpersonal communication skills of the resident.[9] In another study, a modified version of the American Board of Internal Medicine's (ABIM) patient assessment survey was used for self-assessment of residents in surgical and nonsurgical training. The study indicated that the tool was both internally consistent and reliable.[10] A family medicine residency program, utilized Communication Assessment Tool (CAT), developed by Makoul et al. to assess patient's perceptions about physician's interpersonal and communication skills.[11]

■ BREAKING BAD NEWS

Bad news can be defined as the information that drastically and negatively affects the patient's idea of their future.[12] Conveying the news involves communication of the actual news as well as tackling the response of the patient. These responses from patients or their attendants are recipient specific and are highly dependent on their understanding and expectations. Poor communication skills and an inability to deal with emotional outburst of the patient makes breaking the news challenging for the doctors.[6] Several protocols have been devised for this purpose. Still, this essential communication skill is generally learned through trial and error or observation of seniors. These steps can be followed while delivering the news to the patients:
- *Preparation for the interview:* The doctor should mentally rehearse the act of disclosure with probable patient's reactions and techniques of handling these outbursts. The physical settings conducive for the interview should be opted. The factors like maintaining privacy, sitting comfortably, including significant others—maintaining eye-contact and providing enough time for any further queries should be considered while delivering the news.

- *Assessing patient's knowledge and perception:* Doctor should use open-ended questions to understand the perception of the patients about their medical conditions. For example: What have you briefed about your medical condition? Or what is your understanding of the increasing severity of symptoms? This also helps the doctor to assess the patient preparedness for handling the situation which further helps tailoring the information according to the patient.
- *Obtaining patient's invitation for the news*: A majority of patients require full information regarding their disease condition which reduces the anxiety related with revealing the bad news. If the patient does not want the details, offer to answer any questions of the patients or the attendants.
- *Actual breaking of news:* An initial warning prepares the patient for the disclosure of the bad news. The use of nontechnical words, starting at an understanding level of the patient and avoiding excessive bluntness helps in the delivery of the news. The alternative therapeutic goals like management of severity of symptoms, pain control should be brought into perspective.
- *Addressing patient's emotions:* Patients can have variable response to the news ranging from silence to anger or denial. The doctors should have an empathetic response toward the patients by observing patient's emotion, identifying the emotion, assessing the reason for the emotion, and validating the emotions of the patients.
- *Treatment plan and summarize:* It is important to discuss and present the patient with various treatment options available. The patient and their attendants should be involved in the decision-making process guided by the doctors. Summarizing the discussion helps the doctor to emphasize on the further action and assess the understanding at the patient level.

TEACHING COMMUNICATION SKILLS AND MEDICAL CURRICULUM

Communication skill is the backbone of medical practice. The traditional medical teaching imparts the knowledge and practical skills for the treatment of disease but rarely addresses the communication skills which are essential in dealing with the patient.[13] Clinical competence can be enhanced by teaching communication skill and counseling techniques. Medical councils of many countries have incorporated training of communication skills as an integral part of medical teaching program. Medical licensing examinations in USA and UK give due consideration to the assessment of communication skills.[14] In India, ACGME recommends that physicians are required to become effective in communication skills and has laid down certain criteria for the same. Medical Council of India (MCI) in its document "Vision 2015" has emphasized the necessity to enhance the quality and standards of medical education and training.[15]

AETCOM: An Initiative by Medical Council of India

The ethical communication and behavioral skills are seldom given the required importance in the existing medical curriculum. The difficult working conditions like exhaustive working hours, poor work control, administrative responsibilities, and threat of malpractice and lack of work-life balance are major reasons for gradual emotional depletion and reduced professional commitment. The absence of these aspects in the current curriculum does not prepare the graduate to handle these conditions leading to early burnout.[16]

Attitude, ethics, and communication competencies should be an integral part of the medical education imparted to the medical graduates. The MCI took an initiative with a goal to teach correct attitude, communication, and morals to the Indian Medical Graduates as a part of curriculum. The Council has revised and remodeled the Graduate Medical Education Regulations, 1997 with emphasis on curricular reforms. Teaching curricula in various disciplines would be based on a competency-based format with emphasis on domains of attitude, ethics, and communication, as envisaged in the Attitude, Ethics and Communication (AETCOM) module. The MCI has prepared revised Graduate Medical Education Regulations, 2017 and competency-based UG curricula. The MCI has also decided to implement AETCOM in all medical schools across the country. The Council has embarked on an ambitious Faculty Development Program in which medical college teachers are trained to acquire theoretical and practical skills in teaching.

The AETCOM makes affective domain as the heart of teaching module covering emotional values, empathy and development of appreciation leading to betterment in interpersonal and community interaction. The addition of this module throughout MBBS program across medical colleges is a transition into competency-based medical education (CBME). The key elements of the module are knowledge, skill, attitude, and communication which need to be integrated throughout the course. The curriculum includes the foundation of the communication in the first year, bioethics in second year followed by medicolegal issues, ethics, and doctor-patient relationship in the third year (AETCOM). The assessment of competence at the end of year can be assessed through Miller's pyramid model of competence assessment. The pyramid has two components, i.e., (i) cognition assessment with the help of questionnaire, viva-voce and short essay questions and (ii) behavioral practice which can be assessed with the help of objective structured clinical examination and directly observed procedural skills.[17]

■ CONCLUSION

To conclude, good communication skill is a crucial part of medical practice which results in better therapeutic outcome and overall patient and practitioner satisfaction. Difficult patient encounters are not uncommon during practice, which if insufficiently handled could lead to distress as well as malpractice lawsuits. Many doctors find themselves incapable of effectively addressing these challenges which might result in early burnouts. Thus, there is a necessity that communication skills should be taught as a part of medical education to generate practitioners with better clinical competence.

■ REFERENCES

1. Raveesh BN, Nayak RB, Kumbar SF. Preventing medico-legal issues in clinical practice. Ann Indian Acad Neurol. 2016;19(Suppl 1):S15-20.
2. Shafran-Tikva S, Zelker R, Stern Z, et al. Workplace violence in a tertiary care Israeli hospital - a systematic analysis of the types of violence, the perpetrators and hospital departments. ISR J Health Policy Res. 2017;6(1):43.
3. Hobbs FD. Fear of aggression at work among general practitioners who have suffered a previous episode of aggression. Br J Gen Pract. 1994;44(386):390-4.
4. Zeppetella G. Palliative Care in Clinical Practice. Vol. 13. London: Springer-Verlag; 2012. pp. 269.
5. Ranjan P, Kumari A, Chakrawarty A. How can doctors improve their communication skills? J Clin Diagn Res. 2015;9(3):JE01-4.

6. Baile WF, Buckman R, Lenzi R, et al. SPIKES-A six-step protocol for delivering bad news: application to the patient with cancer. Oncologist. 2000;5(4):302-11.
7. Ha JF, Longnecker N. Doctor-patient communication: a review. Ochsner J. 2010;10(1):38-43.
8. Accreditation Council for Graduate Medical Education. Toolbox for the Evaluation of Competence. [online] Available from: http://www.acgme.org. [Last Accessed on August, 2019].
9. Qu B, Zhao YH, Sun BZ. Assessment of resident physicians in professionalism, interpersonal and communication skills: a multisource feedback. Int J Med Sci. 2012;9(3):228-36.
10. Symons AB, Swanson A, McGuigan D, et al. A tool for self-assessment of communication skills and professionalism in residents. BMC Med Educ. 2009;9:1.
11. Myerholtz L, Simons L, Felix S, et al. Using the communication assessment tool in family medicine residency programs. Fam Med. 2010;42(8):567-73.
12. Buckman R. Breaking bad news: why is it still so difficult? Br Med J (Clin Res Ed). 1984;288(6430):1597-9.
13. Choudhary A, Gupta V. Teaching communications skills to medical students: Introducing the fine art of medical practice. Int J Appl Basic Med Res. 2015;5(Suppl 1):S41-4.
14. Duffy FD, Gordon GH, Whelan G, et al.; Participants in the American Academy on Physician and Patient's Conference on Education and Evaluation of Competence in Communication and Interpersonal Skills. Assessing competence in communication and interpersonal skills: the Kalamazoo II report. Acad Med. 2004;79(6):495-507.
15. Medical Council of India. Vision 2015. [online] Available from: https://old.mciindia.org/tools/announcement/MCI_booklet.pdf. [Last Accessed on August, 2019].
16. Bhatia MS, Saha R. Burnout in medical residents: A growing concern. J Postgrad Med. 2018;64(3):136-7.
17. Medical Council of India Regulations on Graduate Medical Education, 1997 (Amended Upto July 2017). [online] Available from: https://www.mciindia.org/documents/rulesAndRegulations/GME_REGULATIONS.pdf. [Last Accessed on August, 2019].

SECTION 4
Medical Records: A Double-edged Sword

Chapter 10 Medicolegal aspects of Informed Consent
Chapter 11 Medicolegal aspects of Medical Records
Chapter 12 Documentation in Healthcare: Standards and Guidelines

CHAPTER 10

Medicolegal Aspects of Informed Consent

VP Singh, Dasari Harish

> *"One cannot know with certainty whether a consent is valid until a lawsuit has been filed and resolved."*
> —The California Supreme Court[1]

■ INTRODUCTION

In the practice of medicine, consent is an essential ingredient for the legitimacy of any treatment offered to the patient. A physician who provides any treatment or performs any surgery/procedure without the patient's consent may be held liable for assault, battery or medical malpractice, depending upon the circumstances. It should be borne in mind that if the doctor cannot prove that he took a valid informed consent of the said patient before examination, investigation or any treatment procedure, etc., it will amount to trespass/assault and make him liable for civil/criminal charges. Consent should be taken directly from the person on whom any medical procedure is contemplated, provided the said person is capable of giving a legally valid consent. The principle of informed consent is based on recognition of the right and responsibility of every competent person, to exercise freely and voluntarily, his/her right to autonomy. It is based on the Latin maxim – "volenti non fit injuria" – he who consents cannot complain.[2]

Consent may be defined as the permission of the patient to undergo a particular treatment/investigative procedure after being adequately informed about the purpose, nature, benefits and risks of the said procedure, as well as any alternative available. It enables the patients to make decisions about the course of their medical care on the basis of information provided to them during the process of informed consent. The basic concept behind informed consent is to enable an adult individual of sound mind to enjoy a right to choose what shall happen to his/her body. The patient has the right to give or withhold consent to the proposed investigation or treatment, even if without the recommended treatment his condition may worsen to the extent that he may die. Most of the physicians consider consent as a legal requirement to protect them in a court of law against medical malpractice lawsuits. For them it is an ambiguous concept, as in spite of taking consent and educating the patient, there may be allegations of improper consent. Physicians must understand that in a given case, Court will accept the consent as valid only if both medical and legal standards have been satisfied completely.

EVOLUTION

To appreciate the importance of informed consent in modern medicine it will be appropriate to review its evolution. During the ancient period of Hippocrates, paternalistic approach was predominant, and there was no concept of taking consent from the patients. Patients were expected to be obeisant, and the only communication with the patients was to persuade them to accept the therapy.[3]

In the nineteenth century, the concept of educating the patient was to motivate compliance with the advice of the physician. Although physicians proposed an idea of informed patient to persuade the patients to accept therapy, they were never the supporters of the concept of consent for treatment.[4] In twentieth century, it was the judicial decisions which provided insights regarding patient's rights of self-determination. According to Faden and Benjamin, "It was case law that introduced the concept of informed consent to medicine in the 20th century using the language of self-determination.[5]

Judicial Decisions Introducing the Concept of Informed Consent

- Schloendorff vs. Society of New York Hospitals[6]
  In 1914, a patient sued his doctor for operating without consent. In this case the patient gave consent to an examination under anesthesia and requested not to do any surgery. The physician found the fibroid tumor and removed it. Justice Benjamin Cardozo gave judgment that,

  Every human being of adult years and sound mind has a right to determine what shall be done with his own body; and a surgeon who performs an operation without his patient's consent commits an assault, for which he is liable in damages.

- Slago vs. Leland Stanford Jr University Board of Trustees[7]
  In 1957, a patient sued his physician for not warning him of the risks of surgery and claimed that, had he known of the risk of paralysis he would not have consented to the surgery. The court ruled that,

  Physicians have the duty to disclose any facts which are necessary to form the basis of an intelligent consent by the patient to proposed treatment.

- Canterbury vs. Spence[8]
  In 1972, a patient sued his physician for not informing the risk and alternatives. In this case, the patient suffered paralysis after laminectomy, and claimed that he had not been warned. The court held that,

  It is the physician's duty to warn patients of risks and alternatives to the treatment.

- Harnish vs. children's hospital medical center[9]
  The complainant, Janine Harnish underwent an operation to remove a tumor in her neck. During the procedure, her hypoglossal nerve was severed, allegedly resulting in a permanent and almost total loss of tongue function. She charged the physicians and hospital with misrepresentation and negligence in failing to inform her before surgery of the risk of loss of tongue function. The doctors pleaded a defense that the patient was not informed about a material and foreseeable risk of the operation (loss of tongue function) due to the apprehension that she would not have consented to the operation. Holding the

doctors and the hospital liable for professional misconduct and malpractice, the court ruled that:

> A physician owes to his patient the duty to disclose in a reasonable manner all significant medical information that he possess or should reasonably possess that is material to an intelligent decision by the patient whether or not to undergo that procedure.

All these judicial decisions from malpractice lawsuits introduced the concept of informed consent, which slowly transformed into a social context to become a moral duty of physicians.

■ OBJECTIVES

To appreciate the true meaning and worth of informed consent in day-to-day practice of medicine, it is essential for the medical practitioners to understand its objective. The purposes of obtaining the informed consent are as follows.

A legal requirement:
Obtaining informed consent before treating a patient is a legal duty of a physician who proposes to treat the patient. Going through the process of informed consent and documenting the same, gives opportunity to the physician to refute the allegations of treating without consent or not informing the risks and alternatives.

Shared decision making-for better clinical results:
Studies have found that well-informed patients who are also involved in decision related to their treatment (shared decision making) show better clinical results. Both patient and physician discuss the preferences and facts related to the decisional process so as to reach a shared decision. This decision might involve a compromise between the parties as they may not consider it to be the best decision, yet both accept it as treatment to be followed. Trying to find a decision, which both parties are committed to agree on, will foster a healthy patient-physician relationship, thus reducing the risk of malpractice litigation in case of poor outcome.

Patient education–as a tool to prevent risk of malpractice lawsuits:
Educating the patent about possibility of complications and the limitations of the treatment option to be followed is a powerful tool to prevent the risk of malpractice litigation. Patients come to physicians with high and often unrealistic expectations, and anything less than a perfect cure will be taken by the patient as unexpected result. Surprise produces anger and anger produces lawsuits.[10] Studies have shown that telling the patients about possibility of complications reduce patient expectation and results in greater satisfaction with whatever result is achieved.[11]

■ MEANING

Consent means an agreement, compliance or permission given voluntarily without any coercion. Sec 13 of Indian Contract Act[12] defines consent as two or more persons are said to consent when they agree upon the same thing in the same sense. Consent should be free and voluntary. For consent to be free, it should not be induced by undue influence, coercion, misrepresentation, mistake or fraud. Informed consent, in medical setting, is a procedure whereby a patient consents to or refuses (informed refusal) a medical intervention based on information provided by a doctor regarding nature and potential consequences of the

proposed medical intervention. A doctor provides information to a competent patient, who after understanding the information, makes a valid decision. The elements of informed consent include:
- Disclosure of information
- Competence
- Understanding
- Voluntariness
- Decision-making

Consent may be express or implied.

Implied Consent

It is a consent given impliedly by the patient by virtue of his actions. When a patient approaches a doctor for consultation, it implies his/her willingness to be examined by the doctor. Similarly when a patient lies on the examination table on doctor's instruction, it indicates implied consent. However, this implied permission cannot be presumed for procedures more complex than general physical examination (inspection, palpation, percussion and auscultation), which do not involve examination of the privates. If the doctor feels that the patient has not properly given implied consent, he should take a clear and unambiguous verbal consent even for such simple procedures. For internal examination (rectal and vaginal) and withdrawal of blood, expressed consent should be obtained.

Express Consent

Consent is said to be express when it is in writing or expressed in words. Verbal consent may be obtained for minor therapeutic as well as diagnostic procedures. If only oral consent is taken it is preferable to document the same in medical record, which may be of help in future if any allegation is made on this issue. Entry of verbal consent in patient's medical record will provide corroborative evidence to support the defense taken by the doctor. In the words of Dr Mark E Bathsta[13] "Document it. If you haven't documented it, you didn't do it." Written consent is a must for any treatment or procedure (therapeutic as well as diagnostic) that has risk of injury to the patient. Written consent affords documentary evidence that consent was actually obtained.

If a patient is unable to give consent due to any reason, proxy consent may be obtained from his/her relative or guardian who is willing to take responsibility on behalf of the patient. However, proxy consent is invalid if the patient is competent to give consent.

■ WHAT MAKES THE CONSENT LEGALLY ACCEPTABLE?

A consent which is taken without full disclosure will not be accepted by the court and may be rejected as an invalid consent. Consent is not just taking the signatures of patient on consent form. It is an ongoing process of communication between the medical professional and the patient, which begins at first meeting and continues through treatment and follow up. The patient must understand the consent as continuing permission of the patient to receive a particular treatment based on adequate information about the nature of proposed treatment, likely benefits and risks, and any alternate available.

Conditions for a Valid Consent

Consent is considered invalid if it is obtained by fraud, undue influence or misrepresentation as to the nature of procedure. For a consent to serve its purpose (medical as well as legal), it must qualify the conditions of a valid consent. A valid consent is one which is voluntary, free, with no coercion, manipulation or persuasion. The conditions for a valid consent are summarized as follows.

Competence

Competence means the ability to perform a task, and in context to consent in healthcare, it means patient's capacity to make decisions about one's own healthcare. The precise criteria for evaluating a patient's competence include his/her ability to understand and appreciate the significance of the information provided, to take decision, to choose and to communicate the choice. To ensure that the patient has assimilated the information, he/she may be asked to paraphrase the information presented to them.[14]

Age for Consent

Unlike many other countries, in India, no legislation specifically apprises the age for consent to medical treatment. Laws for consent in general may be applied to the medical profession also. According to Indian law, majority is achieved at an age of 18 years and any person who is major and of sound mind can give consent for his/her treatment (extrapolation of Sec 87 IPC). A child below 12 years of age cannot give consent (Sec 90 IPC). Parents/guardians can give consent for their medical/surgical treatment. A child between 12–18 years can give consent only for medical examination but not for any surgery/procedure. To perform medical/surgical procedure in patients between 12 and 18 years (except in emergencies when parents cannot be contacted) consent by parents/legal guardian is must (**Box 1**). Such a consent given by parent or guardian, on behalf of patient below 18 years is known as consent by proxy.[15] If a patient is not competent to give consent to treatment, then depending upon the circumstances, legally authorized person may decide on behalf of the patient. Parents or legal guardian may give proxy consent for minors. Decision makers deciding on behalf of a patient should keep in mind what the patient would have decided, had he been competent to do so (on the basis of their knowledge about the patient). In those cases where such knowledge is absent, the decision should be in the patient's best interest.[16]

For medicolegal examination, the age for consent is 12 years and above. In 2014 Ministry of Health and Family Welfare, Government of India[17] published "Guidelines on medicolegal care for survivors/victims of sexual violence." These guidelines have provided the age of consent for medicolegal examination of a survivor of sexual violence as follows:

> The consent form must be signed by the person him/herself if s/he is above 12 years of age. Consent must be taken from the guardian/parent if the survivor is under the age of 12 years.

Voluntariness

For consent to be valid, voluntary participation by the patient is a must. Voluntary participation means that the consent should not be induced by undue influence, coercion,

> **BOX 1** **Sections of Indian Penal Code Related to Consent[18]**
>
> **Sec 87: Act not intended and not known to be likely to cause death or grievous hurt, done by consent of a person above 18 years of age**
> Any act which is not intended and not known by the doer to be likely to cause death, or grievous hurt, will not be an offence if a person, above 18 years of age, gives consent, to suffer that harm even if he suffers any harm which the act may cause, or be intended by the doer to cause
>
> **Sec 88: Act not intended to cause death, done by consent in good faith for person's benefit**
> Any act which is not intended to cause death, will not be an offence even if any harm which it may cause, or be intended or known by the doer to likely to cause, to any person for whose benefit it is done in good faith, and who has given a consent, to suffer that harm, or to take the risk of that harm. Illustration: A surgeon knowing that a particular operation is likely to cause the death, but not intending to cause death and intending in good faith, for patient's benefit performs that operation with patient's consent. Surgeon has committed no offence
>
> **Sec 89: Act done in good faith for benefit of child or insane person, by or by consent of guardian**
> Any act which is done in good faith for the benefit of a person under 12 years of age, or of unsound mind, by or by consent of the guardian or other person having lawful charge of that person, will not be an offence even if any harm which it may cause, or be intended by the doer to cause or be known by the doer to be likely to cause to that person
>
> **Sec 90: Consent known to be given under fear or misconception or given by a person having unsoundness of mind/intoxication or by a person under 12 years of age**
> A consent will be invalid if it is given by a person under fear of injury, or under a misconception of fact, and if the person doing the act knows, or has reason to believe, that the consent was given due to fear or misconception; or consent by a person having unsoundness of mind, or intoxication, is unable to understand the nature and consequence of that to which he gives his consent; or the consent is given by a person under 12 years of age
>
> **Sec 92: Act done in good faith for benefit of a person without consent**
> Any act which is done in good faith, for the benefit of any person even if any harm which it may cause to that person, and even without that person's consent, if the circumstances are such that it is impossible for that person to signify consent, or if that person is incapable of giving consent, and has no guardian or other person in lawful charge of him from whom it is possible to obtain consent in time for the thing to be done with benefit

misrepresentation or fraud. In a clinical set-up voluntariness is vulnerable to be compromised due to various reasons. The imbalance between the knowledge and power between the physician and the patient, a dependent relationship between patient and the healthcare professional, anxious patient due to the disease are some of the factors that may adversely affect the voluntariness of the patient. Even a rational persuasion in good faith by the physician may be construed as undue influence by the patient. Sometimes patients may find it difficult to challenge the doctor's assumption that they would have no objections to the proposed treatment. So it is best to check that the patient has no uncertainties before proceeding with the proposed treatment. A patient has a right to make a decision on the basis of his/her own reasons and values. Healthcare professionals must not confer their own values. Misrepresentation, undue influence, coercion and fraud invalidate the consent, and care must be taken to ensure that the patient makes a decision freely and voluntarily.

It is the right and responsibility of every competent individual to advance his or her own welfare. This is exercised by freely and voluntarily consenting or refusing consent to recommended medical procedures, based on a sufficient knowledge of the benefits, burdens, and risks involved. The ability to give informed consent depends on:

- Adequate disclosure of information
- Patient's freedom of choice
- Patient's comprehension of information
- Patient capacity for decision-making.

By meeting these four requirements, three necessary conditions for valid consent are satisfied: (a) that the individual's decision is voluntary; (b) that this decision is made with an appropriate understanding of the circumstances; and (c) that the patient's choice is deliberate insofar as the patient has carefully considered all of the expected benefits, burdens, risks and reasonable alternatives.[19]

Adequate Information

Consent without necessary information invalidates the consent. The concept of informed consent requires complete disclosure about the necessary information so as to enable the patient to make an informed decision. For many physicians, it is perplexing to judge the adequacy of the information provided to obtain informed consent. It is not necessary or to provide each and every detail of the proposed treatment/procedure. Excessive or technical detail is likely to overload the patient, eventually resulting in a confused patient, and undermining the purpose of providing information. Only that much information that would be expected by a reasonable patient to make an intelligent decision is considered adequate. Any doubts that a patient has should be fully explained. The information to be disclosed should include the following:

- Diagnosis and nature of disease
- Purpose and nature of proposed treatment/procedure
- Benefits and risks of the proposed treatment/procedure
- Alternative treatment available
- Risks involved with refusal to treatment/procedure.

Disclosure of information related to risks is of paramount importance specifically to prevent unrealistic expectations of the patient from proposed treatment/surgery. Avoid statements that might be construed by the patient as guarantee to absolute recovery. Unsatisfied patients may claim that better results were guaranteed. Incomplete disclosure of risks due to the apprehension that a patient will refuse the treatment/surgery is not an acceptable justification for withholding full disclosure.

Duty to Warn a 'Material Risk'

Every physician who proposes to treat a patient has a legal duty to warn the patient about the possible risks of the proposed treatment under the doctrine of informed consent. This duty is confined to the material risk that would affect the decision of a reasonable patient. The material risk in a given case is a risk in which the court is satisfied that, a reasonable patient would be likely to attach significance in deciding whether to accept the proposed treatment/surgery or not.[20] The clinical limitation to this legal duty is that, many a times there are so many risks that it becomes difficult to decide whether a particular risk will affect the decision of given patient in given circumstances or not. There is no clear guideline to decide whether a particular risk will affect the decision of a given patient in a given circumstance or not. It may be safely presumed that, more severe a risk is, the more likely a prudent patient will attach significance to it (even if the risk is remote).

EXCEPTIONS

There are specific circumstances in which it is legally acceptable to forego the requirement of informed consent before starting the treatment. These circumstances may be labeled as *exceptions* to informed consent.

- *Medical emergencies*: In medical emergencies (Sec 92 IPC) where delay caused by waiting for informed consent cannot be afforded at the cost of life of the patient, and also there is no evidence to indicate that the patient would refuse the procedure, it is legally acceptable to start the treatment without informed consent. In Pravat Kumar Mukherjee vs. Ruby General Hospital and Ors,[21] National Commission held that consent is implicit in emergency or critical cases, and there is no question of waiting for consent. In case doctor or a hospital denies treatment or surgery in such cases on the ground that there was no consent, the burden of proving refusal to treatment or surgery despite of informing the consequences thereof is on such doctor or hospital.
- *An incompetent patient*: In circumstances where the patient is incompetent to give consent, and there is no evidence to indicate that the patient would refuse the treatment, it is legally acceptable to start the treatment without informed consent. Incompetence may be due to age (minors) or unconsciousness. In incompetent patients who are not accompanied by any relative or attendant, it is not justifiable to delay the treatment for want of consent.
- *Therapeutic privilege*: In some cases, 'full disclosure' is damaging to the patient. His mental capacity, physical condition, age, etc., have also to be taken into consideration. In such cases, if the doctor considers it necessary, next of the kin of the patient should be taken into confidence and they be appraised of the full situation. Then the treating doctor can withhold certain damaging information from the patient. This is the doctrine of therapeutic privilege and is an exception to professional secrecy. The physician should apply therapeutic privilege with great caution as the concept has the potential of being misused as allegation of invalid consent.

OBTAINING CONSENT: THE PROCEDURE

As it is said, taking consent is not an event rather it's a continuous process, physicians should be well versed with various stages of this process. The information to be disclosed should be well structured, which may be disseminated by various means viz. orally, written material, and audiovisual aids. Discussion should preferably be done by the treating physician himself as he is the one whom the patient/relatives will confide in the most. He is also the most concerned stakeholder who will be charged with the responsibility of defending any malpractice lawsuit. If the information is presented by audiovisual aid or by someone else, the physician should be available at the end of presentation to clear the patient's doubts. It is extremely important as well as challenging to create a balance between information overload and insufficient disclosure. If the information is not understood by the patient, there is a tendency that he/she may feel that the consent form is solely a legal formality to protect the physician, and patient's participation is not truly desired by the physician. The discussion should be unhurried. Patient's concerns should not be ignored; rather he should be encouraged to ask questions. He should also be informed that he has every right to revoke the consent already given, at any later stage.

Documentation of Informed Consent

Once all the information has been presented, and the patient has given well informed decision to consent to treatment/procedure, it is time to document the process of informed consent.

Documentation can be done in the form of consent forms and/or detailed notes in patient's medical record. After giving sufficient time to the patient to read the consent form and/or medical notes, the patient is asked to sign. The signatures should be witnessed by patient's family member and staff of the hospital. If the patient refuses the proposed treatment or procedure, the physician must warn the patient of the risks of refusal, and ask him/her to sign the informed refusal. Similarly, if a patient misses a postoperative appointment or follow up appointment for continuing treatment, the same must be documented along with the risks of delayed treatment, and got signed by the patient.

■ JUDICIAL DECISION ON INFORMED CONSENT

Samira Kohli Case: Landmark Judgment on Informed Consent[22]

In this case, a 44-year-old unmarried female consulted her doctor for prolonged menstrual bleeding. She was advised to undergo a laparoscopy and was made to sign consent form that allowed the surgeon to carry out a "diagnostic and operative laparoscopy" and there was an additional endorsement that a "laparotomy may be needed." When the patient was in the operation theater (and was unconscious), another proxy consent was taken from her mother for a hysterectomy. Her uterus, ovaries, and fallopian tubes were removed. Plaintiff sought damages for the loss of her reproductive organs, irreversible permanent damage, pain, suffering emotional stress and trauma.

The National Commission dismissed the complaint holding that the patient had voluntarily gone to the clinic for treatment and that the hysterectomy had been done with adequate care and caution. An appeal was filed to the Supreme Court. The Apex Court held that, in view of absence of consent by Samira, the performance of hysterectomy and bilateral salpingo-oophorectomy was an unauthorized invasion and interference with the patient's body amounting to a torturous act of assault and battery and therefore a deficiency in service.

Extracts from the Supreme Court's Judgment (Samira Kohli's Case)

- A doctor has to seek and secure the consent of the patient before commencing a 'treatment' (the term 'treatment' includes surgery also). The consent so obtained should be real and valid, which means that:
    - The patient should have the capacity and competence to consent
    - His consent should be voluntary
    - His consent should be on the basis of adequate information concerning the nature of the treatment procedure, so that he knows what he is consenting to.
- The 'adequate information' to be furnished by the doctor (or a member of his team) who treats the patient, should enable the patient to make a balanced judgment as to whether he should submit to the particular treatment or not. This means that the doctor should disclose:
    - The nature and procedure of the treatment and its purpose, benefits, and effect
    - Alternatives, if any, available
    - An outline of the substantial risks
    - Adverse consequences of refusing treatment.

    But there is no need to explain remote or theoretical risks involved, which may frighten or confuse a patient and result in refusal of consent for the necessary treatment. Similarly, there is no need to explain the remote or theoretical risks of refusal to take treatment, which may persuade a patient to undergo a fanciful or unnecessary treatment. A balance

should be achieved between the need for disclosing necessary and adequate information and at the same time avoid the possibility of the patient being deterred from agreeing to a necessary treatment or offering to undergo an unnecessary treatment.
- Consent given only for a diagnostic procedure, cannot be considered as consent for therapeutic treatment. Consent given for a specific treatment procedure will not be valid for conducting some other treatment procedure. The fact that the unauthorized additional surgery is beneficial to the patient, or that it would save considerable time and expense to the patient, or would relieve the patient from pain and suffering in future, are not grounds of defense in an action in tort for negligence or assault and battery. The only exception to this rule is where the additional procedure, though unauthorized, is necessary in order to save the life or preserve the health of the patient and it would be unreasonable to delay such unauthorized procedure until patient regains consciousness and takes a decision.
- There can be a common consent for diagnostic and operative procedures where they are contemplated. There can also be a common consent for a particular surgical procedure and an additional or further procedure that may become necessary during the course of surgery.
- The nature and extent of information to be furnished by the doctor to the patient to secure the consent need not be of the stringent and high degree mentioned in Canterbury but should be of the extent which is accepted as normal and proper by a body of medical men skilled and experienced in the particular field. It will depend upon the physical and mental condition of the patient, the nature of treatment, and the risk and consequences attached to the treatment.

CONCLUSION

In modern medicine, the concept of obtaining informed consent has been well accepted. The patients are treated as partners in the process of providing healthcare. The concept of informed consent goes hand in hand with the concept of quality healthcare. The process of obtaining informed consent should be viewed as an opportunity to build trust between the patient and physician, through patient education, rather than just a legal requirement. Healthcare professionals should appreciate both the medical and legal significance of valid consent. In malpractice lawsuits, many times claim of improper consent is combined to the claim of harm due to medical negligence. Informed consent is more than just a signature on a page. It is a shared process of ongoing discussion between patients and their physicians and is the best tool to bring about the trust and faith of the patient toward his doctor.

REFERENCES

1. Moore vs. Regents of the University of California. 51 Cal.3d 120, 165, 793 P. 2d 479, 271 Cal. Raptr. 147.
2. Bardale R. Principles of forensic medicine and toxicology. Jaypee Brothers Medical Publishers (P) Ltd. 2011.p.20.
3. Miles SH. Hippocrates and informed consent. The Lancet. 2009;374:1322-3.
4. Rush B. On the vices and virtues of Physicians. A lecture delivered November 2, 1801. In: sixteen introductory lectures. Philadelphia: Bradford and Innskeep;1811:123-5. Available: http://18thcenturyreadingroom.wordpress.com/2006/11/20/item-of-the-day-benjamin-rush-on-the-vices-and-virtues-of-physicians-1801.
5. Faden RR, Beauchamp TL. A history and theory of informed consent. New York: Oxford Univ Press. 1986;101.
6. Schloendorff v. Society of New York Hospitals, 211 N.Y. 125;105 N.E. 93.
7. Slago vs. Leland Stanford Jr. University Board of Trustees, 154 Cal. App. 2d 564.
8. Canterbury vs. Spence 464 F.2d 772 (D.C. Cir. 1972.

9. Janine Harnish vs. Children's hospital medical center and others, Available: http://masscases.com/cases/sjc/387/387mass152.html.
10. Bettman JW. Ophthalmology: The art, the law, and a little bit of science. Birmingham, AL: Aesculapius; 1984.
11. Kraushar MF. Informed consent. Risk Prevention in Ophthalmology. Springer. 2008.
12. Indian Contract Act - Act 9 of 1872.
13. Harish D, Sharma BR. Consent in medical practice. Current Medical Journal: North Zone. 2001;(7):36-42.
14. Grisso T, Appelbaum PS. Assessing competence to consent to treatment: a guide for physicians and other healthcare professionals. New York/Oxford: Oxford University Press. 1998.
15. Yadav M. Age of consent in medical profession: A food for thought. JIAFM 2007; 29. Available: http://www.indianjournals.com/ijor.aspx?target=jor:jiafmandvolume=29andissue=2andarticle=014.
16. Elliot C. Patients doubtfully capable or incapable of consent. In: Kuhse H, Singer P, Eds. A companion to bioethics. Oxford: Blackwell. 1998:452-62.
17. Available: www.mohfw.nic.in/showfile.php? lid=2737
18. Indian Penal Code - Act XLV of 1860.
19. Available: http://www.ncbi.nlm.nih.gov/pmc/articles/PMC2598284.
20. Sidaway vs. Board of Governors of Bethlem Royal Hospital and the Maudsley Hospital 1984 QB 493 All Er 1018;1984.
21. II (2005) CPJ 35(NC).
22. Samira Kohli vs. Dr. Prabha Manchanda andAnr.2008 (2) SCC1.

CHAPTER 11

Medicolegal Aspects of Medical Records

Joseph Thomas, Arun Mavaji Seetharam, Rajesh Kumar Sinha

"Nothing is more devastating to an innocent physician's defense against the allegations of medical malpractice than an inaccurate, illegible or skimpy medical record."
— Brad Cohn[1]

■ INTRODUCTION

Medical record is a "clinical, scientific, administrative and legal document related to patient care, in which sufficient data is recorded in the sequence of events to justify the diagnosis and warrant the treatment and the end results." It is a clear, concise, correct, complete, and chronological record of the patient's illness, the course of the disease, the investigations done, the results thereof, the diagnosis, the treatment measures instituted, and the extent of recovery therefrom.[2]

Medical record keeping has evolved into a science of itself and become an important aspect of the management of a patient. It is important for the doctors and medical establishments to properly maintain the records of patients for two important reasons. The first and most important part is that it is very important for the treating doctor to plan the management of a patient under his care. This becomes a better way for the doctor to measure progressive patient care and aids in the continuity of care. This will also be useful in the scientific evaluation and review of patient management issues and to plan treatment protocols. It also helps to evaluate the performance of medical and nursing staff. The proper planning of governmental strategies for future medical care also needs evaluation of properly kept records.[3] Medical records are also of equal importance in the issue of alleged medical negligence. The legal system relies mainly on documentary evidence in a situation where medical negligence is alleged by the patient or the relatives. In an accusation of negligence, this is the most important evidence deciding on the issue "whether the doctor was negligent or not." It is wise to remember that "poor records mean poor defense, no records mean no defense."[3]

With the increasing use of medical insurance for treatment, the insurance companies also require proper medical records, to prove the patient's demand for medical expenses. Improper record keeping can result in declining medical claims.[3]

■ COMPONENT OF MEDICAL RECORDS

Medical records include a variety of documentation of patient's history, clinical findings, diagnostic test results, preoperative care, operation notes, postoperative care, and daily notes of a patient's progress and medications. The doctor is the prime person who has to oversee this process and is primarily responsible for the complete, accurate, adequate, and timely documentation of history, physical examination, treatment plans, operative records, consent forms, medications administered, referral record, discharge records, and medical certificates. As the other healthcare professionals contribute equally in terms of patient care, the medical records should have the proper recording of nursing care, laboratory data, reports of diagnostic evaluations, pharmacy records, and billing processes.

The medical records also contain many other documentary evidences that are indirectly related to patient management such as accounts records, service records of the staff, and administrative records, which are also important during any litigation and malpractice suit. Medical recording needs the concerted effort of all the healthcare professionals involved in patient care. This means that all the staff should be trained in documentation and proper maintenance of patient records.[3]

ELECTRONIC HEALTH RECORDS: AN EMERGING TREND IN INDIA[3-5]

The conventional method of keeping medical records involves paper and folders that pose challenges to the healthcare organization in terms of storage, retention, and maintenance. These records are difficult to retrieve and disseminate to the healthcare professionals and providers in a timely fashion at the point of care. However, it is legally more acceptable as documentary evidence, as it is difficult to tamper with the records without detection.

Many healthcare organizations have adopted electronic health records to overcome these challenges and streamlined the information generation and management processes. The electronic health records support and promote the interdisciplinary charting of patient care in a real-time manner and assist the healthcare professionals in instant access of patient records beyond the geographical boundaries. In the year 2013, Ministry of Health and Family Welfare, Government of India has provided a guideline for the implementation of electronic health record in India. The guideline was further revised in the year 2016 to provide better direction to the Indian healthcare institution in implementing electronic health record. The guideline stresses on ethical, legal, and social issues associated with the use of electronic health record and described under the heading of "Privacy", "Security", and "Trust." The term "privacy" shall mean that only those person(s) including organizations duly authorized by the patient may view the recorded data or part thereof. The term "security" shall mean that all recorded personally identifiable data will at all times be protected from any unauthorized access, particularly during transport (e.g., from the healthcare provider to provider and healthcare provider to the patient). The term "trust" shall mean that person, persons or organizations (doctors, hospitals, and patients) are those who they claim they are.

To maintain the privacy, security, and trust in using electronic health records, the concept of electronic protected health information (ePHI) came into practice, and it refers to "any protected health information (PHI) that is created, stored, transmitted, or received electronically." Electronic protected health information includes any medium used to store, transmit, or receive PHI electronically.

Even though the benefits are tremendous, the cost of implementation and maintenance is high, and due to this reason, the implementation of electronic health records in India was initially only limited to some private superspecialty hospital such as Max Healthcare, Apollo Hospital, Sankar Nethralaya, Fortis, etc., who can afford to maintain the system for longer period of time. These electronic health records work independently only in the implemented hospital and create another challenge with respect to the sharing of patient records with other healthcare institution. The solution of this could be to strengthen the Information and Communication Technology infrastructure at private and public institution and implement a unified electronic health record and link it to Aadhar ID, so that the patient record will be available, irrespective of the patient visit to different hospitals at different time.

Ownership of Data

For data ownership, a distinction is to be made between the physical or electronic records, which are owned by the healthcare provider. These are held in trust on behalf of the patient. The contained data which is the sensitive personal information of the patient is owned by the patient himself/herself. The healthcare provider will have the privilege to change/append/modify any record in relation to the healthcare of the patient as necessary with a complete documented trail of such change. No alteration of the previously saved data will be permitted. A strict audit trail shall be maintained of all activities at all times that may be suitably reviewed by an appropriate authority like system administrator, auditor, legal representatives of the patient, the patient, healthcare provider, privacy officer, court appointed/authorized person, etc. The medium of storage or transmission of such electronic health record will be owned by the healthcare provider. The sensitive personal information (SPI) and personal information (PI) of the patient is owned by the patients themselves. As per the Information Technology Act, 2000 Data Privacy Rules, refer to "sensitive personal data or information" (Sensitive Data) as the subject of protection, but also refer, with respect to certain obligations, to "personal information."

Data Access and Confidentiality

Patients will have the sufficient privileges to inspect and view their health records without any time limit. Patient's privileges to amend data shall be limited to correction of errors in the recorded patient/health details. This shall need to be performed through a recorded request made to the healthcare provider within a period of 30 days from the date of discharge in all inpatient care settings or 30 days from the date of clinical encounter in outpatient care settings. An audit of all such changes shall be strictly maintained. Both the request and audit trail records shall be maintained within the system. Patients will have the privileges to restrict access to and disclosure of individually identifiable health information.

Electronic Health Records Preservation

All records must compulsorily be preserved and not destroyed during the life-time of the person, ever. The digital records must be preserved till such time according to the prevalent law of the land. It is, however, strongly encouraged to ensure that the records are never be destroyed or removed permanently. With rapid decline in costs of data archiving coupled with the ability to store more data that may be readily accessible and maintained permanently.

Data Privacy and Security

Organizations must consider several factors when adopting security measures. In deciding what security measures to adopt, an organization must consider its size, complexity, and capabilities; its technical infrastructure, hardware, and software security capabilities; the cost

of particular security measures; and the probability and degree of the potential risks to the ePHI it stores and transmits. The security standards require healthcare providers to implement reasonable and appropriate administrative, physical, and technical safeguards to:
- Ensure the confidentiality, integrity, and availability of all the ePHI they create, transmit, receive, or maintain.
- Protect against reasonably anticipated threats or hazards to the security or integrity of their ePHI.
- Protect against uses or disclosures of the ePHI that are not required or permitted under the Privacy Standards.
- Ensure their workforce will comply with their security policies and procedures.

■ CONFIDENTIALITY OF MEDICAL RECORDS

Medical records can be used as a personal or impersonal document.
- *Personal document*: This information is confidential and should not be released without the consent of the patient except in some specific situations.
- *Impersonal document*: The record loses its identity as a personal document and patient permission is not required. These records could be used for research purposes.

Confidentiality is an important component of the rights of the patient. The hospital is legally bound to maintain the confidentiality of the personal medical records. The patient can claim negligence against the hospital or the doctor for a breach of confidentiality. However, there are certain situations where it is legal for the authorities to give patient information. They are as follows:
- During referral
- When demanded by the court or by the police on a written requisition,
- When demanded by insurance companies as provided by the Insurance Act when the patient has relinquished his rights on taking the insurance, and
- When required for specific provisions of Workmen's Compensation cases, Consumer Protection cases, or for Income tax authorities.

The impersonal documents have been used for research purposes as the identity of the patient is not revealed. Though the identity of the patient is not revealed, the research team is privy to patient records and a cause of concern about the confidentiality of information. Historically, such research has been exempt from an ethics review and researchers have not been required to obtain informed consent from patients before using their records. Recently, a need has been felt to regulate the use of medical records in research, effectively restricting the manner in which this type of research is conducted. An ethics review is required for using the patient data.[3]

■ CATEGORIES OF MEDICAL RECORDS

The different categories of medical records are as follows:
- Certain records must be given to the patient as a matter of right. Discharge summary, referral notes, and death summary in case of natural death are important documents for the patient. Hence, these have to be given without charge for all including patients who leave against medical advice. The hospital bill cannot be tied up with these sensitive documents that are necessary for continuing patient care. Thus, the above documents cannot be legally refused even when the hospital bill has not been paid.

- Certain records may be issued after the patient or authorized attendant fulfills the due requirements as stipulated by a hospital. This requires a formal application to the hospital requesting for the records. It is necessary that the hospital bills are cleared and the necessary processing fee has been paid. The documents in this group include copies of inpatient files, records of diagnostic tests, operation notes, videos, medical certificates, and duplicate copies for lost documents. It is important that the duplicate copies should be marked appropriately. It is not unusual for an unscrupulous patient to use it for multiple insurance claims without the knowledge of the doctor.
- Certain records cannot be given to patients without the direction of the Court. The outpatient file, inpatient file, and files of medicolegal cases including autopsy reports cannot be handed over to the patient or relatives without the direction of the Court.[3] However, to minimize the workload in courts and for convenience of public at large, some courts have issued directions that "in case any application is received from the person that Post Mortem Report of his relation has been prepared in the hospital, same may be supplied to the party concerned at its own level by the civil surgeon on receipt of application and the fee charged for the same." Similarly "in case any application is received from a person that MLR has been prepared by the hospital, a copy of MLR may be issued to the party concerned at its own level by the civil surgeon on receipt of an application and the fee charged for the same."[6] Some hospitals have prepared their own guidelines for issuing copies of PMR and MLRs only after receiving the application, prescribed fee and NOC from the concerned police station (investigating the case) clearly stating that the issue of copies of the PMR/MLR will not hinder the investigation.[7]

If medicolegal case is being referred to another center for management, copy of records could be given. However, X-rays are given only after a written undertaking by the patient or relatives that these will be produced in the Court as and when required.[3]

GUIDELINES ON MEDICAL RECORD

Medical Council of India Guidelines

The issue of medical record keeping has been addressed in the Indian Medical Council (Professional Conduct, Etiquette and Ethics) Regulations, 2002. The important issues that have been addressed are as follows:
- Maintain indoor records in a standard proforma for 3 years from commencement of treatment (1.3.1 and Appendix 3).
- Request for medical records by patient or authorized attendant should be acknowledged and documents issued within 72 hours (1.3.2).
- Maintain a register of certificates with the full details of medical certificates issued with at least one identification mark of the patient and his signature (1.3.3).
- Efforts should be made to computerize medical records for quick retrieval (1.3.4).

NABH Guidelines[8]

National Accreditation Board for Hospitals and Healthcare Providers (NABH) is a constituent board of Quality Council of India, set up to establish and operate accreditation program for healthcare organizations. The board is structured to set benchmarks for progress of health industry. It has designed healthcare standards and objective elements for hospitals and healthcare providers to achieve in order to get the NABH accreditation. The NABH objectives addressing the issue of medical records are as follows:

The Organization has a Complete and Accurate Medical Record for Every Patient

- Every medical record has a unique identifier, e.g., Unique Hospital Identity number.
- Organization should have written policy authorizing who can make entries in medical records. It could be different category of personnel for different entries, but it should be uniform across the organization, e.g., progress chart by doctors, medication chart by nurses.
- All entries in the medical record should be named, signed, dated and timed. All entries should be documented immediately but no later than an hour of completion of the assessment/procedure. For records on electronic media, the date and time should be automatically generated by the system.
- The personnel making entry in medical record must be identifiable. This could be by writing the full name or by mentioning the employee code, with the help of stamp, etc. In case of electronic records, authorized e-signature provision as per statutory requirements must be kept.
- The record should provide complete, up-to-date and chronological account of patient care. Every medical record should have all the identified sheets filed in proper order. In case a particular sheet is missing, a note to that effect should be put in the medical record.
- Provision should be made for 24-hour availability of the patient's record to healthcare providers to ensure continuity of care. In case the Medical Records Department (MRD) is not open, there should be a system in place by which authorized personnel can open the MRD and retrieve the record.

The Medical Record Reflects Continuity of Care

- The medical record contains information regarding reasons for admission, diagnosis, and plan of care. The final diagnosis must be documented by the treating doctor in all records. In the MRD, all such diagnosis shall be codified as per ICD (latest edition).
- The medical record contains the results of tests carried out and the care provided. The medical record should also reflect any delay in tests and the treatment planned or provided for the patient. This could be taken up for clinical audit.
- Operative and other procedures are incorporated in the medical record.
- When the patient is transferred to another hospital, the medical record contains the date of transfer, reasons for transfer, and the name of the receiving hospital. It is mandatory to mention the clinical condition of the patient before transfer is effected. If the patient has been transferred at his/her request, a note may be added to that effect. If the patient has been transferred by the organization, it shall have an acknowledgement from the receiving hospital. Any element of care carried out during the patient transfer should be documented, where appropriate.
- The medical record contains a copy of the discharge summary duly signed by appropriate and qualified personnel.
- In case of death, the medical record contains a copy of the cause of death certificate. This shall mention the cause, date, and time of death. The organization provides the death certificate as per the international form of medical certificate of cause of death (WHO).

- Whenever a clinical autopsy is carried out, the medical record contains a copy of the report of the same.
- Care providers have access to current and past medical record. The organization provides access to medical records to designated healthcare providers. For electronic medical record system, every faculty shall have a user ID and password.

Documented Policies and Procedures are in Place for Maintaining Confidentiality, Integrity and Security of Records, Data and Information

- The organization shall control the accessibility to the MRD and to its hospital information system. For physical records, it shall ensure usage of tracer card for movement of file in and out of the MRD. It shall have system in place to ensure that only relevant care providers have access to the patient's record. In case of electronic systems, it shall ensure that these cannot be copied at all locations.
- The policies and procedures incorporate safeguarding of data/record against loss, destruction, and tampering. For physical record, the organization shall ensure that there are adequate pest and rodent control measures. For electronic data, there should be protection against virus/Trojans and also a proper backup procedure. To prevent tampering of physical records, access shall be limited only to healthcare provider concerned. In electronic format, this could be done by adequate passwords. In electronic systems, the access should be different for different types of personnel and specific for that user. The organization should have a system to keep track of changes made in medical record or data. In case of physical records and data, there must be a provision to either store in fire-safe cabinets or there must be adequate firefighting equipment.

Documented Policies and Procedures Exist for Retention Time of Records, Data and Information

- The organization shall define the retention period of each category of medical records, OPD, inpatients and medicolegal cases (MLC). It should be according to rules laid down by Medical Council of India (MCI) and respective state authority.
- The policies and procedures are in consonance with the local and national laws and regulations. Some of the related laws in this context are Code of Medical Ethics, 2002, Consumer Protection Act, 1987 and relevant state legislation.
- The retention process provides expected confidentiality and security for both physical and electronic records.
- The destruction of medical records, data and information is in accordance with the laid down policy. Destruction can be done after taking approval of competent authority.

The Organization Regularly Carries out Review of Medical Records

- The medical records are reviewed periodically. The organization should define the periodicity. A standardized checklist can be used for this purpose.
- The review uses a representative sample based on statistical principles. The organization shall define the principles on which sampling is based. The organization shall identify and authorize individuals to conduct review. The review should focus on timeliness, legibility, and completeness of medical records. The review process should include records of both active and discharged patients. The review points out and documents any deficiencies in records. Appropriate corrective and preventive measures are undertaken within a defined period of time and are documented.

There is an Appropriate Mechanism for Transfer (in and out) or Referral of Patients

Documented policies and procedures guide the transfer-out/referral of unstable patients to another facility in an appropriate manner. The organization shall at the outset define as to who an unstable patient is. This shall be defined based on physiological criteria. The documented procedure should address the methodology of safe transfer of the patient in a life threatening situation to another organization. The organization should give a case summary mentioning the significant findings and treatment given. A copy of the same shall be retained by the organization. For admitted patients, a discharge summary has to be given. The same shall also be given to patients going against medical advice. This shall also include patients being transferred both for diagnostic and/or therapeutic purposes.

Patient cared for by the Organization Undergoes an established Initial Assessment

- The organization shall have a format using which a standardized initial assessment of patients is done in OPD, emergency and in-patients. The format shall be designed to ensure that the laid down parameters are captured.
- The organization has defined and documented the time frame within which the initial assessment is to be completed with respect to OPD/emergency/in-patients. The initial assessment for in-patients is documented within 24 hours or earlier as per the patient's condition as defined in the organization's policy. This should cover history, examination including vital signs, and documentation of any drug allergies. It should mention the provisional diagnosis.
- Initial assessments of in-patients should also include nursing assessment and screening for nutritional needs.
- Plan of care shall be documented by the treating doctor or by a member of his team in the patient record. The plan of care should cover preventive aspects of care. In case if it is not able to incorporate at the time of initial assessment, the same shall be done as soon as a definite diagnosis is arrived at. The plan of care should be countersigned by the clinician incharge of the patient within 24 hours.

Patient cared for by the Organization Undergoes a Regular Reassessment

- Patient is reassessed periodically and this is documented in the case sheet. Every patient shall be reassessed at least once everyday by the treating doctor.
- Actions taken under reassessments are documented. At a minimum, the documentation shall include vitals, systemic examination findings, and medication orders.

Laboratory Services are provided as per the Scope of Services of the Organization

Critical result is intimated immediately to the personnel concerned and this shall be documented.

Patient care is Continuous and Multidisciplinary in Nature

Information about the patient's care and response to treatment is shared among medical, nursing, and other care providers, through entries on case sheet or on EMR. Information is exchanged and documented during each shift and during transfer between units/department.

The Organization has a Documented Discharge Process

- The discharge procedures are documented to ensure coordination amongst various departments including accounts so that the discharge papers are complete well within time.
- A discharge summary is given to all the patients leaving the organization, including patients leaving against medical advice and on request. In LAMA (leave against medical advice) cases, the declaration of the patient/attendant is to be recorded on a proper format.
- Discharge summary contains patient's name, UIN, date of admission and date of discharge.
- It contains reasons for admission, significant findings and diagnosis, and patient's condition at the time of discharge.
- It contains information regarding investigation results, any procedure performed, medication administered and other treatment given.
- It contains follow-up advice, medication, and other instructions in an understandable manner.
- It incorporates instructions about when and how to obtain urgent care.

Documentation of *Cardiopulmonary Resuscitation* Event

Documented policies and procedures guide the care of patients requiring cardiopulmonary resuscitation. The events during a *cardiopulmonary resuscitation* (CPR) are recorded and post-event analysis is done by a multidisciplinary committee.

Documentation of Procedures

Procedures are documented accurately in the patient record. The documentation shall mention the name of the procedure, the person who performed the procedure, salient steps of the procedure, key findings, and the post-procedure care. All the documentation shall have name, date, time, and signature. In case the procedure is being done by a person in training, it shall specify the same.

Consent for Donation and Transfusion of Blood and Blood products

Informed consent is obtained for donation and transfusion of blood and blood products. Consent should be taken for every transfusion. With the same consent one can give multiple transfusions in the same sitting. However, if the same is given over 2 days or hours apart, then a separate consent is required. In case of patients who are transfusion-dependent, consent can be taken once in 6 months. However, before every transfusion a verbal approval shall be taken.

Consent for Sedation and Documentation of Procedure

- Pre-anesthesia assessment and plan of anesthesia shall be documented.
- Informed consent for administration of moderate sedation is obtained.
- An immediate preoperative reevaluation is performed and documented. This is essentially a preinduction assessment. Any planned changes to the anesthesia plan shall be documented.
- Intra-procedure monitoring shall be documented. The cardiac rhythm monitored on a monitor during the procedure need not be documented. However, in case of rhythm abnormalities the same shall be documented.
- Patients are monitored after sedation and the same documented.
- During anesthesia vitals monitored should be documented.
- Postanesthesia status is monitored and documented.

- The type of anesthesia and anesthetic medications used are documented in the patient's record. It shall have names of anesthesiologist and other individuals who helped in the procedure. The documentation shall have name, date, time, and signature.
- Adverse anesthesia events are recorded and monitored.

Documentation before a Surgical Procedure
- Surgical patients should have a preoperative assessment and provisional diagnosis documented prior to surgery.
- An informed consent is obtained by a surgeon prior to the procedure.
- In case the procedure is changed intraoperative (and was not planned or an explicit consent taken for the same) a fresh consent needs to be taken.
- A brief operative note is documented prior to transfer out of patients from recovery area. This note provides information about the procedure performed postoperative diagnosis and the status of the patient before shifting and shall be documented by the surgeon/member of the surgical team. If it is documented by a person other than the chief operating surgeon, the same shall be countersigned by the chief surgeon.
- The operating surgeon documents the postoperative plan of care.
- In case of restraints, a documentation of reasons for restraint must be recorded.
- Nutritional assessment and reassessment of patients must be done and recorded. There shall be a written order for the diet and this shall be written in a uniform location in the medical record.

Management of Medication
- The prescription shall have the name of the patient, unique hospital number; name of the drug, dose, route, and frequency of administration of the medicine; name, signature, and registration number of the prescribing doctor.
- Known drug allergies are ascertained before prescribing. It is a good practice to document drug allergies in a prominent manner in the medical record, both OP and IP.
- All the orders for medicines are recorded on a uniform location of the case sheet.
- Electronic records when typed shall again follow the same principles.
- The treatment orders shall be written daily. Phrases like "Continue same treatment" shall not be acceptable.
- Medication orders are clear, legible, dated, timed, named, and signed.
- It contains the name of the medicine, route of administration, dose to be administered and frequency/time of administration.
- Verbal orders shall be countersigned by the doctor who ordered it within 24 hours of ordering.

■ MEDICOLEGAL ASPECTS OF MEDICAL RECORDS

Preservation of Records
There are no standard guidelines regarding how long to retain medical records in India. The hospitals retain the records for varied periods of time. Under the provisions of the Limitation Act, 1963 and Section 24A of the Consumer Protection Act, 1986, which dictates the time within which a complaint has to be filed, it is advisable to maintain records for 2 years for outpatient records and 3 years for inpatient and surgical cases. However, the provisions of the

Consumer Protection Act allows for condoning the delay in appropriate cases. This means that the records may be needed even after 3 years.

It is important to note that in pediatric cases a medical negligence case can be filed by the child after acquiring the age of majority. The Medical Council of India guidelines also insist on preserving the inpatient records in a standard proforma for 3 years from the commencement of treatment. The records that are the subject of medicolegal cases should be maintained until the final disposal of the case even though only a complaint or notice is received. Directorate General of Health Services (DGHS) has published guidelines for preservation of medical records as follows: Inpatient medical records (case sheets) should be preserved for 10 years, medicolegal registers for 10 years, and outpatient records for 5 years.[9]

The provisions of specific Acts like the Pre-Conception Prenatal Diagnostic Test Act, 1994 (PCPNDT), Environmental Protection Act, etc., necessitate proper maintenance of records that have to be retained for periods as specified in the Act. Section 29 of the PCPNDT Act, 1994 requires that all the documents be maintained for a period of 2 years or until the disposal of the proceedings. The PNDT Rules, 1996 requires that when the records are maintained on a computer, a printed copy of the record should be preserved after authentication by the person responsible for such record.[3]

Ownership of Medical Records

By and large medical records are the property of the hospitals and it is the responsibility of the hospitals to maintain it properly. The hospitals and the doctors have to be careful with medical records as these can be stolen, manipulated, and misused for mala fide reasons by any interested parties. It is the primary responsibility of the hospital to maintain and produce patient records on demand by the patient or appropriate judicial bodies.

The patient or their legal heirs can ask for copies of the treatment records that have to be provided within 72 hours. The hospitals can charge a reasonable amount for the administrative purposes including photocopying the documents. Failure to provide medical records to patients on proper demand will amount to deficiency in service and negligence.[3]

Summoning Medical Records by Courts

Medical records are acceptable as per Section 3 of the Indian Evidence Act, 1872 amended in 1961 in a court of law. These are considered useful evidence by the courts as it is accepted that documentation of facts during the course of treatment of a patient is genuine and unbiased. Medical records that are written after the discharge or death of a patient do not have any legal value. Erasing of entries is not permitted and is questionable in Court. In the event of correction, the entire line should be scored and rewritten with the date and time.

Medical records are usually summoned in a court of law in the following cases:
- Criminal cases for proving the nature, timing, and gravity of the injuries. It is considered important evidence to corroborate the nature of the weapon used and the cause of death.
- Road traffic accident cases under the Motor Accident Claim Tribunal (MACT) Act for deciding on the amount of compensation.
- Labor courts in relation to the Workmen's Compensation Act.
- Insurance claims to prove the duration of illness and the cause of death.
- *Medical negligence cases*—these can be in criminal courts when the charge against the doctor is for criminal negligence or under the Consumer Protection Act for deficiency in the doctors' or hospitals' care.

When the court issues summons for medical records, it has to be honored and respected as it is a constitutional obligation to assist in the administration of justice. It is usual to summon a doctor to appear in court to testify and to bring all the medical documents. The records can also be produced in court by the medical records officer of the hospital. The court may require these documents to be submitted for which a record is issued by the court. However, if the records are required for continuation of the medical treatment of the patient, copies can be kept by the hospital.[3]

■ JUDICIAL DECISIONS RELATED TO MEDICAL RECORDS

There have been many judicial decisions pertaining to medical records from various courts in India and a review of some of the important ones is given in this section. The National Commission had held that there was no question of negligence for failure to supply the medical records to patients unless there is a legal duty on the hospital to give the records. The alleged hospital had provided a detailed discharge summary to the patient.[10] However, the Bombay High Court held that doctors cannot claim confidentiality when the patient or his relatives demand medical records.[11] With the enforcement of the MCI Regulations, 2002 it has been held without confusion that the patient has a right to claim medical records pertaining to his treatment and the hospitals are under obligation to maintain them and provide them to the patient on request. The hospital and doctor were guilty of deficiency in service as case records were not produced before the court to refute the allegation of a lack of standard care.[12] The plea of destroying the case sheet as per the general practice of the hospitals appeared to the court as an attempt to suppress certain facts that are likely to be revealed from the case sheet. The opposite party was found negligent as he should have retained the case records until the disposal of the complaint.[13] Not producing medical records to the patient prevents the complainant from seeking an expert opinion. It is the duty of the person in possession of the medical records to produce it in the court and adverse inference could be drawn for not producing the records.[14] The State Commission held that there was negligence as the case sheet did not contain a proper history, history of prior treatment and investigations, and even the consent papers were missing.[15] The State Commission held that failure to deliver X-ray films is deficient service. The patient and his attendants were deprived of their right to be informed of the nature of injury sustained.[16] The State Commission disbelieved the evidence of the surgeon because only photocopies were produced to substantiate the evidence without any plausible explanation regarding the absence of the original.[17] The allegation of not informing the possibility of vocal cord palsy was negated by the detailed written consent that showed that it was explained properly and consented.[18] The allegation of the patient regarding negligence of the doctor was rejected. The allegation of tampering with the operation notes was negated by the State Commission in a case of intraoperative death as the complainant could not prove the allegation.[19] The hospital was held vicariously liable for the negligent action of the doctor on the basis of the bill showing the professional fees of the doctor and the discharge certificate under the letterhead of the hospital signed by the doctor.[20] The State Commission held negligence on the basis of the records, which seemed to be manipulated.[21] Issues of tampering of medical records need detailed examination in a civil court rather than in Consumer Court.[22] The National Commission in another case held that the hospital was guilty of negligence on the ground that the names of the anesthetist were two progress cards about the same patient on two separate papers that were produced in court.[23] Not maintaining confidentiality of patient information can be an issue of medical negligence. The HIV status of a patient was known to others without the consent of the patient. [24]

CONCLUSION

Medical records are an integral part of medical and medicolegal practice. This is the least bothered and most neglected section in medical practice, especially in developing countries like India. Medical records have proven of great help in medicolegal matters and in cases of negligence suits filed against the medical practitioner and hospitals. Properly kept medical records can save the doctor from many unpleasant situations. In the present age of digitalization, every effort should be made to computerize the medical records. It helps in safe storage and easy retrieval. With the recent recommendations from the government, there is some clarity regarding adoption of electronic medical records.

REFERENCES

1. Cohn B. Pediatrician. Chairman, MIEC Board of Governors, Oakland, California. [online] Available from: http://www.miec.com/Portals/0/pubs/MedicalRec.pdf. [Last Accessed on August, 2019].
2. Joshi SK. Quality Management in Hospitals. New Delhi, India: Jaypee Brothers Medical Publishers (P) Ltd.; 2014.
3. Thomas J. Medical records and issues in negligence. Indian J Urol. 2009;25(3):384-8.
4. Electronic Health Record Standards for India v2.0. Ministry of Health and Family welfare, Government of India, 2016. [online] Available from: https://mohfw.gov.in/sites/default/files/17739294021483341357.pdf. [Last Accessed on August, 2019].
5. Srivastava SK. Adoption of electronic health records: a roadmap for India. Healthc Inform Res. 2016;22(4):261-9.
6. Office Orders issued by CJM Amritsar to Civil Surgeon Amritsar dated 8.6.2007 and 27.7.07.
7. Guidelines for Issue of Copies of Post Mortem Report and Medico Legal Injury Report. [online] Available from: http://gmch.gov.in/public_notice/mlr_guidelines.pdf. [Last Accessed on August, 2019].
8. Guide Book to Accreditation Standards for Hospitals, 4th edition. New Delhi: National Accreditation Board for Hospitals and Healthcare Providers (NABH); 2015.
9. Ministry of Directorate General of Health Services. New Delhi: Ministry of Directorate General of Health Services (MOHFW), GOI; 2002. pp. 79-83.
10. Poona Medical Foundation v. Marutturao Tikare. 1995 (1) CPR 661(NC).
11. Raghunath Raheja v. The Maharashtra Medical Council and Ors AIRc1996 Bombay 198.
12. Kanaiyalal Ramanlal Trivedi v. Dr. Satyanarayan Vishwakarma 1996 (3) CPR 24 (Guj); I (1997) CPJ 332 (Guj); 1998 CCJ 690 (Guj).
13. S.A. Quereshi v. Padode memorial Hospital and Research Centre II (2000) CPJ 463 (Bhopal).
14. Dr. Shyam Kumar v Rameshbhai, Harmanbhai Kachiya, 2002 (1) CPR 320, I (2006) CPJ 16 (NC).
15. Force v. M Ganeswara Rao. 1998 (3) CPR 251; 1998 (1) CPJ 413 (APSCDRC).
16. V P Shanta v. Cosmopolitan Hospitals (P) Ltd 1997 (1) CPR 377 (Kerala SCDRC).
17. Devendra Kantilal Nayak v. Dr. Kalyaniben Dhruv Shah 1996 (3) CPR 56; I (1997) CPJ 103; 1998 CCJ 544 (Guj).
18. C Anjani Kumar v. Madras Medical Mission 1998 (2) CPR (Chennai); I (1998) CPJ 533 (Chennai); 1998 CTJ 504 (CP) (SCDRC); 1999 CCJ 915 (TN).
19. Sethuraman Subramaniam Iyer v. Triveni Nursing Home 1997 (2) CPR 144 (NC); I (1998) CPJ 10 (NC); 1998 CTJ 7 (CP) (NCDRC); 1998 CCJ 1532 (NC).
20. P.P. Ismail v. K.K. Radha 1997 (2) CPR 171 (NC); I (1998) CPJ 16 (NC); (1997) 5 CTJ 685 (CP) (NCRDC); 1999 CPJ 99 (NC).
21. Nihal Kaur v. Director, PGI, Chandigarh. 1996 (3) CPJ 112 [Chandigarh (U.T.) CDRC].
22. Harenbalal Das v. Dr. Ajay Paul, 2001 (2) CPR 498.
23. Meenakshi Mission Hospital and Research Centre v. Samuraj and Anr. I(2005) CPJ 33 (NC)
24. Dr. Tokugha Yeptomi v. Apollo Hospital Enterprises Ltd and Anr III (1998) CPJ 132 (SC).

CHAPTER 12

Documentation in Healthcare: Standards and Guidelines

Utsav Parekh

"I have been involved with the defense of physicians in professional liability claims since 1976. One common thread that has existed in all claims seen over the years is that the medical record is the physician's greatest asset in defending him or her against allegations of negligence. If more physicians realized that clear, legible medical records are their best defense and they documented accordingly, most claims would never be brought, and many claims that are contemplated would not be pursued..."

— **Stephen D. Stimel**

■ INTRODUCTION

Documentation is the process of recording information. In medical profession it includes all types of documents written by doctors, nurses, and allied health professionals in their professional capacity in relation to the provision of patient care.[1] Documentation is the basis for communication between health professionals that informs of the care planned, the care provided, and the outcome of that care as a continuous and contemporaneous record. Comprehensive documentation has a critical role in patient care and as well in case court of law when allegation of negligence arises. Thus, it shall be prudent for the physicians to have a clear understanding of medical documentation.[2] A 5 years study on medical negligence cases depicted that in 31.7% cases improperly maintained medical records were responsible for the problem.[3] Another study showed that inadequate documentation and improper consent were the main factors considered in deciding negligence on part of the doctors in a 5 years study on analysis of medical negligence in South India.[4]

Comprehensive and complete documentation supports the fact that the patient was treated diligently and in caring manner. Thus, it is important for healthcare providers to understand all the factors associated with medical documentation, viz. (1) who is responsible for documentation, (2) what is important to document, (3) when to document, (4) how to document, (5) what not to forget in documentation, and (6) what not to do during or after documentation in different situations and various events in medical practice.

■ MEDICAL DOCUMENTATION

Medical documentation is a record of the care and the clinical assessment, professional judgment and critical thinking used by a health professional in the provision of that care.

It includes all forms of documentation by a doctor, nurse, or allied health professional (physiotherapist, dietician, etc.) recorded in a professional capacity in relation to the provision of patient care. The documentation may include written and electronic health records, audio and video tapes, emails, facsimiles, images (photographs and diagrams), observation charts, checklists, communication books, shift/management reports, incident reports, and clinical anecdotal notes or personal reflections (held by the clinicians personally) or any other type or form of documentation pertaining to the care provided.

Documentation not Directly Related to the Patient

Other documentation not directly related to the patient may be of interest to the employer, a regulatory authority, government, court, funding body, or general public. This may include:
- Policies, procedures, and protocols.
- Critical incident/occupational health and safety reports.
- Statistical and research data.
- Reports related to service and funding agreements.
- Staffing rosters.
- Personnel files.
- Performance appraisals.
- Clinical audits.

■ LEGAL IMPORTANCE OF DOCUMENTATION

Key Role in Litigation Process

Medical records are considered as a useful evidence by the courts as it is accepted that documentation during the course of treatment of a patient is genuine and unbiased. Reviewing the medical documentation is one of the most important processes when it comes to medical litigation. Quality of medical documentation is reflective of the standard of care provided. Both the lawyers (defense and plaintiffs) utilize the medical documents extensively and in a wide variety of ways throughout the course of medical litigation. Medical documentation is the key evidence available to prove/disprove whether reasonable and diligent care was provided or not. The medical documents have great significance, especially during the early stage of case evaluation when limited source of information is available to the doctor's lawyer.[5]

"Proper documentation protects the doctor in a lawsuit from significant stress, time loss, distraction, personal expense and all above the good image."

Standard of "Continuum of Care"

Continuum of care means maintaining continuity of the medical care provided to the patient, especially at the change-of-shift junctures or during the transitions between wards and other facilities within the hospital, when different caregivers are involved, and they share information with each other to assure appropriate continuity of medical care. The continuum of care also includes continuity of care in the transition from hospitalization to discharge, and referral from one hospital to the other. There is a vital need to document up-to-date information and to communicate it among the healthcare providers in order to assure continuity of delivery of appropriate medical care.

Incorrect information, misspell or missing information may result in serious injury or even death of a patient. Sloppy documentation can result in sloppy continuum of care. Failure to document relevant data is itself considered a significant breach of and deviation from the standard of care. What you write can change the course of care and/or can change your physician-patient relationship. A well-documented chart can serve as an independent witness to the care provided.

Regulation Governing Medical Records

In India there is dearth of legislation that exclusively governs medical documentation and records. However, the Indian Medical Council (Professional Conduct, Etiquette and Ethics) Regulations, 2002 has addressed some important aspects related to medical records.[6] It states that every physician shall maintain the medical records pertaining to his/her indoor patients for a period of 3 years from the date of commencement of the treatment. If any request is made for medical records either by the patients/authorized attendant or legal authorities involved, the documents shall be issued within a period of 72 hours and refusal to do so would be misconduct.

Cases Compelling Medical Documents

Legal importance of medical documentation is further established by the fact that medical records may be summoned in the court or required by other agencies as follows:
- Insurance cases/death or injury caused due to compromise of safety.
- Workmen's compensation cases.
- Personal injury suits in case of doctor's negligence.
- Malpractice suits against doctors and/or hospital.
- The Income Tax Act for claiming rebate.
- Criminal cases
- Evidence in the court of law.
- Right to Information Act
- Consumer Protection Act
- Age verification as ordered by the court/government department.
- Registration of birth and death.
- Medical Termination of Pregnancy Act/Pre-Conception and Pre-Natal Diagnostic Techniques Act (MTP/PCPNDT).
- Clinical Establishment Act.

■ BENEFITS OF GOOD QUALITY DOCUMENTATION

- Good quality documentation reflects professionalism and competence. Appropriate documentation has a critical role in the delivery of quality healthcare services.
- It helps in the scientific evaluation of patient profile, helping to plan treatment protocols and in analyzing the treatment results.
- It facilitates in creating a database to evaluate the effectiveness of treatment and a permanent record for the patient's future care.
- Proper documentation ensures continuity of care as it serves as a communication tool among healthcare providers.

- It provides chronological evidence of patient evaluation, treatment, and response to therapy, and a tool to review the quality of the care.
- It assists in reconstructing events and recollecting the circumstances without relying on memory and/or justify/defend care provided.
- Good quality documentation is at the foundation of good defense in cases of alleged medical negligence lawsuits.
- It substantiates the billing.
- They are widely used to facilitate healthcare research.
- It also helps in planning governmental strategies for future medical care plans.

■ ERRORS IN DOCUMENTATION

Vacuum in Clinical Documentation

In clinical practice, there are multiple instances where patient information is not documented or there is lapse in getting the information from the patient. In such a scenario, later on during patient care, vital information may be missing in the medical records of the patient. Lapse in clinical documentation tends to adversely affect the patient safety by increasing the chances of medical errors. If vital information is missed during clinical documentation and subsequently complication arises or there is poor outcome, risk of malpractice litigation is very high. The first and foremost contention that arises in such cases is:

"If something that is not documented, it is not done."

On objective analysis of the documentation of any medical task performed on the patient, there is a possibility of the following two situations:

Situation 1: The task was done and documented.

Situation 2: The task was done but not documented.

In case of situation 2, where the task was done but not documented, led to the initial presumption, "not documented, not done." This type of erroneous assumptions based on missed documentation, indeed, results in medical malpractice litigation. Often, in reality reasonable care has been provided in such cases, and the initial presumption of medical negligence turns out to be erroneous. However, such a finding may not be accepted by the court (due to missed documentation), and is usually of no solace to the doctor involved in the lawsuit. Thus, inference of analysis of the situation 2 is that poor documentation is a medicolegal risk that could have potentially been avoided.

The other assumption arising from missed documentation is that "Not documented means not known", meaning, thereby, that if a piece of information is not expressly documented, the doctor caring for a patient did not know it or consider it when making potentially critical healthcare decisions. For example, if a pressure ulcer assessment is not documented at a particular moment during a hospitalization, one can draw the inference that healthcare providers were unaware about the pressure ulcer while making medical decisions. In such a case if any complication occurs, it could be erroneously attributed to that lack of information, thereby implying negligence on the part of healthcare provider.[5]

Failing to Write a Complete Note

During clinical rounds, verbal orders passed to the nursing staff and the junior doctors may not be completely written in the patient notes. Missing out the documentation of the verbal orders or failing to write a complete clinical note may adversely affect the patient care. In Meenakshi *Mission Hospital and Research Centre vs. Samuraj and Anr.,* it was held that the hospital was guilty of negligence on the ground that the name of the anesthetist was not mentioned in the operation notes though anesthesia was administered by two anesthetists. There were two progress cards about the same patient on two separate papers that were produced in court.[7]

Failing to be Concise

Concise, current, and complete documentation in the medical record is an essential component of quality patient care. The urge amongst clinicians for faster text entry while trying to retain semantic clarity has contributed to the unsystematic structure of progress notes. A progress note is considered as unsystematic when there is difference between the surface form of the entered text and the intended content. For instance, when a clinician enters "BP" instead of "blood pressure", or an acronym such as "ARF" that could mean "Acute Renal Failure" or "Acute Rheumatic Fever." The more unsystematic the progress notes, the less intelligible the notes will become. Some of the common contributors to unsystematic medical records are— abbreviation, misspelling, and punctuation errors.

Timeliness of actions cannot be defended if chronological documentation of the same is not done. Chronological entries present a clear picture of the sequence of care provided and events over time and facilitate better communication amongst and between the care providers. Late entries should be appropriately recorded as soon as possible so as to rectify the absence of entries. Many physicians complain that they do not have the time to write sufficient records! It is suggested that such professionals should ask themselves, "Would you rather spend the time in court for weeks or even months?"

In Nihal Kaur vs. Director, PGI, Chandigarh, the State Commission held negligence on the basis of the records, which seemed to be manipulated. In this case, timeliness of the events could not be defended due to manipulation in the documentation.[8] In *Sethuraman Subramaniam Iyer vs. Triveni Nursing Home,* the allegation of tampering with the operation notes was negated by the State Commission in a case of intraoperative death as the complainant could not prove the allegation. Proper documentation is always beneficial to the doctor.[9]

It is always advisable to write complete name of the patient on each and every medical document, as serious cases of negligence have been reported due to wrong medication due to mixing up of patient's name. Writing common names, and that too shorter ones, such as Raja, Swamy, John, and so on, must be strictly avoided and the full name must be written. In *Mrs. Suman & Ors. vs. Government Multi-Speciality Hospital & Ors.* case, wrong blood was transfused to the patients of the same part of name.[10]

Illegible Medical Documentation

Illegible documentation can have adverse impact on patient care, as it may result in improper medical treatment or dispensing of the wrong medication. If the clinical note is not readable due to penmanship or articulation then it serves no purpose and can do more harm than benefit. In court, the healthcare provider can be asked to read the medical records. Countless times, caregivers have not been able to read aloud what they authored in the medical documents. It is advisable to write legibly in the medical records of the patient, never use whitener, never scratch out, draw a line through the mistake, and any alteration must be countersigned along with date and time.

Medical Council of India Guidelines on Prescription Writing

The clause 1.5 of the Indian Medical Council (Professional Conduct, Etiquette and Ethics) Regulations, 2002 has been amended in 2016 and notified in the Gazette of India on 21.09.2016, which read as:

Use of Generic names of Drugs: Every physician should prescribe drugs with generic names legibly and preferably in capital letters and he/she shall ensure that there is a rational prescription and use of drugs.[11]

Use of Unsafe Abbreviations

Use of unapproved abbreviations has led to many medical errors. Often, patients or relatives do not understand the abbreviations commonly used by healthcare providers. For example, patient/relatives may find it hard to understand nil by mouth (NBM), etc. Avoid use of abbreviations other than those approved and documented in organizational policy. Do not depend upon the chemist and use easily understandable language in prescription like once a day, twice a day, etc. Often patient is readmitted because they did not follow the prescription correctly.

■ CLINICAL DOCUMENTATION GUIDELINES

Good clinical notes document all relevant clinical information. Up-to-date clinical notes with sufficient information are very helpful in ensuring that the proper information is provided to all healthcare professionals involved in the treatment. Completeness and continuity in clinical notes is very important in the current medical environment, where many different healthcare professionals are involved in the treatment of a single patient. Structured information which must be included in the clinical records are presented in **Box 1**.[12]

The advantages and disadvantages of keeping good or poor clinical records, respectively, is summarized in **Table 1**.[12]

Guidelines for clinical documentation were summarized in WHO-SEARO coding workshop.[1] The purpose of these guidelines is to support employers, policy makers, managers

---

BOX 1 | **Structured information to be included in clinical records.**

- Patient demographics
- Reasons for the current visit
- The scope of examination
- Positive examination findings
- Relevant negative examination findings
- Key abnormal test findings
- Diagnosis or impression
- Clear management plan and agreed actions
- Treatment details and future treatment recommendations
- Medication administered, prescribed and any drug allergies
- Written (or oral) instructions and/or educational information given to the patient
- Clear documentation and justification for resuscitation status and ceiling of care (if inpatient)
- Documentation of communications with patient and family/friends (level of awareness of the situation and acceptance of the plans)
- Recommended return visit date

TABLE 1: Advantages of good clinical records and disadvantages of poor clinical records.

Good clinical records	Bad clinical records
• Helps in sharing relevant information and multidisciplinary team communication, and thus avoids unnecessary repetition of investigation tests and improves time management • Helps in coordination of care • Helps in continuity of care • Availability of data for risk assessment • Availability of data for route cause analysis of serious incidents • Beneficial in conducting audits • Provide informative evidence to the court	• Misinform healthcare providers and patients • Unnecessary repetition of tests or other investigations • Prolong hospital admission • Adversely affect the patient care • Increased risk of serious incidents • Increased medicolegal risks

and clinical staff in documentation practices and policies that demonstrate the professional obligation, accountability and legal requirements to communicate patient health information and clinical interventions in the public interest. It describes the purpose of professional documentation, maintaining quality documentation practice, documentation policy, clinical competence in relation to documentation, etc. These guidelines elaborate guiding principles for documentation.

Guiding Principle 1: Comprehensive and Complete Record

The guiding principle depicts the principles for documentation by clinical staff as an integral part of medical practice to ensure safe and effective care and describes how comprehensive and complete documentation should be.

Comprehensive and complete documentation and record keeping
- Clear, concise, complete record of clinical care (including assessment, plan of action outcomes and evaluation of care).
- Factual, accurate, true and honest record.
- Avoid duplication of information.
- Legible, permanent, retrievable, confidential, patient-focused.
- Timely and completed as close as possible after episode of care or event.
- Chronological record of care.
- Prefaced with date and time of care or event (including recording of changes or additions).
- Identifying details of person who provided/documented care inclusive of signatures and designation of person recording information.
- Easily interpreted over time and after significant time has elapsed.
- Avoid use of abbreviations (other than those approved in organizational policy).
- Documentation of critical incidents such as patient falls, harm, medication errors, etc.

Guiding Principle 2: Patient Centered and Collaborative

The guiding principle describes the patient-focused documentation. It also emphasizes on collaborative approach. The information may be gathered from various settings within the healthcare system, and clinicians must consider the purpose of documentation and how, by whom and for what purpose the information it to be used.

> **Patient centered documentation and record keeping**
> - Documentation systems and practices appropriate to the specific needs of the patient and context of the care.
> - Appropriate documentation systems to support shared documentation processes.
> - A record of independent and collaborative actions with other health professionals or care providers (e.g., those ordered by another appropriate health professional).
> - Contemporary, secure, resource efficient documentation systems.
> - Documentation systems relevant to the setting in which the care occurs (including patient held records, electronic records and mobile record systems).
> - Individualized, comprehensive and current plan of care.
> - Identifies problems that have arisen and actions taken to rectify/address.
> - Documentation consistent with organization's policy, standards and legislation.
> - Accessible relevant previous/other documentation (including patient history, long- and short-term intervention, diagnostic investigations most recent previous documentation by other clinical staff).
> - Documentation of intervention via telephone (including information obtained and advice given).

Guiding Principle 3: Ensure and Maintain Confidentiality

The guiding principle describes the responsibility of clinician to protect the confidentiality as well as to maintain confidential medical records which is the most essential requirement in the era of electronic record system.

■ KEY POINTS FOR GOOD MEDICAL DOCUMENTATION

In general, the following key points must be considered during the medical documentation:
- *Clear:* Professional documentation by clinical staff is an integral part of practice to ensure safe and effective care. All doctors have professional obligation to form and maintain documents very clearly. Avoid duplication of information. It should be legible and nonerasable.
- *Concise:* Documentation is a record of the care provided, and the judgment and critical thinking used by a health professional in the provision of that care. It should be factual, accurate, true, and honest. Enter date, time, and full name and sign every entry on each page. Put your signature wherever necessary as well as patient's or relative's signature. Be thorough and objective. Only use approved abbreviations. Sometimes clinical staff documents conclusion in place of patient's behavior or circumstances. Example—nurses should avoid statement such as "patient unresponsive" in place of "patient refuses bath" and "patient depressed" in place of "patient shouts."
- *Complete:* Minimum documentation for care provided includes patient identification on each page, how the patient arrived, care that was rendered before arrival, pertinent history, consent, chronological notation of results of physical examination including vital signs and the results of diagnostic and therapeutic procedures and tests. A complete record including completed forms, charts, methods and systems. In *Force vs. M Ganeswara Rao* case, the State Commission held that there was negligence as the case sheet did not contain a proper history, history of prior treatment and investigations, and even the consent papers were missing.[13] In *Anoop Awasthi vs. Dr. T. Kataria* case, it was suggested that the investigation reports must always be in writing except in emergencies.[14]

- *Contemporary:* It suggests doing at the same time. Make entries immediately or soon after care is given or you have findings. If you observe it, listen to it, perform it so, then document it at the earliest. If so, then timeliness and chronology will be maintained itself. If the note is not written on the day of the service, the note must start with "Late note for visit on date of service." Addendum to the chart—addendum is additional entries or appendix to the original records. It is necessary to make an addendum, but before documenting ask yourself if it is a note to enhance the record and provide continuum of care or is it a "cover yourself" note. A progress note written 2 years post care on the day you receive a notice from the lawyer, is not the appropriate time to making an entry.
- *Correct:* Documentation must be accurate. Any incorrect information in the documents would be more harmful during patient care or later on while defending the malpractice lawsuits. Risk management does not advocate to write more, but rather to record the actual facts and findings regarding patient care.
- *Comprehensive:* Documentation acts as evidence of the unique and important contribution of each staff member to healthcare. It forms the basis for evidence of care that can be used for research, legal analysis and determination, allocation of resources and as a primary communication between health professionals. All elements pertaining to patient care should be covered. All aspects of consent or prognosis or treatment, etc. should be explained and recorded in writing. Even document "informed refusal" discussions and document "patients' non-compliance" in the progress record. Any episode of adverse event and your steps toward it should be recorded. If you obtain any info about patient from third party, just record it with his/her details.
- *Collaboration:* Clinical documentation may record diverse information within and across services and settings. Given the diversity of care provided, clinicians must consider the purpose of documentation and how, by whom and for what purpose that information is to be used. Referral notes should be properly addressed. Laboratory and other investigations are appropriately ordered. Documentation is a form of communication: It should be done timely. When an addendum is made it may be necessary to also verbally communicate this information to appropriate caregivers. For example, an addendum reflecting an allergy is not something that should be slipped into the patient's medical record without verbal communication to other caregivers.
- *Patient centric:* Documentation must be patient-focused. It should contain only information relevant to the patient's healthcare. It is important that the patient's response to interventions, not just the intervention itself be described. Medication allergies and adverse reactions are prominently noted. If patient has no allergy, then it is also noted. In *Mrs. Sucheta Sanyal vs. Dr. M. Bhowmik and Anr.*, it was suggested that standard instruction cards about pre- and postintervention precautions should be issued in English or even local language.[15]
- *Confidential:* Clinicians have legislative, professional, and ethical obligations to protect patient confidentiality. It is essential that the confidentiality of that information be safeguarded and shared only as necessary to protect the interests of the person and to ensure the best outcomes of care. This includes maintaining confidential documentation and patient records.
- *Chronological:* Information documented during or immediately after care is provided or an event has occurred is considered to be more reliable and a more accurate record of care or an event than information recorded later, based on memory. Entries in charts and

notes should be in order from very 1st day of patient's admission to last day in hospital. Chronological entries present a clear picture and sequence of care provided and events over time and facilitate better communication amongst and between care providers. If chronology is not maintained, there would be a fear to be exposed at later stage of litigation causing more harm.

■ CRITICAL ISSUES IN MEDICAL DOCUMENTATION

Discharge Notes

Discharge summary is a document that contains vital information, necessary to keep the patient safe after he leaves the hospital. A structured and standard discharge summary form ensures that all the important information is included in the discharge summary. The Joint Commission has established standards outlining the components that each hospital discharge summary should contain. These components are:[16]

- *Reason for hospitalization*:
  - Description of the patient's primary presenting condition; and/or
  - Description of a patient's initial presentation to the hospital admission, including description of the initial diagnostic evaluation.
- *Significant findings*:
  - Primary diagnoses (admission/discharge diagnoses noted in the discharge summary).
- *Treatment provided*:
  - Document the treatment provided to the patient during hospital stay including medical, surgical, invasive, noninvasive, diagnostic, or technical procedures.
- *Patient's condition at the time of discharge*:
  - Discharge summary should include the health status of the patient at discharge.
- *Instructions to the patient*:
  - Medications after the discharge
  - Dietary instructions
  - Precautions to be followed (if any)
  - Plans for follow-up
- *Signature of the treating doctor*:
  - The treating doctor should sign on the discharge summary.

The date and time of all the important events, viz. admission, surgery, discharge, etc., written on the discharge summary proves to be a supportive evidence especially in malpractice lawsuits where the sequence of events is an important point of contention. It is also important to include instructions to be followed by the patient after discharge including dietary advice and date of next follow-up.[17]

It is not uncommon to have patients who get discharged against medical advice. These patients are also entitled to have a discharge summary. It is imperative to record the fact that the doctor advised a course of action with all its implications, if not followed. The fact that the patient understood the implications of discharge against medical advice, but still refused to continue the treatment, must be documented in his medical records. In *Gangapam R Reddy vs. Apollo Hosp*, the discharge summary itself was sufficient to hold that the first operation by the opposite party was done in a most negligent manner.[18] In *Dr. M.L. Deb vs. Rose Mary Lyngdoh* case, the discharge certificate was proved false. The doctor declared live baby brought by its parents as dead and wrote in discharge certificate "brought dead" and was held negligent.[19]

Written Feedback from Patient/Attendants

Taking written feedback at the time of discharge from the patient/attendants is a good practice that can be useful for the hospital in knowing their shortcomings and trying to improve upon based on the feedback. Written feedback can also be used as a documentary proof in legal proceedings. In *B. Gopal Reddy vs. Bollineni Eye Hospital and Research Centre and Ors.* case, the hospital specifically pointed out in defense that the patient as well as his daughter endorsed in the patient feedback register about the excellent performance of the surgery.[20] In *N. Shrivastava vs. S. Shrivastava* case, there was an endorsement in death book in complainant's own handwriting and sign that he has no complaint against the *"Karmacharis"* of the hospital. Commission also stated that doctor should be included as *"Karmachari"* of hospital.[21]

Issuing Medical Certificate

Issuing medical certificates is an integral part of the duty of registered medical practitioners. All medical certificates are legal documents and must be issued cautiously. Casual issuance of medical certificates may be considered as issuance of false certificates, and thus, the doctor shall be liable to punishment and may entail cancellation of his registration with the medical council. The certificate should be based on facts known to the doctor. Copy of the certificate must be kept for record, as the doctor may be summoned by the court to testify the correctness of the certificate. It is mandatory to write identification marks, and get signatures/thumb impression of the patient on the certificate. Always mention your name along with registration number. It should also bear the seal. Writing anywhere on the medical certificate "not valid for legal or court purposes" is legally invalid, and thus such practice must be avoided. As per the directions of the Medical Council of India, all laboratory reports must be signed/countersigned by registered medical practitioners.[22]

The important issue of issuance of medical certificate by registered medical practitioners has been addressed in the Indian Medical Council (Professional Conduct, Etiquette and Ethics) Regulations, 2002 as depicted in **Box 2**.[6]

The Delhi Medical Council has framed guidelines for issuance of medical certificate in its order DMC/DC/F.14/Comp.1107/2/2014/ dated 17th October, 2014 (**Box 3**).[23]

Documenting Adverse Events

An adverse event is a negative consequence of the care provided to the patient that resulted in unintended injury or illness which may or may not have been preventable. A preventable adverse event is an event that could have been avoided in a particular set of circumstances. An unpreventable adverse event is an adverse event that results from a complication that cannot be prevented under the current state of knowledge.

BOX 2 — Medical Council of India (MCI) code of ethics regulations related to issuing of medical certificates.

- Rule 1.3.3: Maintain a register of certificates with the full details of medical certificates issued with at least one identification mark of the patient and his signature
- Rule 7.3: Not displaying registration number in his/her clinic, prescriptions and certificates, etc., issued by him/her can amount to professional misconduct
- Rule 7.7: Signing any professional certificates, reports and other documents that are untrue, misleading or improper can amount to professional misconduct

BOX 3: Guidelines by Delhi Medical Council for issuance of medical certificate.

- Medical certificates are legal documents. Medical practitioners who deliberately issue a false, misleading or inaccurate certificate could face disciplinary action under the Indian Medical Council (Professional Conduct, Etiquette and Ethics), Regulations, 2002. Medical practitioners may also expose themselves to civil or criminal legal action. Medical practitioners can assist their patients by displaying a notice to this effect in their waiting rooms

  It is, therefore, a misnomer to state that medical certificate is "not valid for legal or Court purposes", and should be avoided. Registered medical practitioners are legally responsible for their statements and signing a false certificate may result in a registered medical practitioner facing a charge of negligence or fraud

- The certificate should be legible, written on the doctor's letterhead and should not contain abbreviations or medical jargon. The certificate should be based on facts known to the doctor. The certificate may include information provided by the patient but any medical statements must be based upon the doctor's own observations or must indicate the factual basis of those statements. The Certificate should only be issued in respect of an illness or injury observed by the doctor or reported by the patient and deemed to be true by the doctor

  The certificate should:
  - Indicate the date on which the examination took place
  - Indicate the degree of incapacity of the patient as appropriate
  - Indicate the date on which the doctor considers the patient is likely to be able to return to work
  - Be addressed to the party requiring the certificate as evidence of illness, e.g., employer, insurer, magistrate
  - Indicate the date the certificate was written and signed
  - Name, signature, qualifications and registered number of the consulting registered medical practitioner
  - The nature and probable duration of the illness should also be specified. This certificate must be accompanied by a brief resume of the case giving the nature of the illness, its symptoms, causes and duration. When issuing a sickness certificate, doctors should consider whether or not an injured or partially incapacitated patient could return to work with altered duties

- The medical certificate under normal circumstances, as a rule, should be prospective in nature, i.e., it may specify the anticipated period of absence from duty necessitated because of the ailment of the patient. However, there may be medical conditions which enable the medical practitioner to certify that a period of illness occurred prior to the date of examination. Medical practitioners need to give careful consideration to the circumstances before issuing a certificate certifying a period of illness prior to the date of examination, particularly in relation to patients with a minor short illness which is not demonstrable on the day of examination and should add supplementary remarks, where appropriate, to explain the circumstances which warranted the issuances of certificate retrospective in nature

- It is further observed that under no circumstances, a medical certificate should certify period of absence from duty, for a duration of >15 days. In case the medical condition of the patient is of such a nature that it may require further absence from duty, then in such case a fresh medical certificate may be issued
  - Record of issuing medical certificate—Documentation should include:
  - Patient to put signature/thumb impression on the medical certificate
  - Identification marks to be mentioned on medical certificate
  - That a medical certificate has been issued
  - The date/time range covered by the medical certificate
  - The level of incapacity (i.e., unfit for work, light duties, etc., within scope of practice)
  - Signature/thumb impression of patient

An official serially numbered certificate should be utilized. The original medical certificate is given to the patient to provide the documentary evidence for the employer. The duplicate copy will remain in the Medical Certificate book for records. The records of medical certificate are to be retained with the doctor for a period of 3 years from the date of issue

In case a patient experiences an incident or adverse event while in the healthcare system, it must be ensured that the full details about the event are noted in the patient's record as quickly as possible after the event has occurred, including that the patient and/or individuals designated by the patient have been told about the incident or adverse event. The medical record must reflect objectively, what happened, what information was shared with the patient/attendant along with their response, plan of action or intervention done to address the event.

Documenting Instructions to the Patient

Document all instructions with or about the patient, face-to-face or over the phone. The record serves as log of communication providing insight into what was said, when it was said, specifically to whom it was said and their response. You do not want patient saying, "I never saw a physician the whole time I was in the hospital." You do not want patients blaming you for a bad outcome when their noncompliance played a role in their health.

Documenting Patient's Refusal

If a patient refuses a clinical intervention of any sort, the refusal and any reasons offered must be documented in the clinical record along with the signatures of the patient/attendant, and a witness. Sometimes patient/attendants may totally refuse to sign anywhere, neither approval for consent nor denial of consent. In such a situation, this fact must be specifically documented in prescription, discharge cards and such medical documents. Hospital having video-recording facility should use the same in such situations. In *Reshma Devi Yadav vs. Dr. Mrs. Reeta Bagchi* case, a copy of the referral slip, which the attendants had refused to sign, was produced in the court. The court rejected the allegation on the doctor.[24]

■ CONCLUSION

The doctor-patient relationship is the foundation stone of healthcare system and the practice of medicine. In current era, this relationship has become more formal and structured, and its fiduciary character is at its worst. The society thinks that medical profession is being guided only by the profit motive rather than that of service. In such a distrustful relationship if a challenging situation arises during patient care, chances of allegation of negligence are very high. A malpractice lawsuit can ruin the doctor's career and practice. Similar to the profession of medicine, law is an inexact science, and one cannot predict with certainty an outcome of cases many a time. The axiom "you learn from your mistakes" is too little honored in medicolegal scenarios. The best way to handle medicolegal issues is by preventing them. Effective management of medicolegal risk requires more than simply providing the best possible quality care. Before the care is provided, proper communication is the key to manage the unrealistic expectations of the patients and their families. Always keep in mind that quality documentation has beneficial role in patient care as well as court proceedings. Medical record is the only evidence which stands strong during legal proceedings that informs the care provided to the patient. A clear understanding of a complete and correct documentation helps a physician in issues pertaining to the medical negligence.

REFERENCES

1. Guidelines for Medical Record and Clinical Documentation. WHO-SEARO Coding Workshop. 2007. [online] Available from https://occupationaltherapy2012.files.wordpress.com/2012/03/2007_guidelines_for_clinical_doc.pdf. [Last accessed August, 2019].
2. Ngo E, Patel N, Chandrasekaran K, et al. The importance of the medical record: a critical professional responsibility. J Med Pract Manage. 2016;31(5):305-8.
3. Rayamane AP, Nanandkar SD, Kundargi PA. Profile of medical negligence cases in India. J Indian Acad Forensic Med. 2016;38(2):144-8.
4. Gowda SL, Bhandiwad A, Anupama NK. Litigations in obstetric and gynecological practice: can it be prevented? A probability to possibility. J Obstet Gynaecol India. 2016;66(Suppl 1):541-7.
5. Yankowsky KW. Avoiding unnecessary litigation: communication and documentation. Adv Skin Wound Care. 2017;30(2):66-70.
6. Indian Medical Council (Professional Conduct, Etiquette and Ethics) Regulations, 2002. [online] Available from https://mciindia.org/ActivitiWebClient/rulesnregulations/codeofMedicalEthicsRegulations2002. [Last accessed August, 2019].
7. Meenakshi Mission Hospital and Research Centre v. Samuraj and Anr., I(2005) CPJ (NC) The National Commission.
8. Nihal Kaur vs. Director, PGI, Chandigarh. 1996;3 CPJ 112 (Chandigarh (UT) CDRC).
9. Sethuraman Subramaniam Iyer v Triveni Nursing Home. 1997;2 CPR 144 (NC); I (1998) CPJ 10 (NC); 1998 CTJ 7 (CP) (NCDRC); 1998 CCJ 1532 (NC).
10. Mrs. Suman & Ors. v/s Government Multi-Speciality Hospital & Ors.(5MLCD a34; j85 – March 2012).
11. Medical Council of India vide circular no. MCI-211(2) (Gen.)/ 2017-Ethics/ 104728 dated 21.04.2017.
12. Mathioudakis A, Rousalova I, Gagnat AA, et al. How to keep good clinical records. Breathe (Sheff). 2016;12(4):369-73.
13. Force v. M Ganeswara Rao. 1998;3 CPR 251; 1998 (1) CPJ 413 (AP SCDRC).
14. Anoop Awasthi v Dr. T. Kataria on 18 March 2016- Consumer Case No. 84 of 2002.
15. Mrs. Sucheta Sanyal v Dr. M. Bhowmik & Anr on 5 May 2014- Consumer Case- 25(2002).
16. Joint Commission on the Accreditation of Healthcare Organizations. Hospital Accreditation Standards. Standard IM.6.10, EP 7. [online] Available from: http://www.jointcommission.org/NR/rdonlyres/A9E4F954-F6B5-4B2D-9ECF-C1E792BF390A/0/D_CurrenttoRevised_DC_HAP.pdf. [Last accessed August, 2019].
17. Thomas J. Medical records and issues in negligence. Indian J Urol. 2009;25(3):384-8.
18. Gangapam R Reddy v Apollo Hosp. 2003 (1) CLD 494 (AP SCDRD).
19. Dr. M. L. Deb v Rose Mary Lyngdoh. 2004 (3) CPJ 744, 2004 (3), CPR 29: 2005 (1) CTJ 825 (Meghalaya SCDRC).
20. B. Gopal Reddy v/s Bollineni Eye Hospital and Research Centre & Ors. (6MLCD a1; j1 – January 2013).
21. N. Shrivastava v S. Shrivastava. 2003 (6) CLD 482 (UP SCDRC).
22. Medical Council of India circular No. MCI-211(2) (Gen.)/2014-Ethics/118642, dated 14/06/17.
23. Singhania MA. Guidelines for Issuing a Medical Certificate. [online] Available from: https://medicaldialogues.in/guidelines-for-issuing-a-medical-certificate/. [Last accessed August, 2019].
24. Resham Devi Yadav vs Dr. Mrs. Reeta Bagchi& Ors. 9 MLCD (j132). P. 21-22.

SECTION 5
Litigation Against Medical Practitioners: Let's Take the Bull by the Horns

Chapter 13 Medical Negligence: Meaning, Scope and Legal Interpretation
Chapter 14 How to Defend a Medical Negligence Lawsuit?
Chapter 15 Compensation in Medical Negligence: How much is Justified?
Chapter 16 Professional Indemnity Insurance: Better Safe than Sorry

CHAPTER 13

Medical Negligence: Meaning, Scope and Legal Interpretation

VP Singh, Vivekanshu Verma

> *"To make no mistakes is not in the power of man but from their errors and mistakes - the wise and good learn wisdom for the future."*
> —Plutarch[1]

■ INTRODUCTION

The anguish of medical negligence equally haunts the conscience of medical practitioners as well as the patients. The problem of medical negligence often resurrects as a *cause of action* against the medical practitioners. Most of the patients always have at the forefront of their mind that, 'if complication occurs, it is due to some negligence!' In such a blameworthy environment it is extremely difficult for the medical practitioners to live up to their patient's expectations. It is extremely essential for medical practitioners to have a better understanding of the legal principles related to medical negligence, so that they can live up to the legal expectations and practice their professional skills without any undue stress.

■ WHAT IS MEDICAL NEGLIGENCE?

In everyday usage, the word 'negligence', means absence or lack of care that a reasonable person should have taken in the circumstances of the case. Negligence as a tort is "breach of legal duty to take care which results in damage, undesired by the defendant to the plaintiff."[2] Medical negligence may be defined as, "the act of omission which a reasonably competent medical practitioner, guided by such medical knowledge and practice as is commonly known at the time and at the place where he practices and further guided by such other considerations which ordinarily regulate the conduct of a reasonably competent medical practitioners, would do, or doing something which a reasonably competent medical practitioners would not do." However, deviance from common practice does not necessarily indicate negligence. Similarly a mere accident or error of judgment is also not evidence of negligence.

■ ESSENTIAL COMPONENTS OF MEDICAL NEGLIGENCE

The essential components of medical negligence include: (a) Duty of care toward patient, (b) Dereliction in duty of care, (c) Damage that results to the patient must be reasonably foreseeable, (d) Direct causation (direct relation between the breach in duty of care and the damage).

For any act or omission by a doctor to be considered as medical negligence, all the above mentioned essential components must be proven.

Duty of Care

When a doctor accepts to treat the patient, the doctor-patient relationship is established, and the duty to provide reasonable care starts. Such a duty exists irrespective of the fact whether the doctor charged for his services or provided free treatment, and the doctor can be sued in a civil/criminal court depending upon the facts of the case. However, in case of consumer courts, as per the definition of term, 'service' given by the Sec 2 (1) (o) of the Consumer Protection Act,[3] it does not include the services given free of charge or under 'contract of personal service'. The Supreme Court of India,[4] while explaining the words 'free of charge', observed that the medical practitioners of government hospitals/nursing homes and private doctors/nursing homes broadly fall in three categories:

1. Where services are rendered free of charge to everybody availing the said services
2. Where the charges are required to be paid by everybody availing the services
3. Where charges are required to be paid by persons availing services but certain categories of persons who cannot afford to pay are rendered services free of charge:
    - In case of category (1), doctors and hospitals who render service without any charge whatsoever to every person availing the service would not fall within the ambit of 'service' under Sec 2 (1) (o) of the Act. The payment of token amount for registration purposes would not alter the position in respect of such doctors and hospitals. Thus for category (1), the Consumer Protection Act will not come to the rescue of patients, however, there is no bar from seeking remedy under civil court or criminal court (depending upon the facts of the case).
    - In case of second category, as the services are rendered on payment basis to all the persons, they would clearly fall within the ambit of Sec 2 (1) (o) of the Act.
    - The services rendered by the doctors and hospitals falling in category (3) irrespective of the fact that a part of service is rendered free of charge, would fall within the ambit of 'service' under Sec 2 (1) (o) of the Act.

In certain situations, therapeutic doctor-patient relationship is not established viz., (a) examination for insurance purposes; (b) pre-employment examination; (c) examination in medicolegal cases for assessment of injuries, sexual offenses, etc.; (d) examination in emergency with subsequent referral.[5]

There are situations where the duty of care is imposed upon the doctor as a legal obligation viz. danger to life of any person. The Supreme Court held that, "every doctor, at the governmental hospital or elsewhere, has a professional obligation to extend his services with due expertise for protecting life."[6]

Dereliction in Duty of Care

Nonobservance of due care which is expected from a doctor, in a particular situation tantamount to 'dereliction of duty of care'. The Supreme Court of India laid down that when a doctor is consulted by a patient, the former, namely, the doctor owes to his patient certain duties which are:[7]

- Duty of care in deciding whether to undertake the case
- Duty of care in deciding what treatment to give
- Duty of care in the administration of that treatment.

Ignoring any of these duties, constitute 'dereliction of duty of care'. The care required is that of a reasonable physician.

Damage

A doctor is not liable for every injury suffered by a patient. The liability of a doctor arises when the injury has resulted due to his conduct, which has fallen below that of reasonable care. Damage to the patient must be clearly recognizable by the law, and should have resulted due to dereliction of duty of care by the treating doctor. In case there is no dereliction of duty, the doctor will not be liable. The burden of proof lies on the patient to prove that the damage was due to breach in duty of care by the treating doctor.

Direct Causation

To establish the liability of a doctor for medical negligence, it is must for the plaintiff to prove that there existed a direct relation between the breach in duty of care and the damage. The dereliction in duty must be the actual cause of the damage. There must be a causal link between the conduct of the doctor and the patient's injury. It must be shown that of all the possible reasons for the injury, the breach of duty of the doctor was the most probable cause. It is not sufficient to show that the breach of duty is merely one of the probable causes. Hence, if the possible causes of an injury are the negligence of a third party, an accident, or a breach of duty of care of the doctor, then the plaintiff must prove that the breach of duty of care of the doctor was the most probable cause of the injury.[8] If there are multiple probable causes of injury or sequence of events resulting in injury, it becomes complicated to determine whether dereliction of duty was the actual cause of damage.

■ TYPES OF MEDICAL NEGLIGENCE

Medical Negligence as a Tort

Tort is a civil wrong that results in an injury or harm to the other, and constitute the basis for a claim by the injured party. The primary aim of tort law is to provide relief for the damages incurred and deter others from committing the same harm. Thus medical negligence as tort is the breach of legal duty to take care which results in damage, undesired by the defendant to the plaintiff. The legal remedy for medical negligence under tort law is aimed at providing relief for the damages incurred and to deter others from committing the same harm. It is the amount of damages incurred which determines of the extent of liability in medical negligence under tort law.

Medical Negligence as a Crime

Criminal liability revolves around the maxim *actus non facitreum, nisi mens sit rea,* which means that, "the act alone does not amount to guilt; it must be accompanied by a guilty mind (*mens rea*). The most debatable aspect of criminal negligence is the presumption of *mens rea* in acts constituting negligence. In R vs. Lawrence, Lord Diplock dealt with the concept of recklessness as constituting *mens rea* under criminal law. *Recklessness on the part of the doer of an act presuppose that in the given circumstances, any ordinary prudent individual would have considered that his act could cause such serious harmful consequences that it may be considered as an offence and the risk of occurrence of these serious harmful consequences was not so slight,* to feel justified to treat the act as negligence. The doer of the act is acting recklessly if, before doing the act, he either fails to give any thought to the possibility of there being any such risk or, having recognized that there was such risk, he nevertheless goes on to do it.[9]

To establish the existence of criminal rashness or criminal negligence it must be proved that the rashness was of such a degree as to amount to taking a hazard knowing that the hazard was of such a degree that injury was most likely imminent. The element of criminality is introduced by the accused having run the risk of doing such an act with recklessness and indifference to the consequences. Simple lack of care such as will constitute civil liability is not enough; for purposes of the criminal law, very high degree of negligence is required to be proved. In criminal law, it is not the amount of damages but the amount and degree of negligence that is determinative of liability. To fasten liability in criminal law, the degree of negligence has to be higher than that of negligence enough to fasten liability for damages in civil law.[10]

Negligence *Per Se*

Black's Law Dictionary has defined 'negligence per se' as:

Conduct, whether of action or omission, which may be declared and treated as negligence without any argument or proof as to the particular surrounding circumstances, either because it is in violation of a statute or valid municipal ordinance, or because it is so palpably opposed to the dictates of common prudence that it can be said without hesitation or doubt that no careful person would have been guilty of it. As a general rule, the violation of a public duty, enjoined by law for the protection of person or property, so constitutes.

The Supreme Court of India held that a person who does not have knowledge of a particular system of medicine but practices in that system is a quack. Where a person is guilty of negligence per se, no further proof is needed.[11]

In case of negligence per se, the conduct is automatically considered negligent, and the focus of the suit will be over whether it proximately caused damage to the plaintiff. For the courts to accept negligence per se claim, the plaintiff must show that a law was violated, that the law was intended to prevented the type of injury that occurred, and that the plaintiff was in the class of persons intended to be protected by law.[12]

■ VITAL ISSUES IN MEDICAL NEGLIGENCE

Burden of Proof of Medical Negligence

According to the general principles of law of tort, "the onus of proving negligence lies upon him who alleges it." In case of medical negligence litigation, burden of proof is on patient or the relatives. Burden of proof refers to the obligation of a party to prove its allegations at trial. A charge of professional negligence against the medical professional stands on a different footing from a charge of negligence against the driver of a motor car. The burden of proof is correspondingly greater on the person who alleges negligence against a doctor. It has been held by the Apex Court in catena of judgments that a doctor is not liable for negligence just because someone else of better skill or knowledge would have prescribed a different treatment or operated in a different way. He is not guilty of negligence if he has acted in accordance with the practice accepted as proper by a reasonable body of medical professionals.[4,7,13]

The Supreme Court of India has explained the distinction between the proof of medical negligence required under civil and criminal proceedings. In civil proceedings, a mere preponderance of probability is sufficient, and the defendant is not necessarily entitled to the benefit of every reasonable doubt; but in criminal proceedings, the persuasion of guilt must amount to such a moral certainty as convinces the mind of the Court, as a reasonable man, beyond all reasonable doubts.[14]

In cases where the doctrine of 'res-ipsa-loquitur' (*thing speaks for itself*) applies, the burden of proof shifts from the complainant to the doctor who has to prove that damage did not occur due to his negligence. The doctrine of *res-ipsa-loquitur* assumes negligence from the very nature of an accident or injury, in the absence of direct evidence on how any defendant behaved. An extreme example would be leaving scalpel inside abdomen of the patient during surgery or amputation of the wrong limb. The patient is exempted from the responsibility of proving the negligence of the defendant doctor. However, to invoke this doctrine, a plaintiff has to show that:[15]

- Evidence of the actual cause of the injury is not obtainable
- The injury was not possible in the absence of negligence by someone
- The plaintiff was not responsible for his or her own injury
- The defendant had exclusive control of the instrumentality that caused the injury
- The injury could not occur by any instrumentality other than that over which the defendant had control.

The principle of *res-ipsa-loquitur* has not been generally followed by the consumer courts in India or even by the Apex Court in deciding the cases under the Consumer Protection Act.[13] In Jacob Mathew vs. State of Punjab,[10] the Apex Court held that, "res-ipsa-loquitur is only a rule of evidence and operates in the domain of civil law specially in cases of torts and helps in determining the onus of proof in actions relating to negligence...Inference as to negligence may be drawn from proved circumstances by applying the rule if the cause of the accident is unknown and no reasonable explanation as to the cause is coming forth from the defendant. It cannot be pressed in service for determining per se the liability for negligence within the domain of criminal law. Res-ipsa-loquitur has, if at all, a limited application in trial on a charge of criminal negligence...In criminal proceedings, the burden of proving negligence as an essential ingredient of the offence lies on the prosecution. Such ingredient cannot be said to have been proved or made out by resorting to the said rule."

In Achutrao Haribhau Khodwa and Ors vs. State of Maharashtra and Ors,[16] *facts of the case in nutshell are that*: Chandrikabai was admitted to the government hospital where she delivered a child on 10th July, 1963. She had a sterilization operation on 13th July, 1963. Complications arose thereafter which resulted in a second operation on 19th July, 1963. Her condition did not improve, and ultimately she died on 24th July, 1963. Both Dr Divan and Dr Purandare have stated that the cause of death was peritonitis. *The Supreme Court held that*, "In the present case the facts speak for themselves. Negligence is writ large....In a case like this the doctrine of res ipsa loquitur clearly applies. Chandrikabai had a minor operation on 13th July, 1963 and due to the negligence of respondent no. 2, a mop (towel) was left inside her peritoneal cavity....The formation of pus leaves no doubt that the mop left in the abdomen caused it, and it was the pus formation that caused all the subsequent difficulties. There is no escape from the conclusion that the negligence in leaving the mop in Chandrikabai's abdomen during the first operation led, ultimately, to her death. But for the fact that a mop was left inside the body, the second operation on 19th July, 1963 would not have taken place."

Yardstick used to determine Medical Negligence: The Bolam's Rule
To determine whether the conduct of a medical professional is negligent or not, the Indian courts have widely accepted, the Bolam's rule. This rule has been invariably applied to as touchstone to test the pleas of medical negligence. The Bolam's rule states that:[10]

"Where you get a situation which involves the use of some special skill or competence, then the test as to whether there has been negligence or not is not the test of the man on the top of a Clapham Omnibus, because he has not got this special skill. The test is the standard of the ordinary skilled man exercising and professing to have that special skill. A man need not possess the highest expert skill; it is well established law that it is sufficient if he exercises the ordinary skill of an ordinary competent man exercising that particular art."

In Maynard vs. West Midlands Regional Health Authority, it was held that, "it is not enough to show that there is a body of competent professional opinion which considers that decision of the defendant professional was a wrong decision, if there also exists, a body of professional opinion, equally competent, which supports the decision as reasonable in the circumstances. It is not enough to show that subsequent events show that the operation need never have been performed, if at the time the decision to operate was taken, it was reasonable, in the sense that a responsible body of medical opinion would have accepted it as proper."[17]

In Hunter vs. Hanley, it was held that, "in the realm of diagnosis and treatment there is ample scope for genuine difference of opinion and one man clearly is not negligent merely because his conclusion differs from that of other professional men. The true test for establishing negligence in diagnosis or treatment on the part of a doctor is whether he has been proved to be guilty of such failure as no doctor of ordinary skill would be guilty of if acting with ordinary care. Differences of opinion and practice exist, and will always exist, in the medical as in other professions. A court may prefer one body of opinion to the other, but that is no basis for a conclusion of negligence. A judge's preference for one body of distinguished professional opinion to another also professionally distinguished is not sufficient to establish negligence in a practitioner whose actions have received the seal of approval of those whose opinions, truthfully expressed, honestly held, were not preferred."[18]

Reasonable Care

It is a legal requirement that a medical practitioner will bring to his task a reasonable degree of skill and knowledge and must exercise a reasonable degree of care. Reasonable degree of care and skill is the care and competence which an ordinary competent member of the profession (who professes to have those skills) would exercise in the circumstance in question. Important points regarding reasonable degree of skill and care required by a medical practitioner are as follows:[10]

- The practitioner must bring to his task a reasonable degree of skill and knowledge, and must exercise a reasonable degree of care.
- Neither highest nor a very low degree of care and competence (judged in the light of the particular circumstances of each case) is required by the law.
- A medical practitioner is not liable in negligence because someone else of greater skill and knowledge would have prescribed different treatment or operated in a different way.
- A medical practitioner is not guilty of negligence if he has acted in accordance with a practice accepted as proper by a responsible body of medical men skilled in that particular art, even though a body of adverse opinion also existed among medical men.
- Deviation from normal practice is not necessarily evidence of negligence. To establish liability on that basis it must be shown that:
  - There is a usual and normal practice
  - The defendant has not adopted it
  - The course in fact adopted is one no professional man of ordinary skill would have taken had he been acting with ordinary care.

- While assessing the practice adopted by the doctor, the standard of care, is to be judged in the light of knowledge available at the time (of the incident), and not at the date of trial.
- When a charge of negligence arises out of failure to use some particular equipment, the charge would fail if the equipment was not generally available at that point of time on which it is suggested as should have been used.
- A mere accident or an error of judgment on the part of a professional is not negligence per se. Higher the acuteness in emergency and higher the complication, more are the chances of error of judgment. At times, the professional is confronted

■ CRIMINAL LIABILITY OF MEDICAL PROFESSIONALS

Doctors never intend to kill their patients, and thus do not possess the guilty state of mind (*mens rea*), required to be proved for criminal liability. However, if a doctor's conduct can be proved as 'gross negligence' or 'recklessness', then *mens rea* shall be presumed, and the doctor will be held liable for criminal negligence.

If a patient dies due to 'gross' negligence of the doctor, then the latter is liable to be punished under Sec 304 A of the Indian Penal Code (causing death by a rash or negligent act). Supreme Court of India held that, the degree of negligence required to be proved against a doctor in case of criminal negligence (especially u/s 304 A IPC) should be so high that it can be described as 'gross negligence' or 'recklessness', not merely lack of necessary care.[19]

The Supreme Court distinguished between negligence, rashness, and recklessness. A negligent person is one who inadvertently commits an act of omission and violates a positive duty. A person who is rash knows the consequences but foolishly thinks that they will not occur as a result of her/his act. A reckless person knows the consequences but does not care whether or not they result from her/his act. Any conduct falling short of recklessness and deliberate wrongdoing should not be the subject of criminal liability.[11] Thus a doctor cannot be held criminally responsible for a patient's death unless it is shown that she/he was negligent or incompetent, with such disregard for the life and safety of his patient that it amounted to a crime against the State.[20]

Certain provisions of Indian Penal Code (Sec 87, 88, 89 and 92 IPC) provide immunity against criminal prosecutions to the doctor who acts in good faith and for the patient's benefit. However, such immunity is available if the doctor acted in good faith and for the patient's benefit. If a doctor who consciously or knowingly did not use sterilised equipment for an operation cannot be said to have acted in good faith.

Guidelines: Prosecution of Doctors for Criminal Rashness or Criminal Negligence

In Jacob Mathew's case,[10] the Supreme Court of India laid down certain guidelines for the future which should govern the prosecution of doctors for offences of which criminal rashness or criminal negligence is an ingredient.
- A private complaint may not be entertained unless the complainant has produced prima facie evidence before the Court in the form of a credible opinion given by another competent doctor to support the charge of rashness or negligence on the part of the accused doctor.
- The investigating officer should, before proceeding against the doctor accused of rash or negligent act or omission, obtain an independent and competent medical opinion preferably from a doctor in government service qualified in that branch of medical practice, which can normally be expected to give an impartial and unbiased opinion applying Bolam's test to the facts collected in the investigation.

- A doctor accused of rashness or negligence, may not be arrested in a routine manner. Unless his arrest is necessary for furthering the investigation or for collecting evidence or unless the investigation officer feels satisfied that the doctor proceeded against would not make himself, available to face the prosecution unless arrested, the arrest may be withheld.

■ CONCLUSION

Medical science is not an exact science. Circumstances do occur when in spite of providing due care and diligence, error in judgment occurs and the patient gets harmed. In such circumstances, it is extremely important to ensure that the doctor-patient relationship is not affected. Physicians must realize that providing best possible care is not sufficient, as the patients may still remain unsatisfied. Proper counseling of the patients and shared decision making is the need of the hour. In today's world of consumerism, blaming is a fairly common response to dissatisfaction associated with the healthcare received. If a patient blames negligence against a physician in a court of law, there is a pre-existing bias against a doctor. When outcome of the standard followed by the doctor is already known, evaluation of the standard followed is subject to biased opinion (outcome bias). Similarly a hindsight bias may affect the medical expert evaluating the medical negligence, who may falsely believe that, he could have predicted the outcome in advance and would have acted differently to prevent it.[21] In such a scenario it is extremely important for medical practitioners to understand the underlying legal principles applied to evaluate the complicated issue of medical negligence.

■ REFERENCES

1. Lucius Mestrius Plutarchus, a Roman Historian. Available: *https://www.goodreads.com/quotes/166102-to-make-no-mistakes-is-not-in-the-power-of.*
2. Blyth vs. Birmingham Waterworks Co. Exchequer, 11 Exch. 781.
3. Consumer Protection Act, Act 62 of 2002.
4. IMA vs. VP Shantha. AIR 1996 SC 550.
5. Tiwari S. Medicolegal Problems. Indian Pediatrics 2005;(42):575-6.
6. Parmanand Katara vs. Union of India. AIR 1989 SC 2039.
7. Dr. Laxman Balakrishna Joshi vs. Dr. Trimbak Bapu Godbole and Anr. 1969 SCR(1)206.
8. Joga Rao SV. Medical negligence liability under the consumer protection act: a review of judicial perspective. Indian J Urol. 2009;25 (3):361-71.
9. 1981 (1) All ER 974 HL.
10. R vs. Lawrence. AIR 2005 SC 3180.
11. Poonam Verma vs. Ashwin Patel and Ors. 1996; SCC(4):322.
12. Porat A. Symposium: Third restatement of torts: expanding liability for negligence per-se. Wake Forest Law Review. 2009;44:979-96.
13. Smt. Savitri Singh vs. Dr. Ranbir PD Singh and Ors. 2004 CPJ 25 (Bihar).
14. Syad Akbar vs. State of Karnataka. 1980 SCC(1)30.
15. Proving fault in medical malpractice cases. Available:*http://injury.findlaw.com/medical-malpractice/proving-fault-in-medical-malpractice-cases.html.*
16. AIR 1996 SC 2377.
17. Achutrao Haribhau Khodwa and Ors vs. State of Maharashtra and Ors. 1985 1 All ER 635 (HL)
18. Maynard vs. West Midlands Regional Health Authority. 1955 SLT 213.
19. Hunter vs. Hanley. (2004) 6 SCC 422.
20. R vs. Adomako (1994) 3All ER 79.
21. Thomas BH, Sydney WA. Hindsight bias and outcome bias in the social construction of medical negligence: a review. JLM 2009;16:846-57.

CHAPTER 14

How to Defend a Medical Negligence Lawsuit?

VP Singh, MC Gupta

"The key is not the will to win...everybody has that. It is the will to prepare to win... that is important."

—Bob Knight[1]

■ INTRODUCTION

No patient comes to a hospital with intention to sue his physicians. Similarly, physicians have no intention to harm their patients. However, the bitter truth is that in spite of good intentions, medical malpractice litigation is on the rise. Advances in medicine have not only improved the quality of patient care, but there has also been increase in unrealistic expectations from the physicians. Anything less than a complete cure is unsatisfactory. A patient with high expectations is inclined to blame his her physician for the unexpected outcome. A malpractice lawsuit is not just a legal challenge for physicians, but also a professional and psychological outrage.[2] Often, physicians are not familiar with the process of litigation. Fear of the unknown can be more haunting for a busy medical practitioner. Being sued for medical negligence is a major stressful event in physician's life. Most of the physicians head into the process of legal proceedings totally unaware of what is next to follow. It is imperative that physicians must keep themselves well informed and actively participate in their case. Physicians cannot totally assume that their destiny or attorney will save them.

■ PATTERN OF COMPLAINTS AGAINST MEDICAL PRACTITIONERS

In India, patients can seek relief against the medical professionals from multiple agencies at the same time. The complaints may be filed simultaneously at various levels—State Medical Council, Consumer Courts, and Police Station (allegation of criminal negligence). The complainant has a fair chance of getting more compensation from the courts, if the State Medical Council has already given a decision against the doctor. Recently, a devastating trend of lodging an FIR in the police station is emerging, particularly, in cases where the patient dies or suffers a serious harm.

■ COMPLAINTS UNDER CONSUMER PROTECTION ACT: STEP-BYSTEP APPROACH[3]

Consumer Disputes Redressal Forums have been established at different levels (*district, state and national level*) under the Consumer Protection Act (CPA) to provide speedy, less expensive and hassle-free dispute redressal to the consumers. Patients can file a complaint to the consumer court in case of deficiency of service or negligent treatment by the medical practitioner or healthcare establishment. It is important for medical practitioners to know the rules and regulations, and the procedures followed by the consumer courts while deciding the medical negligence lawsuit.

The consumer courts function as *quasi-judicial* courts. In terms of Sec 13(4) of the CPA, District Forums have the same power as are vested in a Civil Court. In terms of Sec 27 of the CPA, Consumer Forums can also act like a first class Judicial Magistrate. Depending upon the amount of compensation claimed, the complaint can be lodged at district forum (upto ₹ 20 lakhs), state commission (₹ 20 lakhs to ₹ 1 crore) or the national commission (> ₹ 1 crore). It is not mandatory to engage an advocate. A patient can lodge a complaint himself or through a representative. To defend a lawsuit, the defendant physician may represent the case personally or through an advocate or an authorized agent.

The Complaint

On receipt of a complaint, the consumer court proceeds as per the provisions of section 12, given here:

(3) On receipt of a complaint made under sub-section (1), the District Forum may, by order, allow the complaint to be proceeded with or rejected:

Provided that a complaint shall not be rejected under this section unless an opportunity of being heard has been given to the complainant:

Provided further that the admissibility of the complaint shall ordinarily be decided within 21 days from the date on which the complaint was received.

Once the complaint is admitted, the consumer forum will refer a copy of the complaint to the opposite party directing him to give his written version against the allegations made in the complaint within 30 days or such extended period not exceeding 15 days as may be granted [Sec. 13(2) (a) Consumer Protection Act]. The consumer court asks both the parties to be present on the date of hearing either personally or through their agents.

Inform the Insurance Company

The first thing a physician should do is to inform his indemnity insurance company about the claim. Reporting the claim is a must to have the insurance company cover your legal expenses and also the amount of compensation awarded against you, if any. Inform the insurance company in writing, along with the copy of the complaint received from the court. At this stage, there is no need to provide the details of the treatment given to the plaintiff patient. It is sufficient to just deny the allegations made in the complaint.

Selection of Defence Lawyer

The physician should read the complaint thoroughly to know the allegations leveled against him. He should also review all the relevant medical records, so as to be well versed with the medical issues involved in the case. At the same time find out in your insurance policy whether you have the right to choose an advocate. If other physicians have also been sued (co-defendants) and the same advocate is representing all the physicians, there is a chance of *conflict of interest*, especially, if your co-defendants were negligent. If your hospital is a co-defendant, and the same advocate is defending both, he may consider the defence tactic which is in favor of your hospital and may not consider the approach which is clearly in your favor but at the detriment to the hospital co-defendant. If you feel that there is a conflict of interest between you and your co-defendants, it is better to request your insurance company to arrange for a separate advocate to represent your case. Often, the insurance companies assign you an advocate without asking your opinion. You need to ask whether you have a right to select the advocate. In case you do not have the right to choose your advocate and you trust any specific attorney to represent your case, then you may hire the advocate at your own expense. However, at the same time, you should also keep in mind the terms of your insurance policy so that the contract remains valid and your case is covered by the company. If you hire your own lawyer, the insurance company may give you a certain amount of money towards legal expenses as per their policy.

Preparing the Written Statement

After the complainant files a complaint and after it has been admitted and notice sent by the consumer forum to the opposite party or OP (the doctor or the hospital), the OP has to file a reply to the same. The reply is often referred to as the written statement. Drafting a written statement has a crucial role in deciding the case and it is advisable for the defendant physician to seek advice of his advocate. The physician should read the complaint thoroughly to know the allegations against him. He should also review all the relevant medical records, so as to be well versed with the medical issues involved in the case. After thoroughly reviewing the allegations and medical issues involved in the case, the defendant physician should provide to his lawyer, a draft reply to all the allegations in the complaint. If he finds any weakness/deficiency in the case, it should be discussed with the defence lawyer. The defendant physician can help a lot to achieve a successful outcome of the trial.

It is advisable that the written statement should be accompanied by medical records and relevant medical literature, etc., from textbooks and journals, etc., to support the defence. It is always a good idea to get signed expert opinions supporting the defence version. If these are in the form of an affidavit, so much the better. However, consumer courts usually do not insist on this and an expert opinion on the letter head of a doctor suffices. Further evidence in the form of medical opinions by medical experts (qualified as the defendant physician) may be submitted as an affidavit.

While selecting the medical literature, it should be thoroughly reviewed, as sometimes any scientific information/epidemiological data that appears to be a good defence, might be contradicted in the next paragraph, thus defeating the whole purpose. Teamwork between the defence lawyer, defendant physician, expert witness, and the insurance company goes a long way in preparing a successful defence for physicians.

Rejoinder and Affidavits

After submission of the reply/written statement by the opposite party or OP, the consumer forum asks the complainant to submit a rejoinder or counter-reply to the same, along with his *Evidence in the form of affidavit* (often referred to simply as the evidence) on the next date. While filing his rejoinder, the complainant has an opportunity to rebut the contentions of the OP and to present any further documents in his support. While filing his affidavit of evidence, the complainant has to present his complete case in the form of a sworn affidavit, duly notarized, and this forms the basis of his case. After the complainant has filed his affidavit, the OP is likewise asked to submit his own affidavit. He is at liberty to annex any further documents to his affidavit in order to support his case.

Examination of Witnesses

Unlike the regular civil or criminal courts, the consumer forums usually do not require the experts, who have already submitted their opinion in writing, to appear before them as witnesses for the purpose of being subjected to examination and cross examination. In a medical negligence case, the NCDRC in its order stated, "wherever there is a prayer for cross-examination of the witnesses by the learned advocates for the parties, learned advocates to produce the interrogatories on record and those interrogatories should be replied by the concerned parties on affidavit. Thereafter, the Commission would decide whether any further cross-examination on any point is necessary or not."[4]

Arguments

Arguments are the last stage of proceedings of a consumer court before passing an order. First of all the complainant party *puts before the court, the details of his allegations and grievances supported by the documentary evidence. Then the defendant party presents their side of the case. The members of the Consumer forum/Commission may put queries to get any clarification.*

Arguments should be on the lines reflected in Regulation 13 of the Consumer Protection Regulations, 2005, reproduced here:
1. Arguments should be as brief as possible and to the point at issue.
2. Where a party is represented by a counsel, it shall be mandatory to file a brief of written arguments 2 days before the matter is fixed for arguments.
3. In case of default to file briefs, the cost shall be imposed at the same rates as laid down for grant of adjournments.

While it is a daily job for lawyers to argue in the courts, it may be once in a life time occasion for the physician. If the physician is defending his own case in person without the help of a lawyer, it would be a good idea for him to be well prepared by having a rehearsal wherein somebody acting as a lawyer of the opposite side asks questions to the defendant physician as if the opposite party's attorney is cross examining the physician. Such rehearsal is expected to overcome the weaknesses present in the defence prepared against the plaintiff's allegations and to make the defendant physician well prepared for the actual arguments.

The Order

After the arguments, the consumer court passes the order in which the complaint is either dismissed or the complainant is awarded damages to be paid by the medical practitioner within a specified period of time. The medical practitioner may also be asked to pay costs to the complainant. In case of noncompliance with the orders of the court, the medical practitioner can be punished with imprisonment varying from 1 month to 3 years, or a fine ranging from ₹ 2000 to ₹ 10,000 or both. The order is sent to both the parties by registered post free of cost.

Appeal

If the complainant or the defendant is not satisfied with the order of the lower court, he can appeal against the order within 30 days from the receipt of the order to the higher court in hierarchy (State Commission or National Commission, as applicable). Only one appeal is allowed under the CPA. If the appeal filed before the state commission is lost, the appellant has a further chance of going to the National Commission by way of filing a revision petition. The final court for adjudication is the Supreme Court whom a party may approach by way of appeal against a complaint decided by the National Commission or by way of a Special Leave Petition (SLP). The drafting of appeal should be done carefully, as the point missed in the appeal will not be considered at a later stage. The appellate court generally considers those points of law in which the lower court has erred. However, important facts of the case may also be considered.

■ FACING THE COURT: MEDICOLEGAL TIPS AND ADVICE

Avoid Talking to the Complainant or his Advocate

Once the case is in the court, do not talk to the complainant or his advocate in a hope to convince them to drop the case. Any communication with the complainant or his advocate outside the legal setting may be misused against you by the opposite party. Your statement might be twisted by the complainant's lawyer to make your intentions look deceitful.[5]

Avoid Fingerpointing

Physician should avoid the blame game among his codefendants. It has been seen that once fingerpointing begins, it takes a bad shape, and invariably the only beneficiary is the complainant. When the defendants blame one another, ultimately someone will be found at fault. The complainant's advocate may play a game to sue everybody in sight and have them turn against each other and someone will fall in trap and found guilty by the court. You might think that pointing finger on your codefendant may help you get out of the case but in reality it may likely ensure your stay in the case as now your codefendants will blame you. However, if you are cornered and you have no option than to reveal the information which may adversely affect your co-defendant, discuss the same with defence attorney before formulating such adverse opinion.[6]

Avoid Alteration or Destruction of Medical Records

Once the case is in the court, any alteration (addition, deletion) or destruction of medical record can lead to disastrous consequences. Many physicians have lost their cases in court of law due to interference with evidence, even when they were otherwise not proved negligent. A physician may think that he may safely make alterations in the medical records as the same was always in his custody and there is no chance that the records could have been photocopied. However, the physician may not realize that the copy of original medical record (prior to alteration), somehow exists somewhere and will resurface during the trial to defeat the defendant physician.

Appearing in a Criminal Case

While there is no procedural requirement that the defendant physician has to answer questions put by the complainant before a consumer court, things are different in a criminal case where a complaint has been filed before the police and the case comes up before a magistrate for trial. In such a case, the defending physician as well as the expert witness may be asked to stand in the witness box and answer questions put up by the lawyer of the complainant. The following tips are suggested for such an occasion:

Avoid answering in Yes or No Manner and Absolute Words

The complainant's advocate may insist upon the defendant physician to reply the question in 'yes' or 'no'. If 'yes' or 'no' does not fairly explain the position, the physician should explain the same, and not limit his answer to just one word. The defendant physician should also try to avoid absolute words like 'always' and 'never'. The complainant's advocate can try to first get an absolute statement from the physician and then show the evidence to counter the physician's statement with a motive to damage his credibility.[7]

Be Calm, Confident, and Professional

Any question asked by the plaintiff's lawyer should be answered by the defendant physician after thoughtful consideration. No matter what is the tactic of plaintiff attorney, there are general rules to be followed while answering the queries. Be calm, confident, and professional but not arrogant. Do not interrupt the questioner as every word used in the question may affect the meaning of the question, and any interruption may cause you to answer incorrectly.

Compound Questions

The complainant's advocate may try to confuse the physician by asking compound questions (multiple queries combined in a single question). Ask for breakdown so that you can answer one part at a time. Take care that you understand the question properly, before giving any answer. In case you are unable to understand the question, ask the complainant's advocate to explain the question.

Tricky Questions

The complainant's advocate may ask a series of questions in order to ultimately prove that the defendant physician missed the diagnosis. For illustration, he may ask:

Q.1: Did you rule out the risk of 'myocardial infarction' before performing the surgery?
Ans: Yes I did it.
Q.2: Did you do ECG?
Ans: No.
Q.3: Then how can you say, that you ruled out myocardial infarction?
Ans: ECG was not indicated.
Q.4: Did you know that the plaintiff died due to acute myocardial infarction suffered 1 day after the surgery?
Ans: Yes.
Q.5: Is ECG not commonly used in the diagnosis of myocardial infarction?

The complainant's advocate will continue such series of questions and will try to confuse you to ultimately tell you that you 'missed' the diagnosis. The defendant physician can better control such attack of questions by asking the complainant's advocate at every stage to explain what he means by phrases like 'ruled out' the diagnosis, 'missed' the diagnosis. After getting the definition of such terms used by the complainant's advocate, the defendant physician must clear the confusion created by explaining the medical condition of the patient (complainant) and the line of management followed by him.

Narrative Questions

The complainant's advocate may make a long statement before asking the actual question. In such a situation, if the defendant physician answers the question, the court may presume that he agreed to the whole statement made by the complainant's advocate. In such a situation, where a question is preceded by a statement, ask for clarification of the statement and the actual question asked.

Open-ended Questions

The complainant's advocate may try to prompt the physician to volunteer the information not called for in the question by asking open-ended questions. If the physician volunteers some information, there is a possibility that the complainant's advocate will try to use the volunteered statement against the physician. It is advisable to give 'brief' and 'relevant' replies to open-ended questions.

During a long and burdensome cross examination, the physician may make a mistake or misstatement. The physician should get the incorrect statement corrected by the court at the earliest. The complainant's advocate may quickly challenge you on your mistake before you have an opportunity to correct it. In that case, admit your error graciously so as to maintain your credibility.[8]

■ CONCLUSION

In spite of providing the best possible care to their patients, and practicing the risk management strategies, there is still a possibility that medical negligence litigation may occur. Although malpractice lawsuit is a haunting nightmare for the medical practitioners, most of the physicians are usually unfamiliar with the process of litigation. It is imperative that physicians must keep themselves well informed about the stages of court proceedings and how to handle the overbearing problem of litigation head on by following well-prepared step-by-step approach.

■ REFERENCES

1. Available: *http://izquotes.com/quote/244489*.
2. Brunken JD. Five ways doctors can better prepare for, survive malpractice lawsuits. Available: *www.physicianspractice.com/blog/five-ways-doctors-can-better-prepare-for-survive-malpractice-lawsuits*.
3. Consumer Protection Act-Act 62 of 2002.
4. Smt. Indrani Bhattacharjee vs CMO Prakka Super Thermal Power and Ors (O.P. No. 233 of 1996) Available: *http://www.consumercom.nic.in/op23396.html*.
5. Surviving a deposition. Available: *http://adrr.com/law1/survive.htm*.
6. Seibel RC, Eckenrode JT. Defending medical malpractice lawsuits, trying the "gray area" cases. Available: *www.eckenrode-law.com/resources/defending_med_malpractice.pdf*.
7. Babitsky S, Mangraviti J. Advice for experts facing cross-examination. Available: *www.economica.ca/ew04_2p1.htm*.
8. Brenner IR. How to survive a medical malpractice lawsuit: the physician's roadmap for success. West Sussex UK: Wiley-Blackwell, 2010.

CHAPTER 15

Compensation in Medical Negligence: How Much is Justified?

VP Singh, Mukesh Yadav

> *"When will our consciences grow so tender that, we will act to prevent human misery rather than avenge it?"*
> —Eleanor Roosevelt[1]

■ INTRODUCTION

The Supreme Court's verdict of granting ₹ 11.41 crore compensation in Kunal Saha's case[2] has shocked the medical fraternity. There is an apprehension amongst the medical fraternity that the Apex Court has set an alarming standard regarding the quantum of compensation and the effect of this judgment may result in a culture of awarding sky-rocketing compensation in medical negligence cases. There is a feeling of insecurity amongst doctors, which may stop them from taking decisions at crucial moments fearing that, *if things go wrong, they would be dragged to court.* The Indian Medical Association urged the Supreme Court to review its decision in Kunal Saha's case. *The IMA National president Dr Jitendra B Patel told the media, The IMA is not against punishment to the guilty but is of the view that the quantum of punishment is such that it might become restraining for others to join this profession.*[3]

■ COMPENSATION IN MEDICAL NEGLIGENCE

In cases, where medical negligence has been established by Court of law, the guilty must be held liable depending on the degree of negligence. A gross negligence may be penalized as per the criminal law, and at the same time, *exemplary* compensation may also be awarded. In cases where negligence is not gross, only compensation is awarded as per the civil law.

The huge sum of compensation awarded by the Supreme Court in Kunal Saha's case of medical negligence has once again resurrected the issue of just compensation to be decided by the courts.[2] Doctors and their lawyers argue that, "the multiplier method as applicable in no-fault motor vehicle accident cases should also be used for determining the quantum of compensation to be paid in medical negligence cases. For uniformity, objectivity and effective disposal of medical negligence cases, multiplier method is appropriate." However, the counter version that opposes the multiplier method in medical negligence cases is that, "loss of human life in a no-fault motor vehicle accident and due to medical negligence are two very different issues, and must be dealt in different manner. The same method (multiplier method) cannot be used for determining the quantum of compensation in medical negligence cases."

Multiplier Method: Can it be Used in Medical Negligence Cases?

Multiplier's method is well accepted to determine the quantum of compensation in deaths due to no-fault accidents under motor vehicles law. It ensures uniformity and consistency. The Supreme Court discussed this method in detail in *Sarla Verma's case*.[4]

In this method, the quantum of compensation is determined using two numbers:
1. The multiplier
2. The multiplicand

The multiplicand is the amount of every year's loss of earning minus the amount the victim would have spent on himself, and the other number, the multiplier is the difference between the average life, as per the life-expectancy data available, and the age of the deceased minus the number of years for which he would be unproductive, and also taking into account any other risk factors of bad health, accident, etc., which would have shortened the productive age without any negative contribution of medical negligence.

Multiplier's formula for determination of compensation
- Loss of earning per year = Y
- Average life of a similar person as the deceased = A
- Age of the deceased = D
- Multiplier will not be (A–D), but much less than this number
- Multiplier = M
- Compensation = Y x M and not [Y x (A–D)]

In Susamma Thomas's case[5] the Supreme Court stated that, basically only three facts need to be established by the claimants for assessing compensation in the case of death:
- Age of the deceased
- Income of the deceased
- Number of dependents.

The issues to be determined by the Tribunal to arrive at the loss of dependency are:
- Additions/deductions to be made for arriving at the income.
- Deduction to be made towards the personal living expenses of the deceased.
- Multiplier to be applied with reference of the age of the deceased.

If these determinants are standardized, there will be uniformity and consistency in the decisions. To have uniformity and consistency, tribunals should determine compensation in cases of death by the following well-settled steps:

Step 1: Ascertaining the Multiplicand

The income of the deceased per annum should be determined. Out of the said income a deduction should be made in regard to the amount which the deceased would have spent on himself by way of personal and living expenses. The balance, which is considered to be the contribution to the dependent family, constitutes the multiplicand.

Step 2: Ascertaining the Multiplier

Having regard to the age of the deceased and period of active career, the appropriate multiplier should be selected. This does not mean ascertaining the number of years, he would have lived or worked but for the accident. Having regard to several imponderables in life and economic factors, a table of multipliers with reference to the age has been identified by this Court. The multiplier should be chosen from the said table with reference to the age of the deceased.

Step 3: Actual Calculation

The annual contribution to the family (multiplicand) when multiplied by such multiplier gives the 'loss of dependency' to the family. Thereafter, a conventional amount in the range of ₹ 5,000 to 10,000 maybe added as loss of estate. Where the deceased is survived by his widow, another conventional amount in the range of ₹ 5,000–10,000 should be added under the head of loss of consortium. But no amount is to be awarded under the head of pain, suffering or hardship caused to the legal heirs of the deceased. The funeral expenses, cost of transportation of the body (if incurred) and cost of any medical treatment of the deceased before death (if incurred) should also added.

Multiplier's Method is not Applicable in Medical Negligence Cases

In *Nizam Institute case*,[6] the Supreme Court did not apply the multiplier method and awarded a compensation of ₹ 1 crore plus interest. The Court held that:

> "*The kind of damage that the complainant has suffered, the expenditure that he has incurred and is likely to incur in the future and the possibility that his rise in his chosen field would now be restricted, are matters which cannot be taken care of under the multiplier method.*"

While deciding against the multiplier method for medical negligence cases, the court explained that, the compensation must be just and adequate, it is extremely difficult to understand their plight, a person who has lost almost complete control over his body, there is a feeling of helplessness and resignation for the person in the entire family. The multiplier method can never do justice in determining adequate and just compensation. The court held that:

> "*The adequate compensation that we speak of, must to some extent, be a rule of the thumb measure, and as a balance has to be struck, it would be difficult to satisfy all the parties concerned .... The case of an injured and disabled person is, however, more pitiable and the feeling of hurt, helplessness, despair and often destitution enures everyday. The support that is needed by a severely handicapped person comes at an enormous price, physical, financial and emotional, not only on the victim but even more soon his family and attendants and the stress saps their energy and destroys their equanimity ....We, have, therefore computed the compensation keeping in mind that his brilliant career has been cut short and there is, as of now, no possibility of improvement in his condition, the compensation will ensure a steady and reasonable income to him for a time when he is unable to earn for himself.*"

In *Kunal Saha's case*[2] also the Supreme Court rejected the multiplier method for determining the quantum of compensation. The court observed:

> "*The multiplier method was provided for convenience and speedy disposal of no fault motor accident cases. Therefore, obviously, a no fault motor vehicle accident should not be compared with the case of death from medical negligence under any condition. The aforesaid approach in adopting the multiplier method to determine the just compensation would be damaging for society for the reason that the rules for using the multiplier method to the notional income of only ₹ 15,000 per year would be taken as a multiplicand. In case, the victim has no income then a multiplier of 18 is the highest multiplier used under the provision of Ss. 163 A of the Motor Vehicles Act read with the Second Schedule . . . . Therefore, if a child, housewife or*

other non-working person fall victim to reckless medical treatment by wayward doctors, the maximum pecuniary damages that the unfortunate victim may collect would be only ₹ 1.8 lakh. It is stated in view of the aforesaid reasons that in today's India, Hospitals, Nursing Homes and doctors make lakhs and crores of rupees on a regular basis. Under such scenario, allowing the multiplier method to be used to determine compensation in medical negligence cases would not have any deterrent effect on them for their medical negligence but in contrast, this would encourage more incidents of medical negligence in India bringing even greater danger for the society at large."

In *Kunal Saha's case*, the Supreme Court further expressed that the strait jacket formula of multiplier's method cannot be applied in medical negligence cases. The Court observed:

"This Court is skeptical about using a strait jacket multiplier method for determining the quantum of compensation in medical negligence claims. On the contrary, this Court mentions various instances where the Court chose to deviate from the standard multiplier method to avoid over-compensation and also relied upon the quantum of multiplicand to choose the appropriate multiplier...this Court requires to determine just, fair and reasonable compensation on the basis of the income that was being earned by the deceased at the time of her death and other related claims on account of death of the wife of the claimant..."

■ HOW MUCH COMPENSATION IS JUST AND ADEQUATE?

In Sarla Verma's case,[4] the Supreme Court clarified just compensation. The court explained:

"Just compensation is adequate compensation which is fair and equitable, on the facts and circumstances of the case, to make good the loss suffered as a result of the wrong, as far as money can do so, by applying the well-settled principles relating to award of compensation. It is not intended to be a bonanza, largesse or source of profit. Assessment of compensation though involving certain hypothetical considerations, should nevertheless be objective. Justice and justness emanate from equality in treatment, consistency and thoroughness in adjudication, and fairness and uniformity in the decision making process and the decisions. While it may not be possible to have mathematical precision or identical awards, in assessing compensation, same or similar facts should lead to awards in the same range. When the factors/inputs are the same, and the formula/legal principles are the same, consistency and uniformity, and not divergence and freakiness, should be the result of adjudication to arrive at just compensation."

In medical negligence cases, damages (compensation) are given to the aggrieved party with intention to relieve the injured party for loss or injury as far as possible by the award of money. Aggravated compensation may be awarded for the non-pecuniary losses such as pain, anguish, grief, etc. The court may award a punitive compensation where it feels that the compensatory damages will not achieve sufficient deterrence and the defendant must be further punished. The consumer courts have discretion for awarding the quantum of compensation, depending on the fact whether the purpose of the damages is compensatory, exemplary or punitive. No uniform guidelines are followed by the courts to determine the quantum of compensation. There is always a chance that exercise of discretion may lead to arbitrariness. The exercise of discretion must be in a reasonable manner so that the decision is just, equitable and prudent.

National Consumer Disputes Redressal Commission observed that for the purpose of Consumer Protection Act, the word *compensation* has a wide connotation as has been provided by the Supreme Court in Ghaziabad Development Authority versus Balbir Singh (2204) 7 CLD

861 (SC). The word *compensation* appearing in Sec 14 (i) (d) of the Act has been explained by the Supreme Court as under:

> *"The word compensation is of a very wide connotation. It may constitute actual loss or expected loss and may extend to compensation for physical, mental or even emotional suffering, insult or injury or loss. The provisions of the Consumer Protection Act enable a consumer to claim and empower the Commission to redress any injustice done. The commission or the forum is entitled to award not only value of goods or services but also to compensate a consumer for injustice suffered by him. The Commission/Forum must determine that such sufferance is due to malafide or capricious or oppressive act. It can then determine amount for which the authority is liable to compensate the consumer for his sufferance due to misfeasance in public office by the officers. Such compensation is for vindicating the strength of law."*

■ IMPACT OF HIGH QUANTUM OF COMPENSATION

Rapidly rising medical malpractice lawsuits have become an issue of increasing concern for physicians. Given the apprehensions of unbearable compensation the Indian doctors will definitely try to follow risk management strategies. The impact of high quantum of compensation may occur in the following manner:

- *Quality healthcare (The desired effect)*: Physicians and healthcare establishments will be more cautious in providing reasonable care to their patients. This will slowly improve the patient safety and quality of healthcare in India.
- *Defensive medicine*: Physicians will start practicing defensive medicine. Such medical practice is done primarily to avert the future possibility of malpractice suits rather than to benefit the patient. Defensive medicine occurs when doctors order extra tests, procedures, or visits (positive defensive medicine) or avoid certain patients or procedures (negative defensive medicine).
- *Medical malpractice insurance*: Physicians will seek financial security against potential malpractice liability by getting professional indemnity insurance. There is high probability that the cost of malpractice insurance will be passed on to the patients, thus resulting in expensive healthcare in India.

■ MEDICAL LIABILITY—A FUTURE CRISIS: LEARNING FROM THE OTHER COUNTRIES

One should learn from one's experience, but there is no good reason to keep reinventing the wheel. Someone else's experience can be a far better teacher. Many other countries have already experienced what Indian healthcare system may have to face in future, *the Medical Malpractice Liability Crisis*. Indian healthcare leaders and policy makers need to brainstorm the effective ways to counter the crisis in the offing.

The Crisis

In United States of America, the *medical malpractice liability crisis* resulted in drastic increase in insurance premiums and reduced access for patients to specialty care. The crisis was not in the malpractice, as there had not been much increase in frequency of cases, but a crisis of higher amount of compensations.[7] In 2001-2002, the national average jury awards in medical liability cases almost doubled from $3.9 million to $6.2 million. The majority of increase was in noneconomic damages (*pain and suffering component*). The severity of malpractice claims (higher compensations) contributed to increase in insurance premiums. As per a report by the US General Accounting office, "because insurers base their premium rates on their expected costs, their anticipated losses will therefore be the primary determinant of premium rates. With greater payouts, the malpractice insurance premiums increased, and fewer companies offered medical malpractice insurance. The US. House of representatives Joint Economic Committee reported that US medical malpractice liability system neither effectively compensates persons injured from medical negligence nor encourages addressing system errors to improve patient safety.[8]

A report by US Department of Health and Human Services placed the blame of rapid rise in healthcare costs on the shoulder of the legal system. The report stated that, "The excesses of the litigation system are an important contributor to *defensive medicine*. As multimillion-dollar jury awards have become more commonplace in recent years, these problems have reached crisis proportions. Increasingly extreme judgments in a small proportion of cases and the settlements, they influence are driving this litigation crisis."[9]

■ CRISIS REFORM MODELS

The inefficient liability system and rising healthcare cost in the United States led to a countrywide debate over tort system. The legislative response to the growing crisis of medical malpractice insurance aimed to bring about reforms of the system.

Caps on Noneconomic Damages

The placement of caps on noneconomic damages in medical malpractice cases was the first tort reforms effort that occurred in mid 1970s when California was undergoing a medical malpractice crisis. California passed tort reform known as *Medical Injury Compensation Reform Act 1975* (MICRA). Under MICRA, there is no limit on economic damages suffered as a result of any medical negligence. Economic damages may be defined as objectively verifiable monetary losses, including medical expenses, loss of earnings, burial costs, loss of use of property, costs of repair or replacement, costs of obtaining substitute domestic services, loss of employment and loss of business or employment.[10] Noneconomic damages may be in the form of 'pain and sufferings' or 'loss of consortium' with a spouse.

The main provisions of MICRA are as follows:
- Non-economic damages are capped at $250,000.
- Awards for economic damages of > $50,000 can be paid in either a lump sum or over time.
- Disputes can be settled through binding arbitration.
- Attorneys' fees are limited to a certain percentage of the settlement.
- Claims have to be filed within one year of the discovery of the injury or 3 years after the event took place.
- A written notice of intent to sue must be filed at least 90 days in advance to give both the sides an opportunity to reach an out-of-court settlement.

A study reviewed the empirical literature on the effects of damages caps and concluded that, most of the studies show that damages caps reduces liability insurance premiums. The study further concluded that, "Although courts should be cautious in rejecting empirical evidence that caps are effective, legislators should consider that damages caps are not the panacea and that limitations on the recovery of damages for seriously injured victims of malpractice may not be justified by the possibility of lower healthcare cost."[11]

No-fault Compensation

According to the no-fault compensation system, a patient who sustains an avoidable medical injury can apply directly for compensation without litigation. An expert medical board reviews the case and decides on compensation. Several overseas countries like Sweden, New Zealand, and Denmark have adopted no-fault compensation system for medical malpractice injuries, removing these from tort system altogether.[12] This administrative compensation system is based on the concept that:
- Compensation can be given to the injured party even without finding fault or negligence.
- Most medical errors are due to system errors or inherent risks in the practice of medicine.

No-fault compensation system is beneficial to the injured parties as more patients can get compensation, claims are processed faster and more money can go to the affected parties rather than to the attorneys as litigation cost. As the physicians are not sued, they can provide better care. Absence of fear of litigation amongst the medical fraternity can play a significant role in preventing the practice of *defensive medicine*, thus stabilizing the cost of healthcare. No-fault compensation system as a part of malpractice *crisis reform*, would move away from the blame-based system, and encourage the efforts to create safer healthcare system.[13]

Health Courts

Medical negligence is a complex medicolegal issue that is difficult for the judges to decide. There is a chance that legal experts get confused between adverse events and negligence. Establishing *Health Courts* for dealing with medical malpractice cases can be a potential remedy to the costly and inefficient tort system. Proposals that medical malpractice cases be removed from the tort system and processed in an alternative system as administrative compensation in health courts was revived by the Harvard school of public health.[12]

Health courts are proposed specialized courts which use the especially trained adjudicators, and independent expert witnesses to decide the medical negligence cases. Such administrative compensation system already exists in New Zealand, Sweden and Denmark.[14]

The main features of health courts are as follows:[12]
- Medical negligence cases are decided outside the regular court system by especially trained judges.
- Decisions regarding compensation are based on a *standard of care* that is broader than the negligence standard. Preventability of the injury is duly considered. The claimant must show that the injury would not have occurred, if best practices had been followed or an optimal healthcare system had been in place. However, they need not show that care fell below the standard expected of a reasonable practitioner.
- Compensation decisions are based on *avoidability standards* rather than negligence. Patients who are avoidably injured include all the patients whose injuries were avoidable but not due to negligence as well as those who were negligently injured. The *avoidability standard* expands the eligibility for compensation to a wider group of patients than are eligible under the negligence standard, thus improving the capacity of the compensation system to serve the masses.
- Health court system presents greater possibilities for cost control than the tort system does. Although more claims would be filed, the average size of award would be considerably lower. Controlling compensation costs is fairly difficult in the tort system, which is decentralized.

- Health court system can be beneficially used for preventing injuries and promoting patient safety. Compensation for injuries can be linked to preventing them. Sharing information about injuries with systems that facilitate analysis and learning promotes a culture of safety in medicine. A health court system could also provide a mechanism for collecting, and analyzing information on avoidable injuries. Claims researchers extract information about the nature of the adverse event, the surrounding clinical circumstances, and how the accident could have been avoided.

In *tort system*, the patient must allege negligence to obtain compensation. In such a system, even when physicians feel that an event could have been prevented, they rarely admit to negligence. Being accused of negligence induces a strong sense of guilt amongst physicians. Many physicians are reluctant to share information about adverse events with either patients or reporting systems.[15] In Health Court system, the involvement in an avoidable adverse event does not carry the same degree of stigma as negligence does. This alternate compensation system has the advantage of alleviating the barriers to disclosing adverse events.

■ CONCLUSION

Once medical negligence is established by a court of law, liability is to be fixed on the basis of degree of negligence. For fair justice, uniform and objective method should be used for determining the just and adequate quantum of compensation. The multiplier method used in motor vehicle law has not been accepted as suitable by the Supreme Court for medical negligence cases.

Very high quantum of compensation will surely have a deterrent effect on average medical professionals, hopefully resulting in improved patient care. However, there is an apprehension that if high quantum compensation becomes a common practice in the future, it may lead to *medical liability crisis* which other countries are already struggling to overcome. High cost of tort system may result in unbearable cost of healthcare. The possibility of *defensive medicine* and high premium *medical malpractice insurance* cannot be denied. The consumer courts should regulate the quantum of compensation with the actual scenario of the case rather than being tied up by a set of variable precedents and theoretical concepts. Aggravated compensation may justify a single case in hand but to create a culture of affordable, ethical and safe healthcare, reformative measures in medical profession are essential. Future medical liability reforms should focus on a speedy and meaningful compensation system that encourages patient safety and at the same time does not also bear heavy an economic burden on healthcare system that already is in a bad shape.

■ REFERENCES

1. Anna Eleanor Roosevelt (1884–1962) was a renowned American politician. Available: *http://en.wikipedia.org/wiki/Eleanor_Roosevelt*.
2. Balram Prasad vs Kunal Saha (2014) 1 SCC 384.
3. IMA asks SC to review landmark medical negligence verdict. February 12, 2014. Available: *www.thehealthsite.com/news/indian-medical-association-asks-sc-to-review-landmark-medical-negligence verdict*.
4. Sarla Verma and Others vs Delhi Transport Corporation and Another. 2009;6:SCC 121.
5. General Manager, Kerala SRTC vs Susamma Thomas. 1994;SCC(2)176.
6. Nizam Institute of Medical Sciences vs Prasanth S Dhananka and Others. 2009;6SCC 1.
7. Budetti PP, Waters TM. Medical malpractice law in the United States. Menlo Park, CA: The Henry J Kaiser Family Foundation. 2005.

8. Weinstein SL. Medical Liability Reform Crisis 2008. Clin Orthop Relat Res. 2009;467:392-401.
9. Confronting the new health care crisis: improving healthcare quality and lowering costs by fixing our medical liability system. July 24, 2002.U.S. Department of Health and Human Services. Available: http://aspe.hhs.gov/daltcp/reports/litrefm.pdf.
10. Medical Injury Compensation Reform Act MICRA under attack by trial attorneys. Available: *http://www.calchamber.com/GovernmentRelations/IssueReports/Documents/2014-Reports/Medical-Injury-Compensation-Reform-Act.pdf*.
11. Nelson LJ, Morrisey MA, Kilgore ML. Damages caps in medical malpractice cases. Milbank Q. 2007;85(2):259-86.
12. Mello MM, Kachalia A, Studdert DM. Administrative compensation for medical injuries: lessons from three foreign systems. Issue Brief (Commonw Fund). 2011;14:1-18.
13. Sohan DH. Negligence, genuine error, and litigation. International Journal of General Medicine. 2013;6:49-56.
14. Anthony Robert. Can Health Courts Cure the Malpractice System? Physicians Practice journal 2010;20(1). Available: *http://www.physicianspractice.com/articles/can-health-courts-cure-malpractice-system*.
15. Hupert, N, Lawthers AG, Brennan TA, Peterson LM. Processing the tort deterrent signal: a qualitative study. Social Science and Medicine. 1996;43(1):1-11.

CHAPTER 16

Professional Indemnity Insurance: Better Safe than Sorry

Rajendra S Bangal

> *"Being financially secure opens up the fullness of choice, and leads to the search for a deeper experience in life."*
> —**Dr Paul Schervish**[1]

■ INTRODUCTION

In India, the incidence and severity of lawsuits against medical professionals and healthcare establishments has been on the rise for the last few years. More and more patients (customers!) believe that they have suffered as the professional services did not live upto their expectations. Kunal Saha's case of medical negligence has shocked the medical fraternity, in which the Supreme Court granted a compensation of ₹ 11.41 crore.[2] There is a feeling of financial insecurity amongst doctors due to such high quantum of compensation. Regardless of the outcome of the professional liability lawsuit, legal cost of defending a lawsuit alone may be financially crippling particularly in cases that linger on for years. While practicing *medicine* in such set of circumstances, it is imperative for the medical professionals to protect themselves from financial crisis by getting professional indemnity. This chapter is intended to educate the medical professionals about all the necessary information related to indemnity insurance.

■ PROFESSIONAL INDEMNITY INSURANCE

Indemnity means compensation for damages or loss. Indemnity in the legal sense may also refer to an exemption from liability for damages. The concept of indemnity is based on a contractual agreement made between two parties, in which one party agrees to pay for potential losses or damages caused by the other party. A typical example is an insurance contract, whereby one party (the insurer) agrees to compensate the other (the insured) for any damages or losses, in return for premiums paid by the insured to the insurer.

Professional indemnity insurance policy is meant for professionals like architects, engineers, doctors, lawyers, chartered accountants, and medical practitioners to cover liability falling on them as a result of errors and omissions committed by them whilst rendering professional service. In healthcare sector *Professional Indemnity* policies are available to the following:[3]

- Doctors and medical practitioners—which covers registered medical practitioners such as physicians, surgeons, cardiologists, pathologists, dental surgeons, etc.

- Medical establishments (error and omission policy)—which covers legal liability falling on the medical establishment such as hospitals and nursing homes, as a result of error or omission committed by any named professional or qualified assistants engaged by the medical establishment.

Even today, a large percentage of doctors either do not know about the indemnity policy or even, if they know, have not yet secured themselves under the policy. Though indemnity policy is not a compulsory policy like vehicle insurance, still it is strongly recommended that all doctors should get themselves sufficiently insured on the everyday, they obtain their registration to practice, and maintain the continuity of coverage till at least a few years after they stop their practice.

What does it Cover?

The term *legal liability* means responsibilities which can be enforced by law. Legal Liability may be classified into criminal liability and civil liability. Only civil liability claims are payable under this policy. Liability arising out of any criminal Act or Act committed in violation of any law or ordinance is not covered. The terms and conditions of every professional indemnity insurance may vary slightly, however, often it covers the following:[4]

- The policy covers all sums which the insured professional becomes legally liable to pay as damages to third party in respect of any error and/or omission on his/her part committed whilst rendering professional service (If the court finds the doctor guilty of medical negligence and orders him to compensate the patient, the insurance company will pay the ordered amount to the patient/relative on behalf of the insured doctor).
- Legal cost and expenses incurred in defence of the case, with the prior consent of the insurance company, are also payable, subject to the overall limit of indemnity selected.
- The policy offers a benefit of retroactive period on continuous renewal of policy whereby claims reported in subsequent renewal but pertaining to earlier period after first inception of the policy, also become payable.
- Group policies can also be issued covering members of one profession. Group discount in premium is available depending upon the number of members covered.
- The policy is effective and applicable for the liability incurred by the doctor anywhere in India. If the doctor has obtained his indemnity policy from an insurance company located in Maharashtra, operates in Delhi, and is held guilty of negligence and ordered to pay compensation by the Delhi State Consumer Dispute Redressal Commission, then the insurance company in Maharashtra will pay the amount on behalf of the insured doctor.
- Policy regarding *out of court settlement* varies from one insurance company to another. Recently some private insurance companies have come up with 'out of court settlement' as an inbuilt feature in their indemnity policy. Out of court settlements are not routinely covered by the insurance company, though if a proper case is made out, and if it is shown convincingly that it is in the interest of the insurance company as well to do so, it may be possible to settle the case out of court.

What it does not Cover?

The policy will not pay for claims arising out of:[5]
- Liability arising out of any criminal act or act committed in violation of any law or ordinance.
- Services rendered under the influence of intoxicant or alcohol.
- Any procedure carried out under general anesthesia unless performed in a hospital

- Intentional non-compliance of any statutory provision,
- Any third party public liability
- Any condition caused by or associated with AIDS
- Arising out of all personal injuries such as libel, slander, false arrest, wrongful eviction, wrongful detention, defamation, etc., and resultant mental injury, anguish or shock
- Infringement of plans, copy-right, patent, name, trademark, registered design
- Liability assumed by the insured by agreement and which would not have attached in the absence of such agreement.
- Deliberate, wilful or intentional noncompliance of any statutory provision.
- Non-compliance with technical standards commonly observed in professional practice, laid down by law, or regulated by official bodies
- Loss of pure financial nature such as loss of goodwill or loss of market
- Any dishonest, fraudulent criminal or malicious act or omission
- Fines, penalties, punitive or exemplary damages.
- Professional services rendered by the insured prior to the Retroactive Date in the Schedule.
- Deliberate, conscious or intentional disregard of the insured's technical or administrative management of the need to take all reasonable steps to prevent claims.
- Injury to any person under the contract of employment or apprenticeship with the insured their contractor(s) and/or Sub-Contractor(s) when such injury arises out of the execution of such contract.
- War and nuclear perils.

Factors Influencing the Amount of Insurance

The following aspects may be considered, amongst others, while deciding on the amount of insurance:[6]

- The type of professional involvement (i.e., whether he is a family practitioner, a specialist, superspecialist, full-time practitioner or honorary consultant),
- The nature of specialization (Physician/ Surgeon/Anesthesiologist/Plastic Surgeon/ Dental Surgeon, etc.)
- Geographical location of practice (rural/ urban/slums/elite area)
- Type of patient population (literate/ illiterate/Indians, NRIs, foreign national)
- The quality and standard of patient care in the hospital (accredited hospitals)
- Availability of qualified and trained medical/ paraclinical/nursing staff
- One's willingness to adhere to ethical and legal requirement while practicing
- Preparedness to provide the claimed services (scope of services defined and declared by the hospital)
- Pecuniary jurisdictions of the consumer courts (At present the pecuniary jurisdiction of district consumer forums is up to ₹ 20 lakhs. So, it is advisable that the minimum sum insured (even by a family physician) should at least be ₹ 20 lakhs. Other specialists and superspecialist may apply for higher sums depending on other factors).

In case of any event likely to give rise to a liability claim as described above, insurance company should be informed immediately and acknowledgement received. One should also insist on obtaining the claim number. In case, any legal notice or summons is received, it should be sent to the insurance company. The company has the option of arranging the defence of the case. The event giving rise to the claim should have occurred during the period of insurance or retroactive period and the claim first made in writing against the insured during the policy period.

Precautions to be taken while obtaining the indemnity insurance cover:
- Provide all factual, correct and truthful information to the insurance company. Any inaccuracy, nondisclosures or incorrect statement/information in the form might result in your claim getting rejected, whenever it occurs.
- Always inform correct information about your previous claims, number of beds, qualifications of staff, unqualified staff, etc.
- Always preserve a copy of your complete proposal form for future reference. Do not rely on the insurance companies to preserve your proposal form.
- Verify the correctness of the contents of the policy copy once you receive it. In case of any errors, get it corrected immediately.
- Always check and confirm the retroactive date mentioned in the policy issued every year. If wrong get, it corrected.
- As the claims under indemnity policy are almost always retrospective, so preserve all the copies of your previous and current policies in order to prove the continuous coverage.
- Always renew the policy well in advance. Do not rely on your insurance agents for renewals.

■ SOME IMPORTANT INFORMATION

AOO: AOY Ratio

In Professional Indemnity Policy, the sum insured is referred to as limit of indemnity. This limit is fixed per occurrence and per policy period which is called Any One Occurrence (AOO) limit and Any One Year (AOY) limit, respectively. The ratio of AOO limit to AOY limit can be chosen from the following:
- 1:1
- 1:2
- 1:3
- 1:4

  That means, if a doctor has got insured under indemnity policy for ₹ 20 lakhs with a ratio of 1:1, and if the court orders him to compensate the patient for ₹ 18 lakhs, then the insurance company will pay that amount to the patient. On the other hand, if the doctor is insured for the same amount of 20 lakhs with a ratio of 1:4, then in any one year only ₹ 5 lakhs (20/4) will be available for him for one occurrence. The insurance company will pay ₹ 5 lakhs for 4 incidences in one year, if they occur.
- It is advisable to opt for 1:1 ratio. Because in this scenario, the entire insurance amount is available to settle the claim. If a second claim arises in the same insurance year, then the amount available will be the total sum insured minus the amount paid for the previous claim, e.g., a doctor is insured for ₹ 20 lakhs. If he gets a court order to compensate the patient for ₹ 12 lakhs, then the entire ₹ 12 lakhs will be paid by the insurance company. If there is a second case in the same insurance year and this time the court orders to compensate for ₹ 8 lakhs, then this claim too will be entirely settled by the insurer. However, if this same doctor had opted for 1:4 ratio, then for both claims the insurance company's liability to pay would have been ₹ 5 lakhs for each claim, even though the doctor has insured himself for ₹ 20 lakhs.
- Thus, it is advisable to opt for 1:1 ratio, even though the insurers provide a discount (lower premium) for higher ratios, i.e., higher the ratio higher the discount.

Premium Rates (Individuals)

The premium rates are quoted as 'Rupees per Mille', which means 'per one thousand'. For example, physicians, except those doing invasive procedures such as angioplasty, have to pay 1.0 per mille, i.e., ₹ 1 per every thousand rupees insured. Thus premium for ₹ 10,00,000 (Ten lakhs) sum assured would be ₹ 1000 per year. For surgeons, it is ₹ 2 per Mille, i.e., ₹ 2000 per year for ₹ 10 lakhs. For plastic surgeons and anesthetists, it is ₹ 3000 for ₹ 10 lakhs sum assured. For general practitioners, it is ₹ 500 per year for ₹ 10 lakhs. These rates may vary from insurer to insurer.

Premium Rates (Clinical Establishments)

- Basic insurance is: ₹ 3 per thousand sum insured. So, for ₹ 10 lakhs the basic premium will be ₹ 3000.
- Add to this ₹ 5 per every indoor patient, i.e., number of admissions in the previous year. So, if you have 500 indoor patients in the previous year, a premium amount of ₹ 2500 will be added to the basic premium. [₹ 3000 + ₹ 2500 = ₹ 5500]. It is advisable to provide true and correct information about the number of admissions to the insurance company, lest the claim may be rejected on the grounds of nondisclosure/suppression of material facts.
- Add to this ₹ 1 per outdoor patient in the previous year. So, if you had 3000 outpatients in previous year, then ₹ 3000 will be added to the above amount [₹ 5500 + ₹ 3000 = ₹ 8500].
- Plus Service Tax at applicable rate. If it is 12.36%, then ₹ 8500 + ₹ 1051 = ₹ 9551.
- In case your hospital has some staff that is legally and technically unqualified, then do not forget to mention it in the proposal form and add 7.5% of the premium specifically to cover such staff.

These rates may vary from insurer to insurer.

At least till today, in India, the indemnity insurance is provided at a very low premium, as compared to the premiums in US. It is not uncommon in US for a practitioner to apply for a loan at the start of his practice in order to pay the premium of indemnity insurance. Similarly, many senior practitioners in US are forced to retire from practice as they cannot afford the premiums of indemnity insurance (and they also cannot afford to take the risk of practicing without the insurance), which are sometimes as high as 20% of one's annual income. Fortunately, it is not the situation in India, where the premium of indemnity insurance is as low as ₹ 500 to 3000 for a cover of 10 lakhs (Depending on the specialization of practice).

■ RETROACTIVE DATE

It is the date on which the cover incepted for the first time and it will remain the same till the policy is continued uninterrupted. For example, if you get the indemnity cover on 1/1/2008 and continued the policy without break, the retroactive date will remain as 1/1/2008. So even you receive a legal notice/order for compensation in year 2014, for a case you had operated upon in 2010, your claim will be valid. However, if your policy was interrupted even for a few days in the year 2012, your retroactive date will shift to the date of renewal of your policy in 2012 and thus your claim will be rejected.

Consideration of retroactive date is one of the features of this indemnity insurance policy which differentiates it from other insurance policies. In most of the cases, the cause of action (e.g., surgery) occurs during the period of previous policy and the claim (after order of the court) occurs in subsequent policy periods. If there is continuity in the policy from the date of cause of action to the date of court order, then because of the provision of retroactive date, the claim becomes payable. This is also the reason, why all the previous policy documents should be always preserved.[7]

An Ideal Indemnity Insurance Policy: Proposed Components

Though the indemnity policy is a *must have* for all the medical professionals, the protection provided by the policy is far from being adequate. The premiums are low and as such, the insurance companies are disinterested in this insurance, as neither they have any expertise to deal with these matters nor is there any machinery in place to process the claims. As a result, when a claim is intimated to them, doctors generally experience apathy, disinterest and a tendency on the part of insurance company to reject the claim. Hence, there is urgent and great need to formulate a comprehensive mechanism to address all these issues.

Some of the issues that generally arise after a claim occur, can be effectively addressed by opting for group policies and negotiating with the insurers for providing certain additional features which are not provided by the general policy (i.e., to have tailor-made policies). Some of these are:

- Provision to cover expenses incurred for defending complaints before State and Indian medical councils
- Provision for the insurance company directly compensating the patient after the court order, rather than the doctor having to pay first and then getting it reimbursed from insurer.
- Out of court settlements
- Provision to cover the costs incurred for defending cases of medical negligence before criminal courts
- Provision to cover entire defence cost including incidental expenses such as documentation costs, fees for expert evidence, conveyance costs, etc., in addition to the advocate's fees.
- Provision to appoint a pre-approved panel of advocates (by mutual consensus between the insured group and the insurer); decide their professional fees, in order to enable the insured to appoint an advocate at the shortest possible time, when needed.
- Provision to have a single insurance office for processing all claims under this policy for all members of the group.
- Provision for a reduced premium after a doctor stops his practice but only wish to continue the cover in case of any claim that might arise from his acts/omissions committed during his previous years of service (during which period he has paid, the complete premium).

Alternatively, some other mechanism may be devised for financial security against court orders in cases of medical negligence. They may be either on the lines of Medical Defense Union, UK, modified as per Indian needs and scenario or in the form of professional self-insurance schemes, as being tried in Ahmedabad and Kerala, India.

■ CONCLUSION

In cases of allegations of medical negligence, the doctors' reputation is at stake and also much of his quality time is consumed in defending the allegations. Although the policy may indemnify the monetary part, but the reputation and the time lost cannot be indemnified. As of today, professional indemnity policy is an excellent and the only means of security against financial compensations awarded by the courts in cases of medical negligence liability lawsuits.

Doctors should not ignore the magnitude of the ever-growing problem, especially in view of the existing hostile environment and run for the cover. An act or omission, amounting to medical negligence can occur on the first day of one's practice or on the last day of the practice. None of us is immune from it. Hence it is advisable to get financial security by obtaining professional indemnity insurance policy.

Better be Safe than Sorry!

REFERENCES

1. Paul G. Schervish is Director of the Center on Wealth and Philanthropy (CWP) at Boston College. *http://www.pinterest.com/pin/371547037978051492*.
2. Balram Prasad vs Kunal Saha, 2014 1 SCC 384
3. Available: *http://newindia.co.in/Content.aspx?pageid=49*.
4. Kapoor L. Smart doc. 1st edn, September 2005, Published by AMC, Mumbai.
5. Agarwal S, Agarwal SS. Professional indemnity insurance vis-a-vis medical professionals. JIAFM. 2009;31:73-6.
6. *http://www.covermd.com/resources/Medical-Malpractice-Insurance-Rates.aspx*.
7. *http://www.mdanational.com.au/faq.aspx*.

SECTION 6
Medical Laws and Judgments: A Ray of Hope!

Chapter 17 Landmark Judgments Related to Medical Professionals
Chapter 18 Medicolegal Outlook on Transplantation of Human Organs Act
Chapter 19 Medicolegal Outlook on Bio-Medical Waste Management Act
Chapter 20 Medicolegal Outlook on PC-PNDT Act

CHAPTER 17

Landmark Judgments Related to Medical Professionals

VP Singh, Krishnadutt Chavali

> *"Ignorance of the law excuses no man; not that all men know the law, but because 'tis an excuse every man will plead, and no man can tell how to refute him."*
> —John Selden (Jurist)[1]

■ INTRODUCTION

Law is primarily made by legislatures. In India, legislations are enacted by Parliament, State Legislatures and Union Territory Legislatures. In addition, there are also laws known as subordinate legislation in the form of rules, regulations as well as by-laws. When there is no legislation on a particular point, *judicial precedents* may be used, where past decisions of judges are followed in future cases when the facts of the case are similar. Judicial precedent may be defined as a judgment or decision of a court of law cited as an authority for deciding a similar state of fact in the same manner or on the same principle or by analogy.[2] Such decisions become authority or guide for subsequent cases of a similar nature.

Medical law is a vast body of laws related to the rights and responsibilities of medical professionals and their patients. Brief perspective of landmark judgments related to medical professionals and the guiding principles laid by the Apex Court as presented below may be used to understand, *what law expects from medicine*!

■ DR SURESH GUPTA'S CASE[3]

Facts of the Case

- A plastic surgeon operated upon a patient for removing his nasal deformity. The patient died during surgery on 18th April, 1994, and the postmortem was conducted on 21st April, 1994.
- In the postmortem report, the cause of death was: *Asphyxia resulting from blockage of respiratory passage by aspirated blood consequent upon surgically incised margin of nasal septum.*
- A Medical Board gave opinion that, death occurred due to sudden cardiac arrest, the direct cause of which (Cardiac Arrest) cannot be ascertained. However, possible cause of cardiac arrest could be:
    - Hypotension due head-up position
    - Adverse drug reaction
    - Hypoxia

- Death due to Asphyxia resulting from blockage of air passage secondary to antemortem aspiration of blood from the wound is unlikely in the presence of cuffed endotracheal tube of proper size (8.5), which was introduced before the operation and remained in position till the patient was declared dead.
- The team of experts also opined that *presence of fluid and clotted blood in respiratory passage is likely, as it invariably occurs ante-mortem due to aspiration from operation site.* But they also opined that 'presence of fluid and clotted blood in the respiratory passage, as noted in the postmortem report, due to trickling of decomposition bloody fluid and some clot present in the nostril from the site of incision in the nose, cannot be ruled out after the tube is taken out.

The anesthetist (co-accused) died pending the trial. The proceedings, therefore, were abated against him.

Patient's Allegation

The surgeon was guilty of gross negligence in giving an incision at the wrong place and did not take necessary precautions in the course of surgical operation to prevent seepage of blood down the respiratory passage of the patient and the resultant death by asphyxia.

Doctor's Defence

Death due to asphyxia resulting from blockage of air passage secondary to antemortem aspiration of blood from the wound is unlikely in the presence of cuffed endotracheal tube of proper size (8.5), which was introduced before the operation and remained in position till the patient was declared dead.

The presence of fluid and clotted blood in the respiratory passage, as noted in the postmortem report, due to trickling of decomposition bloody fluid and some clot present in the nostril from the site of incision in the nose, cannot be ruled out after the tube is taken out.

The learned counsel on behalf of the doctor referred to Sec 80 and Sec 88 IPC to contend that in various kinds of medical treatment and surgical operation, likelihood of an accident or misfortune leading to death cannot be ruled out.

Relevant Sections of Indian Penal Code

Sec 80. Accident in doing a lawful Act.
Nothing is an offence which is done by accident or misfortune, and without any criminal intention or knowledge in the doing of a lawful act in a lawful manner by lawful means and with proper care and caution.

Sec 88. Act not intended to cause death, done by consent in good faith for person's benefit.
Nothing which is not intended to cause death, is an offence by reason of any harm which it may cause, or be intended by the doer to cause, or be known by the doer to cause, or be known by the doer to be likely to cause, to any person for whose benefit it is done in good faith, and who has given a consent, whether express or implied, to suffer that harm, or to take the risk of that harm.

Sec 304A. Causing death by negligence
Whoever causes the death of any person by a rash or negligent Act not amounting to culpable homicide shall be punished by imprisonment for up to 2 years, or by fine, or both.

Findings of the Court

- The magistrate ordered to proceed with the trial for criminal negligence U/S 304A IPC and recorded following reasons: *Postmortem report clearly mentioned that death was due to the complication arising out of the operation. The deceased was a young man of 38 years having no cardiac problem and because of the negligence of the doctors while conducting minor operation for removing nasal deformity, gave incision at wrong part due to that blood seeped into the respiratory passage due to which the patient died. I am of the opinion that there are sufficient grounds on record to make out a prima facie case against both the accused for commission of offence under Section 304A IPC.*
- The High Court refused to quash the criminal proceedings, with following reasons: *The two doctors who conducted the postmortem examination have taken an emphatic stand which they have reiterated even after the Medical Board opinion, that death in this case was due to 'asphyxia resulting from blockage of respiratory passage by aspirated blood consequent upon surgically incised margin of nasal septum. This indicates that adequate care was not taken to prevent seepage of blood down the respiratory passage which resulted in asphyxia.'*
- The High Court, however, recorded that, the Metropolitan Magistrate was obviously wrong, in the absence of any medical opinion, in coming to a conclusion that the surgeon had given a cut at wrong place of the body of the patient leading to blood seeping into the respiratory passage and blocking it resulting in his death.
- The Supreme Court, while giving the judgment on August 4, 2004, declared that: No case of recklessness or gross negligence has been made out against the doctor to compel him to face the trial for offence under section 304A of the IPC. It allowed the appeal and set aside the impugned orders of the Magistrate and the High Court, and quashed the criminal proceedings pending against the accused doctor.
- From the medical opinions produced by the prosecution, the cause of death is stated to be 'not introducing a cuffed endotracheal tube of proper size so as to prevent aspiration of blood from the wound in the respiratory passage'. This act attributed to the doctor, if accepted to be true, can be described as negligent on account of lacking due care and precaution. For this act of negligence, he may be liable in tort but his carelessness or want of due attention and skill cannot be described to be so reckless or grossly negligent as to make him criminally liable.

Supreme Court's Observation on Criminal Negligence

- Criminal prosecution of doctors without adequate medical opinion pointing to their guilt would be doing great disservice to the community. A doctor cannot be tried for culpable or criminal negligence in all cases of medical mishaps or misfortunes.
- For fixing criminal liability on a doctor or surgeon, the standard of negligence required to be proved should be so high as can be described as *gross negligence or recklessness*. It is not merely lack of necessary care, attention and skill.

   Justice Arijit Pasayat and CK Thakker, on September 9, 2004, referred the question of medical negligence for determination by a larger Bench of the Supreme Court observing that the words gross, reckless, competence, indifference, etc., did not occur anywhere in the definition of negligence under Sec 304A of the IPC, and hence, they could not agree with the judgment delivered in the case of Dr Suresh Gupta.

   The issue was decided in the Supreme Court in the case of Jacob Mathew's case. The court directed the central government to frame guidelines to save doctors from unnecessary harassment and undue pressure in performing their duties. It ruled that until the government framed such guidelines, the above-mentioned guidelines would prevail... (For further details, please read *Jacob Mathew's case*).

■ JACOB MATHEW'S CASE[4]

Facts of the Case

On February 15, 1995, an end-stage cancer patient was admitted in a hospital. On February 22, 1995 at about 11 PM, the patient felt difficulty in breathing. The patient's son contacted the duty nurse, but no doctor turned up for 20–25 minutes. Then Dr Jacob Mathew and Dr Allen Joseph came and an oxygen cylinder was connected to the mouth of the patient, but the breathing problem increased further. The oxygen cylinder was found to be empty. There was no other gas cylinder available in the room. Gas cylinder from the adjoining room was brought but there was no arrangement to make the gas cylinder functional, In the process, 5–7 minutes were wasted. By this time, the patient died. A criminal complaint was lodged against the doctors who were subsequently charged with Sec 304A IPC for causing death due to rash and negligent act.

Patient's Allegation

Complainant's allegation was that, *death of my father has occurred due to the carelessness of doctors and nurses and nonavailability of oxygen cylinder and the empty cylinder was fixed on the mouth of my father and his breathing was totally stopped hence my father died.*

Doctor's Defence

Doctor's defence was that patient was suffering from cancer in an advanced stage. He was only required to be kept at home and given proper nursing care, food, and solace coupled with prayers. His sons were very influential persons, and could, therefore prevail over the doctors and hospital management and got the patient admitted. The patient was treated with utmost care and caution and given all the required medical assistance, but what was ordained to happen did happen.

Findings of the Court

The prosecution of the accused appellant under Section 304A/34 IPC was quashed. The Supreme Court categorically held for this act of negligence doctor may be liable in tort, his carelessness or want of due attention and skill cannot be described to be so reckless or grossly negligent as to make him criminally liable. It is a case of nonavailability of oxygen cylinder either because of the hospital having failed to keep available a gas cylinder or because of the gas cylinder being found empty. Then, probably the hospital may be liable in civil law (or may not be) but the accused appellant cannot be proceeded against under Sec 304A IPC.

The Supreme Court gave the guidelines regarding prosecution of medical professionals for criminal negligence:
- A private complaint may not be entertained unless the complainant has produced prima facie evidence before the court in the form of a credible opinion given by another competent doctor to support the charge of rashness or negligence on the part of the accused doctor.

- The investigating officer should before proceeding against the doctor accused of rash or negligent act or omission, obtain an independent and competent medical opinion preferably from a doctor in Government service qualified in that branch of medical practice who can normally be expected to give an impartial and unbiased opinion in regard to the facts collected in the investigation.
- A doctor accused of rashness or negligence may not be arrested in a routine manner simply because a charge has been leveled against him unless his arrest is necessary for furthering the investigation or for collecting evidence or unless the investigation officer feels satisfied that the doctor proceeded against would not make himself available to face the prosecution unless arrested, the arrest may be withheld.
    - The above judgment gives relief to the medical profession. However, no immunity is conferred. These guidelines prescribe opinion from a proper Government doctor before proceeding against a doctor in a criminal negligence case.

■ SUPREME COURT'S OBSERVATION ON NEGLIGENCE

Negligence as a Tort

- Negligence is the breach of a duty caused by the omission to do something which a reasonable man, guided by those considerations which ordinarily regulate the conduct of human affairs would do, or doing something which a prudent and reasonable man would not do.
- Actionable negligence consists in the neglect of the use of ordinary care or skill toward a person to whom the defendant owes the duty of observing ordinary care and skill, by which neglect the plaintiff has suffered injury to his person or property.

Negligence as a Tort and as a Crime

- The jurisprudential concept of negligence differs in civil and criminal law. What may be negligence in civil law, may not necessarily be negligence in criminal law.
- For negligence to amount to an offence, the element of mens rea must be shown to exist. For an act to amount to criminal negligence, the degree of negligence should be much higher, i.e., gross or of a very high degree.
- Negligence which is neither gross nor of a higher degree may provide a ground for action in civil law but cannot form the basis for prosecution.
- In criminal rashness or criminal negligence, the rashness is of such a degree that taking a hazard even knowing that the hazard is of such a degree that injury is most likely imminent. The consequences entailed in the risk may not be wanted, and indeed the actor may hope that they do not occur, but this hope nevertheless fails to inhibit him from taking the risk.

Negligence by Professionals

The only assurance which a medical professional can give to his patient is that:
- He is possessed of the requisite skill in the branch of profession which he is practicing
- While undertaking the performance of the task entrusted to him, he would exercise his skill with reasonable competence.

Judged by this standard, a professional may be held liable for negligence on one of two findings:
1. Either he was not possessed of the requisite skill which he professed to have possessed
2. He did not exercise, with reasonable competence in the given case, the skill which he did possess.

Standard of Care Required by a Medical Practitioner

- The practitioner must bring to his task a reasonable degree of skill and knowledge, and must exercise a reasonable degree of care.
- Neither the very highest nor a very low degree of care and competence, judged in the light of the particular circumstances of each case, is what the law requires.
- A person is not liable for negligence because someone else of greater skill and knowledge would have prescribed different treatment or operated in a different way.
- He is not guilty of negligence, if he has acted in accordance with a practice accepted as proper by a responsible body of medical men skilled in that particular art, even though a body of adverse opinion also existed among medical men.
- Deviation from normal practice is not necessarily evidence of negligence. To establish liability on that basis, it must be shown that:
  - There is a usual and normal practice
  - The defendant has not adopted it
  - The course adopted is one that no professional man of ordinary skill would have taken had he been acting with ordinary care.
- A medical practitioner was not to be held liable simply because things went wrong from mischance or misadventure or through an error of judgment in choosing one reasonable course of treatment in preference to another.

■ MARTIN D'SOUZA'S CASE[5]

Facts of the Case

In March 1991, the respondent patient suffering from chronic renal failure was referred by the Director, Health Services to the Nanavati Hospital, Mumbai for kidney transplant. On 24.4.1991, the respondent patient reached Hospital, and was under the treatment of the appellant doctor. At that stage, he was already undergoing hemodialysis twice a week. The respondent wanted to undergo kidney transplantation by Dr Sonawala who was out of India for 1 month.

When the respondent patient approached the appellant doctor, he was suffering from high fever, but refused to get admitted despite the appellant doctor's advice. Hence, a broad spectrum antibiotic was prescribed to him.

The respondent attended the Hemodialysis Unit of the hospital but did not get himself admitted. At that time, his fever remained between 101–104°F. The appellant doctor repeatedly advised him to get admitted to hospital but the respondent refused.

The respondent finally agreed to get admitted to hospital due to his serious condition. Urine culture and sensitivity reports showed severe urinary tract infection due to *Klebsiella*. The report also showed that the infection could be treated by Amikacin and Methenamine Mandelate only and the infection was resistant to other antibiotics. Methenamine mandelate cannot be used in renal failure. Later on, the blood culture report showed a serious infection of the bloodstream (*Staphylococcus*).

Amikacin injection was administered to the respondent for 3 days, since the urinary infection was sensitive to Amikacin. Cap. Augmentin (375 mg) was administered three times a day for the blood infection and the respondent was transfused one unit of blood during dialysis. At this stage, the respondent insisted on immediate kidney transplant even though the appellant doctor had advised him that due to his blood and urine infection no transplant could take place for 6 weeks. The respondent, despite the appellant's advice, got himself discharged from hospital. Since the respondent was suffering from blood and urinary infection and had refused to come for hemodialysis on alternate days, the appellant suggested Injection Amikacin (500 mg) twice a day. Certain other drugs were also specified to be taken under the supervision of the appellant when he visited the dialysis unit.

Patient's Allegation

The respondent alleged that the appellant was negligent in prescribing Amikacin to the respondent in a dosage of 500 mg twice a day for 14 days. As such dosage was excessive and caused hearing impairment. It is also the case of the respondent that the infection he was suffering from was not of a nature as to warrant administration of Amikacin to him.

He filed a complaint before the National Consumer Disputes Redressal Commission, New Delhi claiming compensation of an amount of ₹ 12 lakhs as his hearing had been affected.

Doctor's Defence

The appellant submitted before the Commission that Amikacin was prescribed to the respondent patient only after obtaining blood and urine culture reports, which showed the respondent resistant to other antibiotics. Even the witness of the respondent (Dr Sareen) conceded that he would have prescribed Amikacin in the facts of the case.

Findings of the Court

The Commission allowed the complaint of the respondent and awarded ₹ 4 lakh with interest @12% from 1.8.1992 as well as ₹ 3 lakh as compensation as well as ₹ 5000 as costs.

However, the Supreme Court held, "In our opinion the judgment of the Commission cannot be sustained and deserves to be set aside. Considering the facts of the case, we cannot hold that the appellant was guilty of medical negligence. It is evident from the fact that the respondent was already seriously ill before he met the appellant. There is nothing to show from the evidence that the appellant was in any way negligent, rather it appears that the appellant did his best to give good treatment to the respondent to save his life but the respondent himself did not cooperate. A patient who does not listen to his doctor's advice often has to face the adverse consequences.

Supreme Court's Observation

The Supreme Court directed that:
- Whenever, a complaint is received against a doctor or hospital by the Consumer fora or by the Criminal Court then before issuing notice to the doctor or hospital the Consumer Forum or Criminal Court should first refer the matter to a competent doctor or committee of doctors, specialized in the field relating to which the medical negligence is attributed,
- Only after that doctor or committee reports that there is a prima facie case of medical negligence should notice be then issued to the concerned doctor/hospital.
- We further warn the police officials not to arrest or harass doctors unless the facts clearly come within the parameters laid down in Jacob Mathew's case, otherwise the policemen will themselves have to face legal action.

In V Kishan Rao's case the Supreme Court clarified that, Martin D'Souza's Case wrongly interpreted the Jacob Mathew's case (For further detail, please read V Kishan Rao's case).

■ V KISHAN RAO'S CASE[6]
Facts of the Case
The appellant (the original complainant) got his wife admitted in Nikhil Superspecialty Hospital (Respondent No. 1) on 20.07.2002 as his wife was suffering from fever (intermittent in nature, with chills). He alleged that certain tests were conducted by the respondent No. 1 but malaria was not detected.

It was also alleged that his wife was not responding to the medicine given. On 22.7.2002, saline was given to her. Complainant had seen some particles in the saline bottle which was brought to the notice of the authorities of the hospital, but to no effect. Then on 23.7.2002 complainant's wife had respiratory trouble which was brought to the notice of the authorities of the respondent No. 1 who gave artificial oxygen to the patient. According to the complainant at that stage artificial oxygen was not necessary but without ascertaining the actual necessity of the patient, the same was given. Complainant submitted that his wife was not responding to the medicines and her condition was deteriorating. The patient was finally shifted to Yashoda Hospital from the respondent No. 1.

At the time of admission in Yashoda Hospital, blood test detected malaria parasite (*P. falciparum*), Widal test was negative. Patient was admitted in acute condition with history of fever for 8 days and having been admitted 5 days ago in Nikhil Hospital and given Inj Monocef, Inj Cifran and Inj Cholroquine. Upon arrival patient was unconscious, no pulse, no BP, pupils dilated. Immediately, patient was intubated and connected to ventilator. Inj Atropine, inj Adrenaline and inj Soda bicarb were given, DC shock also given. Rhythm restored at 1:35 PM. At 10:45 PM, patient developed bradycardia and inspite of all the resuscitative measures, patient could not be revived and declared dead at 11:30 PM on 24.7.2002.

Patient's Allegation
The complainant's allegation was that his wife was not given proper treatment and the respondent No.1 was negligent in treating the patient.

Doctor's Defence
It was argued that no expert opinion was produced by the complainant that treatment was given by the hospital was wrong or the hospital was negligent.

Findings of the Court
- District Forum, came to a finding that there was negligence on the part of the respondent No.1 and ordered that the complainant is entitled for compensation of ₹ 2 lakhs.
- The State Commission held that there was no negligence of the doctor. It also recorded a finding that no expert opinion was produced by the petitioner to prove the negligence.
- National Consumer Disputes Redressal Commission upheld the finding of the State Commission.
- The Supreme Court set aside the orders passed by the State Commission and the National Commission and restored the order passed by the District Forum. The respondent no. 1 was directed to pay the compensation to the appellant as granted by the District Forum. The appeal was allowed with costs.

- The Supreme Court held that the expert evidence is not required and District Forum rightly did not ask the appellant to adduce expert evidence. It is not a case of complicated issues relating to medical treatment.

Supreme Court's Observation on Expert Medical Opinion
The Supreme Court held that:
- *Before forming an opinion that expert medical opinion is necessary, the fora must come to a conclusion that the case is complicated enough to require the opinion of an expert or that the facts of the case are such that it cannot be resolved by the members of the fora without the assistance of expert opinion.*
- It is not required that in all cases medical negligence has to be proved on the basis of expert evidence. In these matters no mechanical approach can be followed. Each case has to be judged on its own facts.

Supreme Court's Observation on Martin D'Souza's Case
- In *Jacob Mathew's case*, the direction for consulting another doctor for opinion before proceeding with criminal investigation was confined only in cases of criminal complaint and not in respect of complaints filed before the Consumer fora where medical negligence is treated as civil liability for payment of damages.
- The two Judge bench in *Martin D'souza* wrongly equated a criminal complaint against a doctor or hospital with a complaint against a doctor before the Consumer fora.
- The directions of the court in *Martin D'Souza* for referring the opinion of another doctor in criminal cases as well as complaints before the consumer fora is inconsistent with the directions given in Jacob Mathew's case (larger bench), and the principles laid in the Consumer Protection Act. Such directions cannot be treated as a binding precedent.

■ CONCLUSION
Knowledge of law applicable to medical practice is one of the most effective tools for ethical and safe practice of medicine. Ignorance of law of the land is no excuse, and the same can be wiped out only by spreading legal awareness amongst the people. To have a clear insight into the legal expectations from medical practitioners while discharging their professional duties, thorough understanding of medical laws is a must. Supreme Court judgments related to medical professionals are the guiding principles for the physicians to practice their profession in a legally acceptable manner.

■ REFERENCES
1. Available: www.brainyquote.com/quotes/quotes/m/mahatmagan134775.html# OtjHAcYullqJulul.99
2. Tufal A. Judicial Precedent. Available: www.lawteacher.net/PDF/Judicial%20Precedent.pdf.
3. Dr Suresh Gupta vs Govt. of NCT of Delhi and Anr 2004 CTJ 901(SC).
4. Jacob Mathew vs State of Punjab. AIR 2005 SC 1385.
5. Martin F. D'Souza vs Mohd Ishfaq. 2009;3 SCC 1.
6. V Kishan Rao vs. Nikhil Superspeciality Hospital and Another. 2010;5 SCR. 1.

CHAPTER 18

Medicolegal Outlook on Transplantation of Human Organs Act

Sunil Shroff, Sumana Navin, Hemal Kanvinde, Sujatha Niranjan, Christopher Barry

"Without the Organ Donor, there is no Story, no Hope, no Transplant. But when there is an Organ Donor, Life springs from death, sorrow turns to Hope and a terrible loss becomes a Gift."
—United Network for Organ Sharing[1]

■ INTRODUCTION

India passed legislation called the Transplantation of Human Organs Act (THOA) in 1994 and was amended in 2011. Due to the 1994 Act, brain death became legally defined as death and organ donation after brain death was allowed for the first time. New rules have been formulated in 2014.

Organ transplantation can be done either from a living person—who can donate a kidney, part of a liver and part of a lung; or from a brain dead patient—who can donate multiple organs. The Transplant law:
- Regulates removal, storage, and transplantation of human organs and tissues
- Seeks to prevent commercial dealings in human organs and tissues
- Mandates request for organ donation for all ICU patients.

The THO rules can be broadly divided into three aspects:
1. Rules regulating living donation
2. Rules regulating deceased donor programs
3. Rules regulating hospitals and requirements for certification.

■ TRANSPLANTATION OF HUMAN ORGANS AND TISSUES RULES 2014

The new rules formulated in 2014 (The Transplantation of Human Organs and Tissues Rules 2014) have made punishment for organ commerce in living donation very severe. Certain amendments to encourage donation include *required request* in the event of brain death, having a clause of *organ donation in the driving licence* and allowing *swap donation* between two or more families. The new law has 21 forms compared to 13 forms previously (**Table 1**). Significant changes in the new rules are as follows (**Table 2**).

TABLE 1: Comparison of the forms in the old and new rules.

Content	Transplantation of Human Organs and Tissues Rules, 2014	Transplantation of Human Organs Rules, 1995
Consent form—Prospective related donor	Form 1 (Organ/Tissue)	Form 1 (A) (Organ)
Consent form—Prospective spousal donor	Form 2 (Organ/Tissue)	Form 1 (B) (Organ)
Consent form—Prospective unrelated donor	Form 3 (Organ/Tissue)	Form 1 (C) (Organ)
Medical fitness of living donor—Registered medical practitioner (Related/spousal/unrelated)	Form 4	Form 2
Genetic relationship of living donor with recipient - Head of the laboratory	Form 5	Form 3
Certificate from Registered Medical Practitioner for spousal living donor	Form 6	Form 4
Donor pledge form	Form 7 Organ(s)/Tissue(s)	Form 5 Organ(s)
Consent form—By near relatives for organ donation after brain death—Adult donors	Form 8	Form 6
Consent form for unclaimed body in a hospital or prison	Form 9	
Brainstem death certificate	Form 10	Form 8
Joint application (Donor and Recipient) for approval for transplantation (living donor)	Form 11	Form 10
Application for registration of hospital to carry out transplantation	Form 12 (Organ/Tissue except cornea)	Form 11 (Organ)
Application for registration of hospital to carry out organ/tissue retrieval other than cornea	Form 13	
Application for registration for tissue banks other than cornea	Form 14	
Application for registration of eye bank, corneal transplantation and eye retrieval center	Form 15	
Certificate of registration for performing organ/tissue transplantation/retrieval and/or tissue banking	Form 16	Form 12
Certificate of renewal of registration—Office of appropriate authority—Organ(s)/Tissue(s) retrieval/Transplantation/banking	Form 17	Form 13
Certificate by the authorization committee—Unrelated/Swap/Foreign nationals	Form 18	
Certificate by competent authority—For Indian near relative (Other than spouse)	Form 19	
Verification certificate in respect of domicile status of recipient or donor—Tehsildar or any other authorized officer	Form 20	
Certificate of relationship between donor and recipient in case of foreigners—by the Embassy concerned	Form 21	

TABLE 2: Significant changes related to deceased organ donation in THOTR 2014 as compared to THOA 1994.

	THOA 1994	THOTR 2014
Declaration of brain death	Restricted to hospitals registered for organ transplantation	Allowed in any hospital with ICU
Requirement of neurophysician/neurosurgeon	Mandatory for declaration of brain death	No mandatory, if not available
Counseling for organ donation	Not mandatory	Mandatory
Medicolegal donations	Complicated	Simplified
Donor maintenance and organ retrieval charges	Not clear	To be borne by the recipient or institution or Govt. or NGO
Transplant coordinators in hospitals	Optional	Mandatory; qualifications specified

- Declaration of brain death and organ retrieval was earlier permitted only in hospitals approved for organ transplantation. Now, it is allowed from any hospital having intensive care facility equipped with ventilators. However, such hospitals need to apply for sanction as nontransplant organ retrieval centers (NTORC).
- Earlier, the presence of neurologist or neurosurgeon was mandatory in the 4-number team for declaration of brain death. As per the provisions of the new rules, when a neurologist or neurosurgeon is not available in a hospital, any physician, anesthetist or intensivist, nominated by the medical administrator in charge of the hospital, and approved by the appropriate state authority, can be the member of the board of medical experts for certification of brain death.
- Earlier, it was not mandatory to approach the families of patients with brain death for organ donation. As per the new rules, it is mandatory for the treating doctor to ascertain whether the potential donor had pledged to donate organs during lifetime and to approach the relatives for organ donation, irrespective of previous pledge.
- In patients with medicolegal requirements, like in all patients with head injury due to road traffic accidents, the procedure for clearance from police and postmortem authorities had been simplified. After the consent to donate organs from a brainstem dead donor is obtained from the family, the registered medical practitioner of the hospital is required to make a request to make a request to the police to facilitate timely retrieval of organs or tissue from the donor and a copy of such a request is simultaneously sent to the disignated post mortem authority. Following retrieval of organs, the surgeon issues a certificate listing out the organs retrieved to the postmortem authorities, who are required to carry out the autopsy expeditiously, even beyond office hours.
- Earlier there was no clarity regarding the donor maintenance or organ retrieval charges. It has now been clarified that the cost of donor maintenance, retrieval of organs and tissues, their tranportation and preservation, may be borne by the recipient or institution or government or nongovernment organization as decided by respective state or union territory.
- Earlier the requirement of transplant coordinators was not mandatory. It is now essential for hospitals carrying out organ transplantation to employ trained transplant coordinators and their qualifications have been specified.

Medicolegal Aspects of Living Donation and Transplantation

Since THOA (1994) was passed, there have been problems with its implementation process. The rules regulating living donation were meant to curb commerce in organs, especially kidneys. Unfortunately, this has not happened. Often, there has been a circus of sorts, which has left the government always ducking in defence. The bugbear has been Sec 9(3) of chapter II of THOA which states that:

"If any donor authorizes the removal of any of his human organs before his death under Sec 3(1) for transplantation into the body of such recipient, not being a near relative as is specified by the donor, by reason of affection or attachment towards the recipient or for any other special reasons, such human organ shall not be removed and transplanted without the prior approval of the Authorization Committee."

Some of the significant points pertaining to living donation in the Act and amendment are provided below.

- In the case of living donation, the Registered Medical Practitioner (RMP) must certify:
  - The donor's consent
  - The donor is fit to donate
  - All forms pertaining to the donor-recipient relationship (i.e., relative, spouse, or unrelated) are in order.
- The Central Government, in cooperation with each State Government, will nominate Authorization Committees (AC) which shall ensure that all transplant donors and recipient applicants have complied with the requirements of THOA.
- One State level Authorization Committee (AC) and, depending on regional transplant volumes, one or more Hospital Based or District Level ACs that will comprise a Chief Medical Officer/Medical Director, two senior medical practitioners, two community members of high esteem, a Health Secretary, and Health Director. No members of the transplant team shall be part of the AC.
- All living unrelated donor transplant cases and foreign national cases must be reviewed by the AC for approval. If the donor, recipient, and transplant institution are from different states, then issuance of 'no objection certificate' (NOC) is mandatory from the state in which the donor or recipient legally reside. The transplant institution must receive approval from the AC.
  - All the unrelated donors who are presented to the committee readily express *reason of affection or attachment towards the recipient*. The committee often turns a blind eye knowing well that this might not be the case and clears the papers to proceed for the transplantation. In most instances, an unofficial monetary transaction follows between the two parties. All goes well until a donor who does not get the promised sum makes a complaint to the police. Neither the complainant, nor the police realize that selling a kidney is as much an offence as buying the organ.
  - All the three parties in this kind of medicolegal muddle have an undeniable responsibility. The implementation process of the act is more complex than was ever envisaged by the pundits who put the framework together.
- The Central and State Governments appoint "Appropriate Authorities" (AA) whose function is to grant, suspend, or cancel transplant center and tissue bank privileges based on compliance with THOA standards. Periodic inspections by the AAs of transplant centers and tissue banks will be undertaken to ensure that THOA standards are being followed. The AA has the authority to investigate and act upon any deviations from THOA rules.

- All tissue banks must be duly registered and approved by the AA. The AA may issue "show cause" (registration suspension) notices to hospitals or tissue banks that are found to be in violation of THOA rules.
- Every transplant center must be registered as such in order to perform transplant activity. The AA will determine an institution's capabilities in performing transplant activities. Each authorized transplant center must maintain its own website that regularly updates the numbers and details of each of its transplants.
- In certain cases, special state orders exist regarding transplantation. These special orders issued by the states of Andhra Pradesh, Tamil Nadu, Maharashtra and Kerala may be viewed by referring to the following website links: *http://www.dmrhs.org/tnos/orders-of-tn-govt;http://www.jeevandan.gov.in/PDF's/GOMS184.pdf;* *http://knos.org.in/pdf/go_ms_36_2012.pdf*

Medicolegal Aspects of Deceased Organ Donation and Transplantation

Rules regulating the deceased donor program in the act need to protect the interests of a brain dead donor and at the same time facilitate the process of donation to ease the shortage of organs. In this regard, the delays that result in the organ donation process (especially in medicolegal cases that require postmortem procedures) can be very traumatic to the families and some simplification is required.

A doctor is authorized to remove an organ from a brain dead patient only if the:
- Patient is certified as brain dead
- Proper authorization has been obtained from the family (person lawfully in possession of the dead body) of the brain dead patient
- Clearance from the police officer and forensic doctor has been obtained in case of a medicolegal case.

A board of four medical experts is required to certify brain death:
1. The medical administrator in charge of the hospital where brain death has occurred
2. An authorized specialist, nominated by #1 above and approved by the AA
3. A neurologist, neurosurgeon, anesthetist, intensivist, physician or surgeon
4. The RMP treating the patient.

The board must not contain any members from the recovering transplant team.

The certification of brain death requires to be done twice with a minimum time interval of 6 hours between the two certification processes. The new rules (2014) state that when a neurologist or neurosurgeon is unavailable, then an anesthetist or intensivist, physician or a surgeon nominated by the medical administrator in charge of the hospital shall be a part of the panel of doctors that certifies brain death.

Since most of the brain death cases are due to accidents, an inquest followed by an autopsy becomes a norm. These cases are medicolegal cases (MLC) and the victim of the accident can become an organ donor.

In Tamil Nadu for the year 2013, 72% cases of organ donation were from MLC and 84% of these MLC were due to road traffic accidents, according to the annual report from the Tamil Nadu Organ Sharing Registry.[2] In recent years, tier-II cities in Tamil Nadu are contributing to the deceased donor numbers. An editorial that appeared in the Indian Transplant Newsletter[3] attributed this to the increased awareness about the success of deceased organ donation

among the doctors and the public due to positive media support, better infrastructure and presence of grief counselors.
Protocol followed in Tamil Nadu for deceased organ donation:
- First certification of brainstem death
- Counsel the relatives for organ donation
- Intimate the Police and Forensic Expert
- Second certification of brainstem death
- Authorization for removal of organs from Forensic expert—No objection for harvesting the organs from the cadaver (Indicates that the organs authorised for removal are not necessary for confirmation of cause of death)
- Proceed with organ harvesting
- Send the body for autopsy.

In Tamil Nadu, those centers which are authorized Organ transplant centers can do the postmortem examination in their own premises using experts who have a reasonable experience in doing medicolegal postmortems.

The issue in MLC is the time at which the post-mortem (PM) is performed. Whereas in some states the PM is done at the time of retrieval, in others it is done only during daytime and in some cases it is waived. In the new rules of 2014 the postmortem examination is permitted at the time of organ retrieval and the forensic doctors can be requested to make their notes from the medical report of the organ/tissue retrieval.

The amended THOA also permits license for hospitals to be designated as only *organ retrieval centers* without payment of any fees. These are nontransplanting hospitals that may have the necessary infrastructure and can help with only organ retrieval. Once retrieved the organs are to be used by transplanting hospitals. It is expected that such centers would identify brain death cases and improve the numbers of organs that can be retrieved. In the state of Kerala in 2013, of the 36 deceased organ donors, 13 originated from such nontransplanting organ retrieval hospitals, according to the Annual report of the Kerala Organ Sharing Registry.[4] The 2014 rules also provide for the establishment of a system of reimbursement of expenses for such organ retrieval centers.

■ FUTURE CHALLENGES

The deceased donor program can become a viable alternative to living donation in India only if a mechanism is put in place to make the program more visible. This can only happen by education, first of our own medical fraternity and then of the Indian public. There are innumerable ways of accomplishing this objective, but what is essential is continuous engagement.

The current deceased organ donor rate in India is only 0.26 per million population. The number of deceased organ donors and transplants in the year 2012 and 2013 in India from different states is given in **Tables 3** and **4**.

To improve the organ donation rate the THOA amendment has mandated the appointment of a trained transplant coordinator in all licensed transplant centers. The transplant coordinator will initiate the processes to intimate the certifying doctors about a brain death case, obtain consent from next of kin, and proceed to coordinate for organ recovery.

Of utmost importance is the early identification and certification of brain death in the ICUs of all hospitals. This needs to be made mandatory in all hospitals accompanied by regular audits. In the year 2008, the Government of Tamil Nadu had made this mandatory in three of its

TABLE 3: Deceased donor organ transplantation (2012).

State	No. of deceased donors	Kidney	Liver	Heart	Lung	Pancreas	Small intestine
Tamil Nadu	83	148	80	16	8	0	0
Maharashtra	29	49	19	0	0	0	0
Karnataka	17	32	13	1	0	0	0
Andhra Pradesh	13	21	12	2	1	1	0
Kerala	12	24	2	0	0	0	0
Gujarat	18	30	16	0	0	0	0
Delhi NCR	12	24	6	0	0	0	1
Punjab	12	24	0	0	0	0	0

TABLE 4: Deceased donor organ transplantation (2013).

State	Tamil Nadu	Andhra Pradesh	Kerala	Maharashtra	Delhi	Gujarat	Karnataka	Puducherry
Donor	131	40	35	35	27	25	18	2
* ODR (pmp)	1.8	0.47	1.05	0.31	1.61	0.41	0.29	1.6
Heart	16	2	6	0	-	0	1	0
Lung	20	2	0	0	-	0	0	0
Liver	118	34	23	23	23	20	16	0
Kidney	234	75	59	53	40	54	29	4

* ODR (pmp): Organ donation rate (per million population)

hospitals by issuing a special Government order (GO (Ms) No 6 of 2008). And this has reflected in the increase in deceased multiorgan donations coming from Tamil Nadu, according to an article in the British Medical Journal that appeared in 2013.[5]

In addition, a 'mandated choice' clause for organ donation on the Indian driving license makes for greater visibility. The new THOA rules mention that a person can make known his/her wish for organ donation in documents like the driving license. The amended act has introduced more stringent punishment for those indulging in commercial trade of organs. New forms for living donation have been incorporated to make the procedure more foolproof, but implementation remains a challenge.

The 2014 amendment to the law has laid down guidelines for establishing national, regional and state networks for organ allocation and sharing. It also states that an organ transplant registry, organ donation registry and tissue registry will be established. Transplant outcomes will be documented. All this will help in greater accountability and transparency both in living as well as deceased organ donation.

■ CONCLUSION

Health and education are state subjects in India, for individual states. The THOA act allows states to adopt the law or change some of the rules to ensure that the donation rate in their states goes up and illegal organ trade stops. To bridge the gap between shortage of organs and increasing number of organ failure patients the various state health departments in the country needs to work with the hospital, NGO's and the public to promote both the living and deceased organ donation and transplantation programme. The current 2011 amended law and the 2014 rules plug in all the loop-holes that were resulting in organ trade in India. It also has some very proactive clauses to promote deceased donation transplantation. The challenge will be in implementing the law in its framework and in the right spirit to make sure that a highly ethical programme evolves. Lives can be saved provided a concerted inclusive effort is made that involves all the stakeholders in the program.

■ REFERENCES

1. Available: *http://unos.org/docs/Annual Report.* 2009.pdf.
2. Amalorpavanathan J, Shroff S, Karunakaran C E, Castro R. Annual Report from Tamil Nadu Organ Sharing Registry for the year 2013. Chennai.
3. Shroff S, Sumana N. Editorial desk, Contribution of Tier–II cities Key factor in success of deceased organ donation in Tamil Nadu. Indian Transplant Newsletter. 2013-2014;13(40).
4. Pisharody R, Gracious N, Shroff S and Castro R. Annual Report of the Kerala Organ Sharing Registry for the year 2013, Kerala.
5. Srinivasan S. Has Tamil Nadu turned the tide on the transplant trade? BMJ 2013; 346:f2155 *http://www.bmj.com/content/346/bmj.f2155.*

CHAPTER 19

Medicolegal Outlook on Bio-Medical Waste Management Act

VP Singh, Pardeep Singh

> *"Environmental pollution is an incurable disease. It can only be prevented."*
> —**Barry Commoner**[1]

■ INTRODUCTION

Hospital waste generated during the process of healthcare activities carries a potential for polluting the environment. Proper handling and disposal of hospital waste as per the provisions of *environment law* is the responsibility of every healthcare establishment. The present scenario of hospital waste management in Indian hospitals is dismal. Some healthcare establishments are dumping the hospital waste into municipal solid waste resulting in adverse effect on environment and human health. As the environmentalists and the courts are taking a serious note on the issue of hospital waste, there is an emerging concern among the Indian healthcare establishments that the hospital waste is managed properly. Awareness regarding safe management of bio-medical waste is a must for the generators, operators, and decision makers.

■ BIO-MEDICAL WASTE

Bio-medical waste means any waste, which is generated during the diagnosis, treatment or immunization of human beings or animals or in research activities pertaining thereto or in the production or testing of biologicals, and including categories mentioned in Schedule I of Bio-medical Waste (Management & Handlings) Rules. The bio-medical waste may be categorized as follows:[2]
- *Nonhazardous waste:* Approximately 75–85% of the bio-medical waste is nonhazardous. This includes waste comprising of food remnants, wash water, paper cartons, packaging material, etc.
- *Hazardous waste*: The remaining 15–25% waste which is hazardous may be categorized as follows:
  - *Infectious waste*:
    - Dressings and swabs contaminated with blood, pus, and body fluids
    - Laboratory waste including laboratory culture stocks of infectious agents

- Potentially infected material: Excised tumors and organs, placenta removed during surgery, extracted teeth, etc.
- Potentially infected animals used in diagnostic and research studies
- Sharps, which include needle, syringes, blades, etc.
- Blood and blood products
  - *Toxic waste*:
    - *Radioactive waste*: It includes waste contaminated with radionuclides. These are generated from in vitro analysis of body fluids and tissue, in vitro imaging, and therapeutic procedures.[3]
    - *Chemical waste*: It includes disinfectants (hypochlorite, glutaraldehyde, phenolic derivatives, and alcohol-based preparations), X-ray processing solutions, associated reagents, and base metal debris (dental amalgam in extracted teeth).
    - *Pharmaceutical waste*: It includes anesthetics, sedatives, antibiotics, analgesics, etc.[4]
    - It is important to take care that nonhazardous waste should also be handled cautiously so that it does not mix up with the hazardous waste. If both these wastes mix together then the nonhazardous waste will also become hazardous.

■ LAW ON BIO-MEDICAL WASTE MANAGEMENT[5]

Pursuant to the directives of the Supreme Court, the Ministry of Environment and Forests, Government of India in exercise of the powers conferred by Sections 6, 8, and 25 of the Environment (Protection) Act, 1986 framed *"Bio-Medical Waste (Management and Handlings) Rules" in 1998.* The objectives of these rules are to regulate the disposal of bio-medical wastes and to ensure the safety of the staff, patients, public, and the environment. These rules were amended twice in 2000 and 2003. To further improve the collection, storage, processing, treatment, and disposal of the bio-medical waste thereby, reducing the bio-medical waste generation as well as its impact on the environment, The Central Government, Ministry of Environment, Forest & Climate Change published the rules called *"Bio-Medical Waste Management Rules, 2016"* vide the notification no. G.S.R. 343(E) in the government gazette, dated 28th March 2016.

■ BIO-MEDICAL WASTE MANAGEMENT RULES, 2016[6]

Application of the Rules

1. These rules shall apply to all persons who generate, collect, receive, store, transport, treat, dispose, or handle bio-medical waste in any form including hospitals, nursing homes, clinics, dispensaries, veterinary institutions, animal houses, pathological laboratories, blood banks, ayush hospitals, clinical establishments, research or educational institutions, health camps, medical or surgical camps, vaccination camps, blood donation camps, first aid rooms of schools, forensic laboratories, and research labs.
2. These rules shall not apply to:
   a. Radioactive wastes as covered under the provisions of the Atomic Energy Act, 1962 (33 of 1962) and the rules made there under;
   b. Hazardous chemicals covered under the Manufacture, Storage and Import of Hazardous Chemicals Rules, 1989 made under the Act;

c. Solid wastes covered under the Municipal Solid Waste (Management and Handling) Rules, 2000 made under the Act;
d. The lead acid batteries covered under the Batteries (Management and Handling) Rules, 2001 made under the Act;
e. Hazardous wastes covered under the Hazardous Wastes (Management, Handling and Transboundary Movement) Rules, 2008 made under the Act;
f. Waste covered under the e-Waste (Management and Handling) Rules, 2011 made under the Act; and
g. Hazardous microorganisms, genetically engineered microorganisms, and cells covered under the Manufacture, Use, Import, Export and Storage of Hazardous Microorganisms, Genetically Engineered Microorganisms or Cells Rules, 1989 made under the Act.

Important Definitions

- *Occupier* means a person having administrative control over the institution and the premises generating bio-medical waste, which includes a hospital, nursing home, clinic, dispensary, veterinary institution, animal house, pathological laboratory, blood bank, healthcare facility, and clinical establishment, irrespective of their system of medicine and by whatever name they are called;
- *Authorisation* means permission granted by the prescribed authority for the generation, collection, reception, storage, transportation, treatment, processing, disposal or any other form of handling of bio-medical waste in accordance with these rules and guidelines issued by the Central Government or Central Pollution Control Board as the case may be;
- *Authorised person* means an occupier or operator authorised by the prescribed authority to generate, collect, receive, store, transport, treat, process, dispose or handle bio-medical waste in accordance with these rules and the guidelines issued by the Central Government or the Central Pollution Control Board, as the case may be;
- *Bio-medical waste* means any waste, which is generated during the diagnosis, treatment or immunisation of human beings or animals or research activities pertaining thereto or in the production or testing of biological or in health camps, including the categories mentioned in Schedule I appended to these rules;
- *Bio-medical waste treatment and disposal facility* means any facility wherein treatment, disposal of bio-medical waste or processes incidental to such treatment and disposal is carried out, and includes common bio-medical waste treatment facilities (CBWTFs).

Duty of an Occupier

It shall be the duty of every occupier to:
- Take all necessary steps to ensure that bio-medical waste is handled without any adverse effect to human health and the environment and in accordance with these rules;
- Make a provision within the premises for a safe, ventilated, and secured location for storage of segregated bio-medical waste in colored bags or containers in the manner as specified in Schedule I, to ensure that there shall be no secondary handling, pilferage of recyclables or inadvertent scattering or spillage by animals and the bio-medical waste from such place or premises shall be directly transported in the manner as prescribed in these rules to the CBWTF or for the appropriate treatment and disposal, as the case may be, in the manner as prescribed in Schedule I;

CHAPTER 19: Medicolegal Outlook on Bio-Medical Waste Management Act | 215

- Pre-treat the laboratory waste, microbiological waste, blood samples, and blood bags through disinfection or sterilisation on-site in the manner as prescribed by the World Health Organization (WHO) or National AIDS Control Organisation (NACO) guidelines and then sent to the CBWTF for final disposal;
- Phase out use of chlorinated plastic bags, gloves, and blood bags within 2 years from the date of notification of these rules;
- Dispose of solid waste other than bio-medical waste in accordance with the provisions of respective waste management rules made under the relevant laws and amended from time to time;
- Not to give treated bio-medical waste with municipal solid waste;
- Provide training to all its healthcare workers and others, involved in handling of bio-medical waste at the time of induction and thereafter at least once every year and the details of training programs conducted, number of personnel trained, and number of personnel not undergone any training shall be provided in the Annual Report;
- Immunise all its healthcare workers and others, involved in handling of bio-medical waste for protection against diseases including hepatitis B and tetanus that are likely to be transmitted by handling of bio-medical waste, in the manner as prescribed in the National Immunisation Policy or the guidelines of the Ministry of Health and Family Welfare issued from time to time;
- Establish a bar-code system for bags or containers containing bio-medical waste to be sent out of the premises or place for any purpose within 1 year from the date of the notification of these rules;
- Ensure segregation of liquid chemical waste at source and ensure pre-treatment or neutralization prior to mixing with other effluent generated from healthcare facilities;
- Ensure treatment and disposal of liquid waste in accordance with the Water (Prevention and Control of Pollution) Act, 1974 (6 of 1974);
- Ensure occupational safety of all its healthcare workers and others involved in handling of bio-medical waste by providing appropriate and adequate personal protective equipment;
- Conduct health check up at the time of induction and at least once in a year for all its healthcare workers and others involved in handling of bio-medical waste and maintain the records for the same;
- Maintain and update on day-to-day basis the bio-medical waste management register and display the monthly record on its website according to the bio-medical waste generated in terms of category and colour coding as specified in Schedule I;
- Report major accidents including accidents caused by fire hazards, blasts during handling of bio-medical waste, and the remedial action taken and the records relevant thereto, (including nil report) in Form I to the prescribed authority and also along with the annual report;
- Make available the annual report on its website and all the healthcare facilities shall make own website within 2 years from the date of notification of these rules;
- Inform the prescribed authority immediately in case the operator of a facility does not collect the bio-medical waste within the intended time or as per the agreed time;
- Establish a system to review and monitor the activities related to bio-medical waste management, either through an existing committee or by forming a new committee and the committee shall meet once in every 6 months and the record of the minutes of the meetings of this committee shall be submitted along with the annual report to the prescribed authority and the healthcare establishments having less than 30 beds shall

designate a qualified person to review and monitor the activities relating to bio-medical waste management within that establishment and submit the annual report;
- Maintain all records for operation of incineration, hydro or autoclaving, etc., for a period of 5 years;
- Existing incinerators to achieve the standards for treatment and disposal of bio-medical waste as specified in Schedule II for retention time in secondary chamber and dioxin and furans within 2 years from the date of this notification.

Prescribed Authority
- The prescribed authority for implementation of the provisions of these rules shall be the State Pollution Control Boards in respect of States and Pollution Control Committees in respect of Union territories.
- The prescribed authority for enforcement of the provisions of these rules in respect of all healthcare establishments including hospitals, nursing homes, clinics, dispensaries, veterinary institutions, animal houses, pathological laboratories, and blood banks of the Armed Forces under the Ministry of Defence shall be the Director General, Armed Forces Medical Services, who shall function under the supervision and control of the Ministry of Defence.

Procedure for Authorization
- Every occupier or operator handling bio-medical waste, irrespective of the quantity, shall make an application in Form II to the prescribed authority, i.e., State Pollution Control Board and Pollution Control Committee, as the case may be, for grant of authorisation and the prescribed authority shall grant the provisional authorisation in Form III and the validity of such authorisation for bedded healthcare facility and operator of a common facility shall be synchronised with the validity of the consents.
- The authorisation shall be one time for non-bedded occupiers and the authorisation in such cases shall be deemed to have been granted, if not objected by the prescribed authority within a period of 90 days from the date of receipt of duly completed application along with such necessary documents.
- In case of refusal of renewal, cancellation or suspension of the authorisation by the prescribed authority, the reasons shall be recorded in writing: Provided that the prescribed authority shall give an opportunity of being heard to the applicant before such refusal of the authorisation.
- Every application for authorisation shall be disposed of by the prescribed authority within a period of 90 days from the date of receipt of duly completed application along with such necessary documents, failing which it shall be deemed that the authorisation is granted under these rules.
- In case of any change in the bio-medical waste generation, handling, treatment, and disposal for which authorisation was earlier granted, the occupier or operator shall intimate to the prescribed authority about the change or variation in the activity and shall submit a fresh application in Form II for modification of the conditions of authorisation.

Advisory Committee
1. Every State Government or Union territory Administration shall constitute an Advisory Committee for the respective State or Union territory under the chairmanship of the

respective health secretary to oversee the implementation of the rules in the respective state and to advice any improvements and the Advisory Committee shall include representatives from the Departments of Health, Environment, Urban Development, Animal Husbandry and Veterinary Sciences of that State Government or Union territory Administration, State Pollution Control Board or Pollution Control Committee, urban local bodies or local bodies or Municipal Corporation, representatives from Indian Medical Association, CBWTF, and non-governmental organisation.
2. Notwithstanding anything contained in sub-rule (1), the Ministry of Defence shall constitute the Advisory Committee (Defence) under the chairmanship of Director General of Health Services of Armed Forces consisting of representatives from the Ministry of Defence, Ministry of Environment, Forest and Climate Change, Central Pollution Control Board, Ministry of Health and Family Welfare, Armed Forces Medical College or Command Hospital.
3. The Advisory Committee constituted under sub-rule (1) and (2) shall meet at least once in 6 months and review all matters related to implementation of the provisions of these rules in the State and Armed Forces Health Care Facilities, as the case may be.
4. The Ministry of Health and Defence may co-opt representatives from the other governmental and non-governmental organisations having expertise in the field of bio-medical waste management.

Monitoring of Implementation of the Rules in Healthcare Facilities

1. The Ministry of Environment, Forest and Climate Change shall review the implementation of the rules in the country once in a year through the State Health Secretaries and Chairmen or Member Secretary of State Pollution Control Boards and Central Pollution Control Board and the Ministry may also invite experts in the field of bio-medical waste management, if required.
2. The Central Pollution Control Board shall monitor the implementation of these rules in respect of all the Armed Forces healthcare establishments under the Ministry of Defence.
3. The Central Pollution Control Board along with one or more representatives of the Advisory Committee constituted under sub-rule (2) of rule 11 may inspect any Armed Forces healthcare establishments after prior intimation to the Director General Armed Forces Medical Services.
4. Every State Government or Union territory Administration shall constitute District Level Monitoring Committee in the districts under the chairmanship of District Collector or District Magistrate or Deputy Commissioner or Additional District Magistrate to monitor the compliance of the provisions of these rules in the healthcare facilities generating bio-medical waste and in the common bio-medical waste treatment and disposal facilities, where the bio-medical waste is treated and disposed of.
5. The District Level Monitoring Committee constituted under sub-rule (4) shall submit its report once in 6 months to the State Advisory Committee and a copy thereof shall also be forwarded to State Pollution Control Board or Pollution Control Committee concerned for taking further necessary action.
6. The District Level Monitoring Committee shall comprise of District Medical Officer or District Health Officer, representatives from State Pollution Control Board or Pollution Control Committee, Public Health Engineering Department, local bodies or municipal corporation, Indian Medical Association, CBWTF, and registered nongovernmental organisations working in the field of bio-medical waste management and the Committee

may co-opt other members and experts, if necessary and the District Medical Officer shall be the Member Secretary of this Committee.

Annual Report

1. Every occupier or operator of CBWTF shall submit an annual report to the prescribed authority in Form-IV, on or before the 30th June of every year.
2. The prescribed authority shall compile, review, and analyse the information received and send this information to the Central Pollution Control Board on or before the 31st July of every year.
3. The Central Pollution Control Board shall compile, review, and analyse the information received and send this information, along with its comments or suggestions or observations, to the Ministry of Environment, Forest and Climate Change on or before 31st August every year.
4. The Annual Reports shall also be available online on the websites of Occupiers, State Pollution Control Boards, and Central Pollution Control Board.

Appeal

1. Any person aggrieved by an order made by the prescribed authority under these rules may, within a period of 30 days from the date on which the order is communicated to him, prefer an appeal in Form V to the Secretary (Environment) of the State Government or Union territory administration.
2. Any person aggrieved by an order of the Director General Armed Forces Medical Services under these rules may, within 30 days from the date on which the order is communicated to him, prefer an appeal in Form V to the Secretary, Ministry of Environment, Forest and Climate Change.
3. The authority referred to in sub-para (1) and (2) as the case may be, may entertain the appeal after the expiry of the said period of 30 days, if it is satisfied that the appellant was prevented by sufficient cause from filing the appeal in time.
4. The appeal shall be disposed of within a period of 90 days from the date of its filing.

Liability of the Occupier, Operator of a Facility

1. The occupier or an operator of a CBWTF shall be liable for all the damages caused to the environment or the public due to improper handling of bio-medical wastes.
2. The occupier or operator of CBWTF shall be liable for action under section 5 and section 15 of the Act, in case of any violation.

Treatment and Disposal

Bio-medical waste shall be treated and disposed of in accordance with Schedule I, and in compliance with the standards prescribed in Schedule II.

Segregation, Packaging, Transportation, and Storage (Table 1)

1. No untreated bio-medical waste shall be mixed with other wastes.
2. The bio-medical waste shall be segregated into containers or bags at the point of generation in accordance with Schedule I prior to its storage, transportation, treatment, and disposal.

3. The containers or bags referred to in sub-rule (2) shall be labeled as specified in Schedule IV.
4. Barcode and global positioning system shall be added by the occupier and common bio-medical waste treatment facility in 1 year time.
5. The operator of CBWTF shall transport the bio-medical waste from the premises of an occupier to any off-site bio-medical waste treatment facility only in the vehicles having label as provided in part 'A' of the Schedule IV along with necessary information as specified in part 'B' of the Schedule IV.
6. The vehicles used for transportation of bio-medical waste shall comply with the conditions if any stipulated by the State Pollution Control Board or Pollution Control Committee in addition to the requirement contained in the Motor Vehicles Act, 1988 (59 of 1988), if any or the rules made there under for transportation of such infectious waste.
7. Untreated human anatomical waste, animal anatomical waste, soiled waste, and biotechnology waste shall not be stored beyond a period of 48 hours: Provided that in case for any reason it becomes necessary to store such waste beyond such a period, the occupier shall act appropriately to ensure that the waste does not adversely affect human health and the environment and inform the prescribed authority along with the reasons for doing so.
8. Microbiology waste and all other clinical laboratory waste shall be pre-treated by sterilisation to Log 6 or disinfection to Log 4, as per the WHO guidelines before packing and sending to the CBWTF.

TABLE 1: Bio-medical wastes categories and their segregation, collection, treatment, processing and disposal options (Schedule I – Part 1).[6]

Category	Type of waste	Type of bag or container to be used	Treatment and disposal options
Yellow	**Human anatomical waste:** Human tissues, organs, body parts, and fetus below the viability period (as per the MTP Act 1971, amended from time to time)	Yellow coloured non-chlorinated plastic bags	Incineration or plasma pyrolysis or deep burial*
	Animal anatomical waste: Experimental animal carcasses, body parts, organs, tissues, including the waste generated from animals used in experiments or testing in veterinary hospitals or colleges or animal houses		
	Soiled waste: Items contaminated with blood, body fluids like dressings, plaster casts, cotton swabs and bags containing residual or discarded blood and blood components		• Incineration or plasma pyrolysis or deep burial* • In absence of above facilities, autoclaving or micro-waving/hydroclaving followed by shredding or mutilation or combination of sterilization and shredding • Treated waste to be sent for energy recovery

Continued

Continued

Category	Type of waste	Type of bag or container to be used	Treatment and disposal options
	Expired or discarded medicines: Pharmaceutical waste like antibiotics, cytotoxic drugs including all items contaminated with cytotoxic drugs along with glass or plastic ampoules, vials, etc.	Yellow coloured non-chlorinated plastic bags or containers	• Expired cytotoxic drugs and items contaminated with cytotoxic drugs to be returned back to the manufacturer or supplier for incineration at temperature >1200°C or to common bio-medical waste treatment facility or hazardous waste treatment, storage and disposal facility for incineration at >1200°C or encapsulation or plasma pyrolysis at >1200°C • All other discarded medicines shall be either sent back to manufacturer or disposed by incineration
	Chemical waste: Chemicals used in production of biological and used or discarded disinfectants	Yellow coloured containers or non-chlorinated plastic bags	Disposed of by incineration or plasma pyrolysis or encapsulation in hazardous waste treatment, storage and disposal facility
	Chemical liquid waste: Liquid waste generated due to use of chemicals in production of biological and used or discarded disinfectants, silver X-ray film developing liquid, discarded formalin, infected secretions, aspirated body fluids, liquid from laboratories and floor washings, cleaning, house-keeping and disinfecting activities, etc.	Separate collection system leading to effluent treatment system	After resource recovery, the chemical liquid waste shall be pre-treated before mixing with other wastewater. The combined discharge shall conform to the discharge norms given in Schedule-III
	• Discarded linen, mattresses, beddings contaminated with blood or body fluid	Non-chlorinated yellow plastic bags or suitable packing material	• Non-chlorinated chemical disinfection followed by incineration or plasma pyrolysis or for energy recovery • In absence of above facilities, shredding or mutilation or combination of sterilization and shredding. Treated waste to be sent for energy recovery or incineration or plasma pyrolysis

Continued

CHAPTER 19: Medicolegal Outlook on Bio-Medical Waste Management Act | 221

Continued

Category	Type of waste	Type of bag or container to be used	Treatment and disposal options
	• **Microbiology, biotechnology and other clinical laboratory waste:** Blood bags, Laboratory cultures, stocks or specimens of microorganisms, live or attenuated vaccines, human and animal cell cultures used in research, industrial laboratories, production of biological, residual toxins, dishes and devices used for cultures	Autoclave safe plastic bags or containers	Pre-treat to sterilize with non-chlorinated chemicals on-site as per National AIDS Control Organisation or World Health Organization guidelines thereafter for Incineration
Red	• **Contaminated waste (recyclable):** Wastes generated from disposable items such as tubing, bottles, intravenous tubes and sets, catheters, urine bags, syringes (without needles and fixed needle syringes) and vaccutainers with their needles cut and gloves	Red coloured non-chlorinated plastic bags or containers	• Autoclaving or micro-waving/hydroclaving followed by shredding or mutilation or combination of sterilization and shredding. Treated waste to be sent to registered or authorized recyclers or for energy recovery or plastics to diesel or fuel oil or for road making, whichever is possible • Plastic waste should not be sent to landfill sites
White (Translucent)	• **Waste sharps including metals:** Needles, syringes with fixed needles, needles from needle tip cutter or burner, scalpels, blades, or any other contaminated sharp object that may cause puncture and cuts. This includes both used, discarded, and contaminated metal sharps	Puncture proof, Leak proof, tamper proof containers	Autoclaving or dry heat sterilization followed by shredding or mutilation or encapsulation in metal container or cement concrete; combination of shredding cum autoclaving; and sent for final disposal to iron foundries (having consent to operate from the State Pollution Control Boards or Pollution Control Committees) or sanitary landfill or designated concrete waste sharp pit
Blue	• **Glassware:** Broken or discarded and contaminated glass including medicine vials and ampoules except those contaminated with cytotoxic wastes	Cardboard boxes with blue colored marking	Disinfection (by soaking the washed glass waste after cleaning with detergent and sodium hypochlorite treatment) or through autoclaving or microwaving or hydroclaving and then sent for recycling
	• **Metallic Body Implants**	Cardboard boxes with blue colored marking	

*Disposal by deep burial is permitted only in rural or remote areas where there is no access to common bio-medical waste treatment facility (CBWTF). This will be carried out with prior approval from the prescribed authority and as per the Standards specified in Schedule-III. The deep burial facility shall be located as per the provisions and guidelines issued by Central Pollution Control Board from time to time.

Continued

Continued

Part 2
• All plastic bags shall be as per Bureau of Indian Standards (BIS) standards as and when published, till then the prevailing Plastic Waste Management Rules shall be applicable
• Chemical treatment using at least 10% sodium hypochlorite having 30% residual chlorine for 25 min or any other equivalent chemical reagent that should demonstrate $Log_{10}4$ reduction efficiency for microorganisms as given in Schedule III
• Mutilation or shredding must be to an extent to prevent unauthorized reuse
• There will be no chemical pretreatment before incineration, except for microbiological, lab, and highly infectious waste
• Incineration ash (ash from incineration of any bio-medical waste) shall be disposed through hazardous waste treatment, storage, and disposal facility, if toxic or hazardous constituents are present beyond the prescribed limits as given in the Hazardous Waste (Management, Handling and Transboundary Movement) Rules, 2008 or as revised from time to time
• Dead fetus below the viability period [as per the Medical Termination of Pregnancy (MTP) Act 1971, amended from time to time] can be considered as human anatomical waste. Such waste should be handed over to the operator of common bio-medical waste treatment and disposal facility in yellow bag with a copy of the official MTP certificate from the obstetrician or the medical superintendent of hospital or healthcare establishment
• Cytotoxic drug vials shall not be handed over to unauthorised person under any circumstances. These shall be sent back to the manufactures for necessary disposal at a single point. As a second option, these may be sent for incineration at common bio-medical waste treatment and disposal facility or treatment, storage, and disposal facilities (TSDFs) or plasma pyrolysis at temperature >1200°C
• Residual or discarded chemical wastes, used or discarded disinfectants, and chemical sludge can be disposed at hazardous waste treatment, storage, and disposal facility. In such case, the waste should be sent to hazardous waste treatment, storage, and disposal facility through operator of common bio-medical waste treatment and disposal facility only
• On-site pre-treatment of laboratory waste, microbiological waste, blood samples, blood bags should be disinfected or sterilized as per the Guidelines of WHO or NACO and then given to the common bio-medical waste treatment and disposal facility
• Installation of in-house incinerator is not allowed. However, in case there is no common bio-medical facility nearby, the same may be installed by the occupier after taking authorisation from the State Pollution Control Board
• Syringes should be either mutilated or needles should be cut and or stored in tamper proof, leak proof, and puncture proof containers for sharps storage. Wherever the occupier is not linked to a disposal facility, it shall be the responsibility of the occupier to sterilize and dispose in the manner prescribed
• Bio-medical waste generated in households during healthcare activities shall be segregated as per these rules and handed over in separate bags or containers to municipal waste collectors. Urban local bodies shall have tie up with the common bio-medical waste treatment and disposal facility to pickup this waste from the Material Recovery Facility (MRF) or from the household directly, for final disposal in the manner as prescribed in this Schedule

SALIENT FEATURES OF BIO-MEDICAL WASTE RULES 2016

Name of the Rules

The earlier rules were named as *Bio-Medical Waste (Management and Handlings) Rules, 1998*. The phrase "handling" has been omitted and the new rules have been aptly named as *"Bio-Medical Waste Management Rules, 2016."*

The Categories of Bio-medical Waste

For the ease and simplification of segregation of bio-medical waste at healthcare facility level, the 10 categories of bio-medical wastes are now categorized into 4 different color categories only. There is single color choice for any category of bio-medical waste.

Widened Scope of the Rules

There has been addition in the establishments to which the rules apply. For example, AYUSH hospitals, research/educational institutes, health camps, medical or surgical camps, vaccination camps, blood donation camps, first aid rooms of schools, forensic laboratories, etc., come under the purview of the new rules. This has widened the scope of its applicability.

The Authorization

The Bio-Medical Waste (BMW) Rules 2016 have simplified the process of authorization by addressing to the hurdles in the process of getting authorization.

The application for authorization shall be disposed within a period of 90 days from the date of receipt of completed application. In case of a pending application beyond the time frame of 90 days, the authorization shall be deemed to have been granted.

Small nonbedded healthcare establishments [(HCEs), e.g., dispensaries, clinics] are required to have "one time authorization", bringing them within the purview of the BMW Rules, 2016. At the same time, these nonbedded HCEs have been taken care of by avoiding unnecessary formality and paperwork renewal.

Duties and Responsibilities

- The BMW Rules 2016 have enlisted 20 points for the duty of the occupier and 17 points for the duty of the CBWTF operator generating/handling the bio-medical waste.
- The list of prescribed authorities and their corresponding duties are also clearly mentioned in the new rule.

Phasing out the Use of Chlorinated Plastic Bags

- As per the BMW Rules 2016, there is a provision to phase out use of chlorinated plastic bags, gloves, and blood bags. These bags shall be in compliance with BIS and till then it should be as per plastic waste management rules, 2011. The phasing out of the chlorinated plastic bags has been decided, considering the environmental hazard resulting due to the emission of toxic gases like dioxin and furan due to inadvertent burning of chlorinated plastics.

Tracking the Bio-medical Waste Bags

The provision of barcode system for bio-medical waste bags or containers has been given 1-year time frame.

With the GPS enabled system, the bio-medical waste bags can be tracked as well. So, the original healthcare institution can be made accountable for untreated, improperly treated or improperly segregated bio-medical wastes.

Newer Technologies Incorporated

The technology and method to be used for treatment and disposal of bio-medical waste is not fixed. Any technology that is environmentally sound and achieves the operating standards may be adopted after approval and authorisation. Hydroclave and plasma pyrolysis for the incineration of bio-medical wastes lead to lesser environmental degradation, negligible health impacts, safe handling of treated wastes, lesser running and maintenance costs, more effective reduction of microorganisms, and safer disposal.

The inclusion of plasma pyrolysis as an additional method of choice as an alternative to incineration is appreciated aloud by environmental agencies and activists who are against the growing number of incinerators in the country. The alternative of deep burial earlier available for remote rural area during the phased implementation of the old rule is still mentioned but applicable only in remote rural areas where no CBWTF is available.

Treatment and Disposal of Bio-medical Waste

- The standard for treatment and disposal of bio-medical waste has been revised.
- The acceptable SPM emission of 150 mg/Nm^3 has been reduced to 50 mg/Nm^3.
- The standard retention time in the secondary chamber has been increased from 1 second to 2 seconds. This change in retention time has been done to reduce the levels of hazardous gases like dioxins and furans.
- If the nearest CBWTF is within 75 km of the healthcare institution, then establishment of new treatment and disposal facility in a healthcare institution is not allowed. However, those healthcare institutions which already have such facility may continue to operate the same but shall have to comply to the operating standards within a maximum time frame of 2 years.
- As per the new rules, whenever a chemical disinfection is applied onsite at the source of generation, only nonchlorinated chemical disinfection is allowed. This provision has been added to address the issue of improper use of chemical disinfection. It is a common practice that when chemical treatment is done with hypochlorite solution, the chemically treated bio-medical waste is negligently sent for incineration, which further adds to the environmental risk of toxic gases through burning of bio-medical waste treated with (and thus containing) chlorine.
- The new rule has a provision that the treated bio-medical waste should not be mixed with other municipal solid waste. All recyclable waste should be sent to the registered or authorized recyclers. These recyclers should have valid authorisation or registration. CBWTF has to keep a record of recyclable waste and be submitted to prescribed authority as part of their annual report.
- As per the new rule, the CBWTF operator has to collect the bio-medical waste even on holidays. The untreated bio-medical waste shall not be stored beyond a period of 48 hours. The occupier of the HCE has to inform the prescribed authority immediately if the CBWTF operator does not collect the bio-medical waste within the intended time or as per the agreed time and take appropriate steps to safeguard human health and environment. The occupier can visit the CBWTF operator and see whether the treatment is done as per the rules. The CBWTF operator needs to inform the prescribed authority immediately regarding the occupiers who are not handing over the segregated bio-medical waste in accordance to the rules.

Occupational Safety of Healthcare Workers

- In the new rules, there is a provision regarding the training and health check-up of all the healthcare workers. Training and health check-up is to be done at the time of induction and yearly thereafter. These details are also required to be mentioned in the annual report as well.
- The occupier is required to ensure occupational safety of all its healthcare workers and others involved in handling of bio-medical waste. He shall provide appropriate and adequate personal protective equipment and effective immunization against diseases likely to be transmitted.

Records of the Bio-medical Waste

- In the new rules, there is a provision of maintenance of records of the bio-medical waste on daily basis in the register and display the monthly record on its website.
- A time frame of 2 years is given to the HCEs to create their own website.

■ PENALTIES UNDER THE ENVIRONMENT PROTECTION ACT[7]

Bio-Medical Waste (Management and Handling) Rules, 1998 and its amendment do not specify any penalty for hospitals and operators of waste disposal facilities if the autoclaves, incinerators, microwaves, etc., do not meet the standards prescribed in the rules. The Environment (Protection) Act, 1986 is a landmark legislation which provides for single focus in the country for protection of environment and aims at plugging the loopholes in existing legislation. Environment (Protection) Act, 1986 has specified penalties for violations of act/rules made thereunder. Thus, even though no specific provision was incorporated in the Bio-Medical Waste (Management and Handling) Rules, 1998, recourse to Environment (Protection) Act for punishing the violators of waste management rules can always be taken.

Penalties for Offences

Section 15 prescribes the penalties for offences under the Act. An imprisonment up to 5 years or a fine of up to ₹1 lakh, or both, shall be imposed for violating the provisions of the Act. An additional fine of up to ₹5,000 shall be imposed for every day of continuing violation. If a failure or contravention occurs for >1 year after the date of conviction, an offender may be punished for up to 7 years imprisonment.

Sections 16 and 17 make corporate officials/Heads of Government Departments liable for the offences under the Act. However if the official/head can establish that the offence was committed without his knowledge or that he has exercised all due diligence to prevent the commission of the offence, then he will not be held liable to any punishment provided in this Act.

Who can File a Complaint Under the Act?

Section 19 provides that any person, in addition to authorized government officials, may file a complaint with a court alleging an offence under the Act. However, the person must have given notice of not <60 days of the alleged offence and the intent to file a complaint with the government official authorized to make such complaints. The citizen's suit provision expands the concept of locus standi in environmental prosecutions. It appears to give power to the public to enforce the Environment Act.

If the Violation is also an Offence Under any Other Legislation

Section 24 provides that, where an offence under this Act is also an offence under any other Act, the offender shall be punished only under the other Act.

■ CONCLUSION

Safe bio-medical waste management is not only a legal duty but also a social responsibility. Lack of awareness, training, and cost factors are some of the hurdles responsible for poor management of hospital waste. Medical professionals and hospital administrators must realize the importance of managing the bio-medical waste in a nonhazardous and legally acceptable manner. Training and continuing education programs for healthcare personnel is an intelligent decision that can play a key role in safe bio-medical waste management in the future.

■ REFERENCES

1. Barry Commoner (An environmentalist). [online] Available: www.brainyquote.com/quotes/quotes/b/barrycommo462461.html [Last accessed February, 2020].
2. National Institute of Communicable Diseases and National AIDS Control Organization, Government of India, Delhi. HIV Testing Manual: Laboratory diagnosis, biosafety and quality control.
3. Environment management for control of hospital infections: Proceedings of 7th conference of hospital infection society, India. 9th January 2003. CMC, Vellore.
4. Wilson HF, Edward BG, Mjör IA. Dental practice and the environment. Int Dent J. 1998;48(3):161-6.
5. Bio-Medical Waste (Management and Handlings) Rules, 1998.
6. Bio-Medical Waste Management Rules, 2016
7. Environment (Protection) Act, 1986.

CHAPTER 20

Medicolegal Outlook on PC-PNDT Act

Chandrashekhar A Sohoni

"The worst manifestation in our country of gender discrimination is female foeticide."
—Smt Pratibha Devisingh Patil[1]

■ INTRODUCTION

In India, discrimination against females and preference of a son over daughter has resulted in disheartening decline in sex ratio. One of the major manifestations of such discrimination has gender-biased sex selection. Proliferation of medical diagnostic technology which enables sex determination reinforces the gender-biased sex selection. Often, doctors are blamed as facilitators for the murder of a girl child in the womb. Due to few black sheep, the whole medical fraternity is being discredited. To curb the social evil of female foeticide, the Government of India enacted Prenatal Diagnostic Techniques (PNDT) Act on 20th September, 1994. In 2003, the act was amended to preconception and Prenatal Diagnostic Techniques (Prohibition of Sex Selection) Act (PC-PNDT Act) for better regulation of the technology used in sex determination. The Act does not prohibit the conduct of prenatal diagnostic technique but it is for regulation and monitoring the conduct of technique. Under the Act, there is a total and strict ban on sex determination tests.

■ PRECONCEPTION AND PRENATAL DIAGNOSTIC TECHNIQUES ACT IN A NUTSHELL

The Act may be divided in four major parts:
1. Registration of ultrasound machine.
2. Record keeping.
3. Monitoring and implementing.
4. Offences and penalties.

Registration of Ultrasound Machine

- Every center (herein referring to diagnostic center, clinic or hospital where an ultrasound machine is going to be used) needs to register the ultrasound machine with the Appropriate Authority at least 3 months in advance. This registration is mandatory irrespective of whether the machine is going to be used for obstetric ultrasound or otherwise. The application should be made in duplicate using the form 'A'. An affidavit needs to be submitted simultaneously by the owner of the machine to the effect that no sex determination shall be performed at the center and the center shall clearly display a notice stating the same. A nonrefundable application fee needs to be paid at the time of registration. The fees were controversially raised in the year 2012 from INR 3,000 to INR 25,000 for a diagnostic center, and from 4,000 to 35,000 for a hospital. A registration certificate is valid for a period of 5 years after which it needs to be renewed. An application for renewal should be made 1 month before the date of expiry of the certificate. The fees payable at the time of renewal of registration is half that of the amount specified for first-time registration. One must note that even computed tomography (CT) and magnetic reronance imaging (MRI) machines require registration with the appropriate authority.

- A center may have more than one ultrasound machine; however, the center has to make sure at the time of registration that the name of manufacturer and model number of all the machines is specified on the registration certificate or on a separate paper to be displayed along with the certificate.
- An ultrasound machine registered with one center cannot be shifted to another center. However, the ultrasound machine can be shifted within the premises of a registered center.
- All those doctors intending to use the ultrasound machine need to have their names entered on the registration certificate or on a separate paper that is to be displayed along with the registration certificate. The concerned ultrasound center needs to submit the names and copies of degree certificates/medical council registration numbers of all such doctors to the appropriate authority for prior approval. Nobody other than the registered doctors is legally permitted to use that specific ultrasound machine for any purpose. Whenever a locum doctor needs to be arranged, prior approval from the appropriate authority needs to be sought by submission of an application specifying the dates of such use, along with the locum doctor's degree certificate/medical council registration number.
- It is mandatory for every ultrasound center to intimate every change of employee, place address and equipment installed to the Appropriate Authority at least 30 days in advance and seek re-issuance of certificate of registration from Appropriate Authority, with changes duly incorporated. Indian Radiology and Imaging Association (IRIA) sought an interim relief from the Delhi High Court as to the time period required for informing the Appropriate Authority whenever locum doctors need to be appointed. As per the interim relief, the period for notifying the appropriate authority about locum doctors has been shortened to 7 days.

Record Keeping

- All case related records, forms of consent, laboratory results, microscopic pictures, sonographic images, recommendations and letters need to be preserved in print for a period of 2 years from the date of performing the procedure or scan. In the event of any legal proceedings, the records must be preserved till the final disposal of legal proceedings, or till the expiry of the said period of 2 years, whichever is later.
- It is mandatory for every center to afford facilities necessary for inspection of the place, equipment and documents by the authorities whenever required.
- The PC-PNDT registration certificate must be displayed in original at the reception and in the ultrasound room. If there are two or more ultrasound machines and hence two or more

ultrasound rooms, then an original copy of PC-PNDT certificate needs to be displayed in-original in each room. A request for multiple copies of original registration certificate can be made to the Appropriate Authority.
- Every center must display a prominent notice in English and the local language to the effect that disclosure of the sex of the foetus is prohibited under law. The names, qualifications and timings of doctors working on the ultrasound machine should be displayed at the reception for public information.
- At least one copy of the PC-PNDT Act and rules must be made available on the premises of the center, and must be provided to the clients on demand.
- Form 'D' is to be maintained by genetic counseling centers.
- Form 'E' is to be maintained by genetic laboratories.
- Form 'F' is to be maintained by ultrasound centers and genetic clinics for pregnant patients.
- The general guidelines for optimally completing form 'F' are as follows:
    ○ All sections of the form should be filled-up. No section should be left blank. It is required to write 'not applicable' or 'no' wherever necessary.
    ○ Past obstetric history of the patient with the number and gender of each child should be mentioned in the form.
    ○ The name of the referring doctor and indication and results of the ultrasound scan must be mentioned on the form.
    ○ The form should be duly signed by the doctor performing the scan.
    ○ As per the rules, it is necessary to explain the procedure to the patient beforehand in her own language. Consent for performing the scan with a declaration that the patient does not want to know the sex of the foetus must be obtained from the patient. The consent must be duly signed by the patient as well as the doctor.
    ○ The doctor performing the ultrasound scan must give a declaration at the end of each ultrasound report that he/she has neither detected nor disclosed the sex of the foetus to the pregnant woman or to anybody.
    ○ A monthly report needs to be submitted to the Appropriate Authority before the 5th day of the next month. Recently, it has also been made mandatory for centers to additionally fill the online form F for all patients on the relevant PC-PNDT website. Despite the website automatically generating a monthly report (based on the data from online form-F), most local authorities insist on submission of both—a manually filled-in monthly report and a print-out of the online-generated monthly report. Ultrasound centers should therefore ensure before submitting the monthly report that the entries in the online-generated monthly report and the physically submitted monthly report tally correctly. A mismatch, even though a result of an inadvertent error, would raise suspicion of foul play.

Monitoring and Implementation

The PC-PNDT act is a remarkable exception in the sense that the implementation of the act has been severe, which is otherwise not a very common scenario in India. Under the PC-PNDT act the Central Government has the power to make rules regarding the following:
- Minimum qualifications for persons employed at a registered centers (herein referring to Genetic counseling center, genetic laboratory, genetic clinic, ultrasound clinic or hospital with ultrasound machine).
- The manner of record-keeping by centers.
- The format of seeking consent of the pregnant woman undergoing the procedure or scan.

- The procedure to be followed by the members of the Central Supervisory Board (CSB).
- Allowances for members other than ex officio members.
  - Code of conduct for employees working at the registered centers.
  - The manner in which reports shall be furnished to the Central Government and CSB by the states and Union Territories.
  - Empowerment of appropriate authority.
  - Period between meetings of Advisory Committee.
- Terms and conditions of appointment to the Advisory Committee.
- Format for application for registration and fees paid for the same.
- Facilities to be provided and standards to be maintained by registered centers.
- The format of registration certificate.
- Guidelines for registration renewal and fees applicable therein.
- The manner in which a center can appeal against the suspension or cancellation of registration by the Appropriate Authority.
- The period of preservation of records by the center.
- Guidelines for seizure of documents and material at the centers.
- Any other matter that is required or prescribed.

Under the PC-PNDT act, the Appropriate Authority has following powers:
- Summoning of any person who is in possession of any information relating to the violation of the act and rules made thereunder.
- Asking for production of any document with reference to the violation of the act and rules.
- Issuing search warrant for any place suspected of indulging in sex determination. The Appropriate Authority or any officer authorized in this behalf may enter and search any ultrasound center at all reasonable times and with assistance if required. The authority or officer can examine any document or material found therein and seize and seal the same if he/she has reason to believe that it is in violation of the said act and rules. The Appropriate Authority or the officer or the government shall not be liable for any type of legal proceedings for an act done in good faith in pursuance of the provisions of the act.
- Any other matter which may be prescribed.

Offences and Penalties

The PC-PNDT Act and the rules have specified the offences and penalties for violations of the provisions of the act and the rules (**Table 1**).

PC-PNDT Act–Controversies and Practical Difficulties:
Safety Measures to be taken by the Doctors

Though the PC-PNDT Act intends well, some of the provisions of the act are so severe that they almost border on the unreasonable. While the act might appear feasible on paper, the practicality of some of its provisions in day-to-day ultrasound practice is questionable. Due to these and other reasons, the PC-PNDT act has raised lot of controversies.
- The inspecting authorities under PC-PNDT act insist on the availability of a valid prescription—a prescription on the letter-head of the referring gynecologist with date, stamp and signature—for every pregnant patient who presents to an ultrasound clinic. However, there is no clarity in the PC-PNDT act as to what constitutes a valid prescription. Does a phone call or a message sent via short messaging service (SMS) or an electronic

CHAPTER 20: Medicolegal Outlook on PC-PNDT Act | 231

TABLE 1: Offences and Penalties for violations of the provisions of the PC-PNDT Act and Rules.

Violations	Section/Rule of The PNDT Act	Penalties
Minor offences: • Nonavailability of copy of the PNDT Act in the registered center • Nondisplay of registration certificate in the center • Nondisplay of Board in the premises in English and Local Language that 'Disclosure of the sex of the fetus is prohibited under law'	Rule No. 17(2) Rule No. 6(2) Rule No. 17(1)	**For minor offences:** Case may be launched in the court of JMIC u/s 25 of the Act. Punishment may extend to 3 months or with fine, which may extend to ₹ 1,000 for first offence. Additional fine upto ₹ 500 per day for the period of contravention for subsequent offence Or Show cause notice u/s 20(1), (2) for temporary suspension of registration Or Under Sec 20(3)
Advertisement relating to preconception and prenatal determination of sex	Sec 22(1), (2)	• U/s 22(3) of the PNDT Amendment Act, imprisonment which may extend to 3 years and with fine which may extend to ₹ 10,000 • Case is to be launched in the court u/s 28 of the Act
Unregistered centers. It includes all such centers where any portable equipment capable of detecting sex before or after conception is used. The owner of such equipment may be having a registered facility somewhere else.	Sec 3	• Any such equipment has to be sealed and seized by the Appropriate Authority concerned. He/She may launch the case in the court u/s 28 of the Act • Register such center after receiving 5 times the registration fee as penalty and after taking a undertaking as per the PNDT Rules-Rule 11(2)
Irregularities in registered center • Owner/employee conducting the ultrasonography not qualified • More ultra sound machines/equipment where as less number register • Minor deficiency in record keeping	Sec 3(2) and Rule 3(b) Under Rule 4.6 and as per Form 'A'. Sr. No. 8 Under Rule 9	The Appropriate Authority or person authorized thereupon may: • Issue show cause notice u/s 20(1) (2) of the Act and with the endorsement of the Advisory Committee, may suspend (for a reasonable period) or cancel the registration, as per the magnitude of the violation • May take Suo Moto Action u/s 20(3) and suspend the registration without issuing show cause notice Note: 1. During the period of suspension of registration, the equipment needs to be sealed and signed and kept with the owner. After cancellation of the registration, the equipment has to be sealed and seized Any body aggrieved by the above decision may appeal to the higher-level Appropriate Authority within 30 days of the action. The appeal shall be disposed of by the higher authority within 60 days of its receipt

Continued

Continued

Violations	Section/Rule of The PNDT Act	Penalties
Record keeping Irregularities in record keeping as per revised form 'F' are a major offence	Sec 4, 29 and Rule-9	Contravention (a major offence) of provision of section 5 and 6 of the Act and punishable u/s 23(1) of the PNDT Act
Sex selection	Sec 3A. 4(5). 6 read with section 2(0)	Violation of section 5 and 6 of the Act and punishable u/s 23 of the Act

Important Note:
1. It is to be noted that an error in completing the form F will be treated as major offence.
2. All offences under the Act are cognizable, nonbailable and noncompoundable (Sec 27).
3. Even if a case has been registered by the police, no court shall take cognizance except when the complaint has been filed by the Appropriate Authority or by the person/group who had served a legal notice of 15 days to the Appropriate Authority already (Sec 28).
4. Action u/s 20 and filing of criminal complaint u/s 28 can go simultaneously (Sec 20).

mail (e-mail) from the gynecologist is not generally accepted as a valid prescription. It is sometimes difficult for a pregnant lady to get a prescription from the gynecologist, especially in case of an obstetric emergency. At such times a radiologist working in a stand-alone ultrasound clinic faces a catch-22 situation. If he refuses to attend to an obstetric emergency, he is guilty of breaching medical ethics; whereas, if he performs an ultrasound scan without a prescription, it is quite likely to raise suspicion in the minds of the inspecting authority under PC-PNDT Act. There is a provision for self-referral by doctors in the form F. However, unlike a gynecologist, a radiologist does not advise patients regarding antenatal care, and hence the question of self-referral does not arise in the case of radiologists. It is not difficult to imagine the anger that would be incited in a pregnant lady and her relatives when an obstetric ultrasound is refused for the lack of a prescription. It is beyond the simple understanding of a lay man as to why a radiologist, a qualified doctor himself, should need a prescription in a particular format from another doctor just to perform a scan. In the year 2014, a doctor was assaulted by the patient's relatives in a small town called Safidon in Haryana state for refusing to perform obstetric ultrasound for the lack of proper documentation on the part of the patient.[2] Few months later, the doctor was shot dead by motorcycle-borne assailants.[2] Short of such extreme reactions, angry exchange of words between the doctor and the patients in ultrasound clinics over documentation formalities before performing obstetric ultrasound are not uncommon.

- In the case where an ultrasound center fails to inform the Appropriate Authority about a doctor who has resigned from work, the name of the doctor continues to officially remain on the PC-PNDT registration certificate till expiry date. In case there is a legal action against an ultrasound center under PC-PNDT Act, all such doctors whose names are officially registered with PC-PNDT would face legal action. Thus, resignation from the post of a sonologist is no longer just an agreement between the employer and the employee; the Appropriate Authority needs to be duly informed about the same. While employers make sure of registering a doctor's name with the Appropriate Authority under PC-PNDT at the time of employment, they may not be as prompt in deregistering the doctor while relieving him of his duties. It is ultimately the doctor who suffers the legal consequences of the same. Hence, doctors working as employees at ultrasound clinics are well-advised to make sure that the Appropriate Authority is duly informed about their resigning from work. If the employer fails to inform the Appropriate Authority in-time, an application along with a copy of the resignation letter (duly accepted by the employer) should be submitted by the doctor to the Appropriate Authority, and a duplicate copy counter-signed by the Appropriate Authority should be preserved as an acknowledgement of the same. Such a document would come to the defense of a doctor just in case the doctor is erroneously summoned at a later date for a PC-PNDT related legal matter involving his previous workplace. In 2012, the Judicial Magistrate First Class directed legal proceedings against five radiologists for noncompliance of PC-PNDT Act at a particular ultrasound center in Pune, Maharashtra.[3] Three of the five radiologists had resigned years before the date of legal action against the ultrasound center. However, the ultrasound center had not informed the Appropriate Authority about the resignations of the said doctors.[3] Thus, it was presumed that the radiologists were still registered with the ultrasound center. When the three radiologists approached the Sessions Court with a criminal revision plea, the court promptly rejected the same. Such is the unforgiving nature of the PC-PNDT Act and hence doctors practicing ultrasound need to be aware of the nuances of the act.

- There have been reports of harassment of doctors by the authorities enforcing the PC-PNDT Act.[4] The PC-PNDT Act has created a sort of licensing body for ultrasound in India. There is always a possibility of corruption wherever there is a licensing body.
- The stringent punishment for documentation errors even before a court trial has been criticized.[4] There have been instances where Ultrasound machines have been sealed by appropriate authority for trivial deficiency in paperwork.[5] An offence under the act being cognizable, nonbailable and noncompoundable, a criminal case can be framed against the radiologist. There is the provision by which the Appropriate Authority reports the erring doctor to the State Medical Council for taking necessary action, including suspension of license. Such a practice of penalizing a person without a fair trial appears undemocratic and violative of Article 21 of the constitution.
- The correlation between such heavy documentation as prescribed by the act, and the improvement of sex ratio, has been questioned.[6] Despite the law being implemented for so many years and doctors being prosecuted, there has not been any considerable improvement in the sex ratio.[6] According to the consensus, the child sex ratio (0–6 years) has shown a decline from 927 in 2001 to 914 in 2011.
- In the presence of a blood test which can detect the sex of the fetus independent of ultrasound, the relevance of such a draconian act for ultrasound has been questioned.[6,7]
- In 2012, the Rajasthan High Court questioned the constitutionality of the PC-PNDT Act due to its arbitrary and discriminatory implementation.[8] The court questioned the state and central government about the appropriateness of prosecuting doctors and ultrasound centers merely on technical grounds, which is in contravention to the Article 14 of the constitution. The court made these comments while entertaining a writ petition filed by an association of sonography centers in the state about harassment of doctors via prosecution for reasons such as not wearing white aprons, not bearing name-plates, etc.
- The act is unique in the sense that the guilt of the defendant-doctor is presumed and the burden of proof is not on the prosecution. In this regard, a radiologist is treated like someone accused of rape or dowry death.[5] In other criminal cases, the burden of proof is on the prosecution.

- The gazette notification on PC-PNDT [Rule 3(3)] restricting radiologists to two centers or hospitals has been publically condemned and labeled as undemocratic and unconstitutional by radiologists and radiology associations.[8] A gazette notification prescribing amendment of the PC-PNDT Act to this effect was issued by the central government on June 04, 2012. The same was challenged before the Bombay High Court in the case *Dr Rajeev Vasant Zankar vs. Union of India and Ors. WP (Lodg) no 1829 of 2012,* wherein the petition was admitted and the division bench through its order dated July 20, 2012 issued an ad-interim stay on the government notification. The government notification was also concurrently challenged in the Delhi High Court in the case *Indian Radiological and Imaging Association vs. Union of India, WP(C) 4009 of 2012.* The Delhi High Court also issued ad-interim stay on Rule 3(3) of the government notification. The Indian Radiological and Imaging Association thereafter filed a fresh civil application seeking clarifications from the Delhi High Court about applicability of the ad-interim stay throughout the country. The Delhi High Court then directed the central government via an order to inform all the states about the ad-interim stay, although the court concurrently stated that an order passed by Delhi High Court may not be binding on other states. As of today, the ad-interim stay on Rule 3(3) is applicable. Radiologists should cite the High Court orders mentioned above if they are quizzed by the local authorities about multiple ultrasound attachments.
- There is a ban on portability of ultrasound machines in India.[9] The Maharashtra state branch of Indian Radiological and Imaging association filed a writ petition challenging the ban; however, it was dismissed by the Bombay High Court in 2011. The ban on portable ultrasound machines has put severe limitations on the use of this very useful modality, in addition to creating a shortage of radiology services.[9] On the one hand, the government is trying to restrict radiologists from practicing ultrasound at more than two centers; on the other hand, it is trying to prescribe a 6-months training programme in ultrasound for MBBS doctors, citing deficiency of qualified radiologists. Such measures are self-contradictory and may arguably be one of the reasons for failure of the child sex-ratio to improve despite strict implementation of PC-PNDT Act.[10]

CONCLUSION

The declining sex-ratio is a serious social threat that stares the Indian Society in the face. This problem is largely a result of the perverted mind-set of the society that views female child with a negative bias. PC-PNDT Act was brought into existence to curb the social evil of female foeticide. While there is no denying of the fact that an act of parliament is essential to prevent female feticide, the PC-PNDT Act is draconian and has resulted in wide-spread apprehension in the medical community due to the prospect of irrational implementation. As the members of a civilized society, it is the duty of doctors to contribute in every possible way to save the girl child. At the same time, it is extremely important for ultrasound practitioners to completely understand and diligently follow the PC-PNDT Act. Even an unintended, technical error under this act can land doctors in grave legal trouble and hence doctors are well-advised to beware.

REFERENCES

1. Smt Pratibha Devi Singh Patil, former President of India at the 17th convocation of Mother Teresa women's univ. 2 Nov. 2007. Available: *http://pib.nic.in/release/rel_print_page.asp?relid=32395*
2. Medicos body condemns killing of doctor in Haryana. Times of India. Available: *http://timesofindia.indiatimes.com/city/chandigarh/Medicos-body-condemns-killing-of-doctor-in-Haryana/articleshow/42310639.cms*

3. Court rejects appeal of 3 radiologists. Times of India. Available: *http://timesofindia.indiatimes.com/city/pune/Court-rejects-appeal-of-3-radiologists/articleshow/44892502.cms*
4. Walia JK. Has the PC-PNDT Act become a source of harassment for doctors? India Medical Times. Available: *http://www.indiamedicaltimes.com/2012/12/04/has-the-pcpndt-act-become-a-source-of-harassment-for-doctors/*
5. Onkar P, Mitra K. Important points in the PC-PNDT Act. Indian J Radiol Imaging. 2012;22:141-3.
6. Patnaik AM, Kejriwal GS. A perspective on PC-PNDT Act. Indian J Radiol Imaging. 2012;22:137-40.
7. Ryu HM, Weismann G. Study published in the FASEB (Federation of American Societies for Experimental Biology) Friday, January 20, 2012.
8. Sharma A. Rajasthan High Court notice to govts over petition of sonography centers. Times of India. Available: *http://timesofindia.indiatimes.com/city/jaipur/Rajasthan-High-Court-notice-to-govts-over-petition-of-sonography-centers/articleshow/15024813.cms*.
9. Khan A. Use of portable ultrasound machines banned. Daily News and Analysis. Available: *http://www.dnaindia.com/pune/report-use-of-portable-ultrasound-machines-banned-1671813*.
10. IRIA derides Gazette Notification on PNDT Act. Express Healthcare. Available: *http://archive.expresshealthcare.in/latest-updates/556-iria-derides-gazette-notification-on-pndt-act*.

SECTION 7
Medicolegal Issues in Various Specialties: Eagle's Eye and Lion's Heart!

Chapter 21 Medicolegal issues in Obstetrics and Gynecology
Chapter 22 Medicolegal issues in Surgery
Chapter 23 Medicolegal issues in Orthopedics
Chapter 24 Medicolegal issues in Ophthalmology
Chapter 25 Medicolegal issues in Pediatrics
Chapter 26 Medicolegal issues in Radiology
Chapter 27 Medicolegal issues in Blood Transfusion Practice
Chapter 28 Medicolegal issues in Dentistry
Chapter 29 Medicolegal issues in Anesthesiology

CHAPTER 21

Medicolegal Issues in Obstetrics and Gynecology

Charu Mittal, PS Mittal

"It is inexcusable that in 21st century motherhood remains so dangerous for so many. It is not only morally wrong but also hampers economic development, and the survival and well-being of families, communities and nations."

Babatunde Osotimehin, Executive Director, UNFPA[1]

■ INTRODUCTION

The bygone era when women accepted obstetrical problems as their fate, and had no choice but to undergo universal domiciliary childbirth, has been largely replaced by the extremely modern healthcare through the specialty of obstetrics and gynecology. Today we practice in the era of antibiotics, institutional deliveries and painless labor. Operative deliveries and traditional surgery exist alongside minimally invasive surgery and robotic surgery. Undisputedly this has reduced suffering, morbidity and mortality of women from obstetric and gynecological causes. However, as every coin has two sides, the development in healthcare is also not without its pros and cons. The technical support is associated with vast investment, leading to expensive healthcare. In India, health insurance coverage is still far from universal.

Access to quality healthcare outside government funded institutions can be a costly prospect for most women. With easy access to internet, a literate woman approaching a specialist is often equipped with piecemeal information which unfortunately many a times is unreliable. This leads to a confused patient who has hundreds of queries even after the specialist explains the disease and the proposed treatment. A modern specialist must be well-equipped to deal with numerous queries, suggest appropriate investigations, and provide the right diagnosis and management. Dealing with less educated patients and their relatives throws up a different set of challenges altogether.

Apart from these clinical and practical challenges the specialist in obstetrics and gynecology must also fulfill requirements of the various laws of our country especially those pertaining to obstetrics and gynecology practice like MTP Act, PC-PNDT Act, etc.

The unpredictable nature of the human body and limitations of medical science can expose any practicing obstetrician and gynecologist to risk of litigation at any time. In depth knowledge of one's subject as well as medico-legal awareness with frequent updating of both is now essential to have a smooth professional practice as well as to deal calmly with occasional difficult situations.

Why Obstetricians are More Vulnerable to Litigation?[2]

Obstetric patients are usually young and seemly free from obvious disease. Hence, relatives find it difficult to accept mishaps. In other branches of medicine, doctors usually handle pathological conditions, which often have a known course, and the patient and relatives are mentally prepared to face adverse outcomes, where as pregnancy and childbirth are perceived as physiological processes.

Obstetricians deal with two lives simultaneously—mother and her developing foetus. While pregnant lady can be evaluated clinically and with necessary investigations, the prediction of well-being of the intrauterine fetus has an inherent potential for error or inability to diagnose certain fetomaternal disorders. Follow-up of an obstetric case lasts up to nearly 11 months (i.e., 40 weeks of gestation plus 6 weeks of postpartum phase). During such a prolonged duration, fetomaternal physiological derangement or any pathological condition may occur, resulting in poor outcome.

Poor outcome in obstetric cases is stressful for the family. Life can become totally disturbed for such family. Relatives are usually not willing or able to understand the situation. Educational status in India is varied and too much or too little knowledge, both can increase the risk for litigation specifically in cases where poor outcome is associated with inefficient and inadequate communication. Obstetric practice can often be very busy in an individual or institutional set-up and risk of errors and omissions is higher when attention is divided among multiple patients and time constraints can make the task more difficult.

Survey of Medicolegal Claims Against Gynecologists

An ACOG (American College of Obstetricians and Gynecologists) survey found that an obstetrician and gynecologist can expect an average of 2.5 liability claims over the course of his or her career[3,4] or around 80% of obstetricians and gynecologists can anticipate being sued one or more times in their career.[5] Another report[6] mentioned that 25.6% of surveyed obstetricians decreased their high-risk obstetric patients while 7.2% totally quit practicing obstetrics. Furthermore 28.5% of those who continue to deliver patients reported increasing the number of cesarean section with 26.4% not performing Vaginal Birth After Cesarean (VBAC). The 85% of suits were found to be filed against 3–6% doctors. It was concluded that doctors who are hurried, uninterested, or unwilling to listen to and answer questions are at risk of suit, even if they practice quality medicine. While those who are perceived as concerned, accessible and willing to communicate are sued far less.

■ MEDICOLEGAL ISSUES IN OBSTETRICS

There are several potential domains in obstetrics which are prone to malpractice lawsuits against the treating doctors. The surgeon must be aware of medicolegal implications related to those risky domains in their day-to-day practice, and deal carefully as per the existing laws while providing accepted standard of care.

Obstetric Cases Vulnerable to Malpractice Lawsuits

Any deviation from the standard approach, especially if associated with poor outcome can lead to legal problems. Common areas of obstetrics vulnerable to malpractice lawsuits are illustrated below:

- Errors or omission in antenatal clinical screening and diagnosis or in ultrasonographic screening and diagnosis
- *Antenatal care for high-risk pregnancy*: Any omissions in investigations or treatment.
- *Maternal injuries during delivery*: Perineal tears during vaginal delivery, operative vaginal delivery, complications during LSCS
- Perinatal death (IUFD, stillbirth, or neonatal death)
- Birth asphyxia/neurologically impaired infant
- Missed ectopic pregnancy or multiple gestation
- Undiagnosed placenta previa or adherent placenta
- Incomplete medical termination of pregnancy
- Perforation during MTP
- Postpartum hemorrhage.

Other areas of litigation are:
- Blood transfusion reactions
- Missed congenital anomalies like severe dwarfism, hypoplastic left heart, severe IUGR
- Failure to suggest appropriate investigations like screening for aneuploidy, color Doppler
- Failure to act on abnormal and suspicious USG findings
- Failure to give proper advice or options for management.

Errors in Antenatal Care: Medical and Legal Implications

Errors in antenatal screening and diagnosis increases the risk of complications which are unexpected and unacceptable to the pregnant lady and relatives, laying the surgeon vulnerable to malpractice lawsuits. Some of the claims associated with errors in antenatal care are illustrated below.

Wrongful Birth

Claim for a *wrongful birth* is brought against a clinician for the birth of an infant with serious or disfiguring disabilities (as opposed to a specific birth injury) such as central nervous system defects (e.g., hydrocephalus, meningomyelocele, encephalocele) or various chromosomal abnormalities (e.g., trisomy 21), Tay-Sachs disease or cystic fibrosis. As in the case of *Keel versus Banach*,[7] the parents alleged that the genetic or hereditary basis for a potentially serious condition was not recognized by the clinician, or that appropriate diagnostic testing was not offered early enough for pregnancy prevention or termination. In these proceedings, the parents must prove that if they had been informed of the potential for a defective fetus prior to pregnancy or of the existence of an abnormality during pregnancy, they would have sought to either avoid pregnancy altogether or to terminate the affected pregnancy. Allegations of wrongful birth emphasize the importance of obtaining a complete family or genetic history and informing pregnant women of the available methods of genetic testing. Currently, at-risk families are often referred to prenatal centers for genetic testing and evaluation by perinatal geneticists. Routine referral to a genetics counsellor for evaluation is not yet considered the standard of care.

Wrongful Life

In *wrongful life* case, there is a claim that negligent prenatal testing on the part of the healthcare provider resulted in the birth of a *damaged* child. Wrongful life differs from wrongful birth in that the claim is brought in the name of the physically or mentally disabled child and not of the parents.[8] Such claims usually involve devastated infants with serious genetic disorders or those born with major injuries as a result of undiagnosed maternal disease or early pregnancy drug exposure. The legal theory for these claims is that the duty of the clinician owed to the unborn child is similar to that owed to the parents.

Wrongful Conception

This usually arises in cases of unwanted pregnancy so the allegations of wrongful conception are brought by the parents of a healthy, normal infant. In this instance, the alleged negligence is in the improper performance of a sterilization operation or the improper provision of contraceptive techniques leading to the birth of an otherwise normal but unwanted child. A common problem is when a woman becomes pregnant even after a postpartum tubal ligation procedure; also a woman who undergoes tubal ligation was already pregnant at the time of surgery.

Wrongful Death

Wrongful death is a cause of action arising when an otherwise normal pregnancy, which may or may not have reached viability, is terminated because of a misdiagnosis, as in the case of *Lollar versus Tankersley*[9] where the lady suffered bleeding in first trimester and approached the obstetrician who diagnosed spontaneous inevitable abortion, advised and performed a D and C, however, pregnancy continued for a further period of 12 days with ultrasound revealing a viable fetus with less amniotic fluid incompatible with life, ultimately it required termination of pregnancy. Another illustration of wrongful death is a case of misdiagnosis of renal agenesis resulting in pregnancy termination.

American College of Obstetricians and Gynecologists now recommends offering antenatal screening for chromosomal abnormalities to all pregnancy patients regardless of age.[10] In addition, the broader availability of nuchal translucency screening establishes an expectation that most patients should be offered the opportunity for first trimester screening. A physician failing to offer such diagnostic testing is at risk for suit.

Ectopic Pregnancy

The nontubal ectopic pregnancy or interstitial and cornual pregnancies are especially problematic because of rarity and are difficult to diagnose. Also the risk of rupture with poor outcome is high. Litigation related to ectopic pregnancy usually results from delayed diagnosis leading to increased morbidity, and performing surgery which can be avoidable if diagnosed early. The *standard of care* followed in treating such cases (i.e., medical/surgical/ type of surgery) may also create legal problems in cases where there is damage to the patient. The surgeon has to justify the *standard* followed on the basis of *good clinical practice*.

Premature Baby

Errors in the diagnosis and management of preterm labor give grounds for malpractice lawsuit due to higher incidence of complications in preterm infants. As the causes of many cases of preterm labor cannot be established, investigations such as fetal fibronectin can help to identify a population at high-risk for preterm labor and delivery. Use of corticosteroid to enhance lung maturity, role of tocolytic and referral for management in a tertiary well-equipped center in such cases may minimize the problem.

High-risk Pregnancy

In high-risk pregnancy, the mother, fetus or neonate is at increased risk of morbidity or mortality. It might pose challenges before, during or after delivery. High-risk pregnancy requires antepartum fetal surveillance through various tests like electronic fetal heart rate monitoring, USG surveillance, AFI study, biophysical profile study, color Doppler study. Proper use of such testing has been established as an essential component of risk management protocol. Deviation from such norms may lead to substandard decision making and poor outcome. Cases of high-risk obstetrics with the potential for unsatisfactory outcome may be dealt with by appropriate counseling and documentation accompanied with adequate precautions. Explanation about the prognosis of mother and baby, along with options of route of delivery may minimize the lawsuits. It is seen that hospitals not equipped with proper facilities to deal with high-risk cases are vulnerable to malpractice lawsuits.

Medical Disorders in Pregnancy

Medical disorder in pregnancy may arise *de novo*. Often obstetricians may differ with the physician's management protocol because most of the physiological changes in pregnant woman makes her management quite different from nonpregnant patients. It would be preferable that both specialists (*obstetrician and physician*) should have a team-based approach in the management of such cases. To manage the medical disorders in pregnancy, as a part of good clinical practice it is better for obstetrician to get routine consultation from a physician. Fixing liability in such cases is a gray area, where physician and obstetrician may be jointly held liable for any damage to the pregnant lady.

Cesarean Section

Obstetric cases related with cesarean section may face malpractice lawsuits with allegations like: *Why cesarean section was performed?* or *Why there was performance of a delayed cesarean section?* Wishful obstetrics refers to trying for unsuccessful attempts at vaginal delivery by allowing another half to one hour of pushing or making one or more pulls with the vacuum. Cases such as threatened scar rupture, cord prolapse, placenta previa, placental abruption, hand prolapse may need quick delivery by operative route but some hospitals are not fully equipped or the staff is not trained to combat an obstetric emergency which may cause a delay in *cesarean section,* resulting in a poor outcome. Such delay or mismanagement of case can lead to legal action.

Vaginal Birth After Cesarean

Vaginal birth after cesarean (VBAC) cases require exta caution like documentation of the counseling related to risks and benefits involved, written informed consent signed by the patient. Immediate availability of obstetrician and operative capabilities are a must. If a patient or relative insists for vaginal delivery then put down their wish on paper and take their signature with an explanation of the full risk to mother and baby. If they refuse to give written consent they may be referred with findings on paper and reason for referral.

Intrauterine Fetal Death/Stillbirths

Intrauterine fetal deaths, and stillbirths are very distressful. Mother and relatives are usually not willing or able to accept the situation. Such cases have a potential for malpractice lawsuits against the obstetrician most commonly due to lack of proper communication, and even if the specialist was not negligent. Past and present medical history with previous antenatal records and USG reports are useful defense. For establishing a nonpreventable etiology of stillbirth most important is the gross and microscopic examination of placenta and a fetal autopsy by an experienced pathologist. In general, autopsy alone can provide a diagnosis in 30% or more of unexplained stillbirths and can occasionally approximate the time of death which can often be a safeguard for the doctor.

Ultrasonography in Obstetrics: Legal Issues

Ultrasound imaging in obstetrics is a standard part of prenatal care, as it yields a variety of information regarding the health of the mother and the fetus, and progress of the pregnancy. The basic obstetric ultrasound examination is very useful to determine the location of a pregnancy, number of fetuses, gestational age, prenatal diagnosis of fetal anomalies, and early diagnosis of placental insufficiency.

Some of the common reasons for malpractice lawsuits related to ultrasound examination include the following:[11]

- Unreasonable expectations of the ultrasound examination on the part of the patient and the referring physician.
- Physician performing the examination has inadequate training or equipment.
- Failure to seek consultation in difficult cases.
- Misinterpretation of the ultrasound examination.
- Inadequate or incomplete study.
- Poor communication with referring clinicians (improper wording, lack of timely communication)
- Failure to maintain ultrasound equipment.
- Failure to supervise healthcare personnel adequately.

Missed diagnosis of fetal anomalies accounts for over a quarter of obstetric suits.[12] Legal problems may arise when the ultrasound is carried out by an obstetrician not having proper medical degree and training. If an obstetrician comments on any congenital anomaly following which the pregnancy is terminated, based on such a ultrasound report and afterward the report is found to be wrong then the obstetrician has to face legal problems. It is better that in such a case the obstetrician should take a second opinion from a qualified radiologist. The best approach is to have a properly trained and qualified ultrasonologist with well-maintained and good quality equipment. In case of any doubt or when a major decision is to be taken on the basis of ultrasound report, a second opinion must be taken as a part of good clinical practice, which is often found helpful in preventing malpractice lawsuits. Potential areas of litigation in USG scanning are missed CNS anomalies, cardiothoracic anomalies, GIT anomalies, severe IUGR.

Obstetric Anesthesia

Obstetric anesthesia is a subspecialty of anesthesiology devoted to peripartum, perioperative, pain and anesthetic management of women during pregnancy and the puerperium. It has become an integral part of practice of most anesthesiologists. Perhaps no other subspecialty of anesthesiology provides more personal gratification and clinical challenges than the practice of obstetric anesthesia. Obstetric anesthesia is generally considered to be one of the higher-risk areas of anesthetic practice. However, in addition to clinical challenges obstetric anesthesia is laden with medicolegal liabilities.[13] Malpractice lawsuit may be against the anesthesiologist for failure to fulfill the duty of care or for damage suffered by the patient due to negligence during the procedure.

Complications of obstetric regional anesthesia (*spinal and epidural*) may be postdural puncture headache, permanent or transient neurologic complications, epidural abscess, epidural hematoma, hypotension, bradycardia (maternal or fetal), cardiac arrest, supine hypotensive syndrome of pregnancy, extensive block, shivering, backache, catheter breakage, local anesthetic convulsion, paresthesia. Complications of general anesthesia can be failed intubation, pulmonary aspiration of the gastric contents, awareness during anesthesia.[14] Fatalities associated with obstetric anesthesia can be categorized as:

- Anesthesia mishaps
  - Overdosage
  - Technical failure
  - Equipment failure
- Surgical mishaps
- Death due to comorbid conditions other than the disease for which anesthesia was given.

Good perioperative evaluation of all patients, detailed review of patient's medical records, and perpetual diligence can decrease the incidence of complications and subsequent medicolegal issues.

■ MEDICOLEGAL ISSUES IN GYNECOLOGY

In the practice of gynecology, there are several potential areas which are vulnerable to malpractice lawsuits. *Some of the specific reasons for litigation against gynecologists are as follows*:

- Improper indication of hysterectomy
- Removal of ovaries without specific informed consent
- Retained swab or foreign body after surgery
- Injuries to adjacent abdominal organs like bladder or bowel
- Postoperative complications like burst abdomen, vesicovaginal fistula (VVF), rectovaginal fistula (RVF)
- Sterilization failure
- Delay in diagnosis of malignancy
- Wrong diagnosis of malignancy in a non-malignant case
- Incomplete surgery done in case of malignancy.

■ MEDICOLEGAL ISSUES IN PERIOPERATIVE PATIENT CARE

Hysterectomy

Hysterectomy is a common operation performed by gynecologists in both government and private healthcare systems. Women who have completed child-bearing, feel contented after the removal of their uterus if the indication is absolute or justified and the patient is relieved from her distressing symptoms. On the other hand, if the patient is young and starts suffering from menopausal symptoms she may regret her decision and may blame the surgeon for such removal. This problem may arise if she underwent oopherectomy too, and more so without proper counseling and valid informed consent. When the ovaries are to be removed, the endocrine role of ovaries, i.e., hormone secretion, must be explained beforehand. The patient must realize the need for removal of ovaries, the risk of persistence or recurrence of the disease and the possibility of another operation if they are conserved. The second operation can be more difficult and may even be risky. Proper counseling will not only convince her to agree to the operation but will minimize if not forestall menopausal symptoms that are likely to follow the removal of the ovaries. Availability of hormone replacement therapy is further reassuring but not a justification for removal of functioning healthy ovaries.

Allegations of assault and claims for compensation against a gynecologist are often seen in such cases. The case of *C Jayapal Reddy versus Yashoda Hospital*[15] illustrates the importance of written informed consent for hysterectomy for fibroid uterus as well as removal of both ovaries in a 36-year-old lady. Compensation was granted as the complaining parents wanted another child which would now require assisted reproductive techniques and surrogacy along with ovum donation.

There are indications where in a young patient, uterus can be removed due to disease of ovary such as tumors, however, in borderline tumors of low malignant potential and with improved techniques and availability of effective radiotherapy as well as chemotherapy, a conservative approach is preferable. Ipsilateral oophorectomy or two stage surgery for such malignancy is justified to preserve the reproductive function. As such in younger age group retention of some functional ovarian tissue is always preferable. Radical surgery in a young patient is an invitation for legal suit. Many such situations end up in a court of law to decide, what should have been done and what should not have been done.

In this era of organ conserving surgery and minimally invasive therapy with the advent of new highly effective drugs, conservative management is the first choice of a patient and same should hold true for the doctor. No lapse is pardonable and no shortcuts are acceptable if litigation against such surgery arises. Hysterectomy as the first approach for *dysfunctional uterine bleeding, pelvic inflamatory disease* or *pelvic pain syndrome* may not be justified. Hysterectomy may be found life-saving in young patients due to unexpected events such as trauma, perforation, uncontrolled pelvic hemorrhage during myomectomy, rupture uterus, uncontrolled *postpartum hemorrhage* during cesarean section or during vaginal delivery. Such emergency hysterectomy can be justified and properly defended in a court of law if there is a documented second opinion with a senior consultant and discussion with relatives.

Common areas of litigation following hysterectomy are: operation without proper documented counseling and consent, error of judgment in extent of operation, inappropriate indication, failure in identification and appropriate management of complications. Injury to vital structures and uncontrolled hemorrhage may occur in hysterectomy leading to legal suits.

Retained Surgical Objects

Retention of surgical objects is a preventable medical error, in which any item is inadvertently left behind in a patient's body in the course of surgery, and the consequences of which may include injury, repeated surgery, excess monetary cost, loss of hospital credibility and in some cases death of patient. Probability of such retention is more in abdominal surgeries.

A retained surgical sponge or swab is also known as a *gossypiboma*, derived from *gossypium* (Latin; cotton) and *boma* (Swahili; place of concealment). Clinically, retained sponges may be asymptomatic or result in a granulomatous response with abscess development, intestinal obstruction, or fistula formation. On radiological examination, gossypiboma may be confused with post-operative collections or tumors. [16,17]

The possibility of 'retained surgical item' should be considered in the differential diagnosis of any postoperative patient presenting with pain, infection, or a palpable mass. Plain radiography, ultrasound, and even magnetic resonance imaging (MRI) have been used for diagnosis, but the computed tomography (CT) scan has emerged as the most reliable method for diagnosing retained items.

Human factors such as exhaustion, lack of tools necessary for an accurate count, and a chaotic environment have been seen to increase the risk of forgetting a tool.[18,19] An inaccurate count can occur when nurses are deprived of sleep, when the operation is particularly difficult, long, and tiring, when the operation is an emergency, or when there are unforeseen changes in the procedure. When a foreign body is erroneously left in a patient the doctrine of *Res ipsa loquitor* or 'the thing speaks for itself', applies. The burden of proof shifts from patient to the surgeon and his/her team. In such cases, often the surgeon may be deemed liable as any of the three settings:

1. **The count was reported by the nurses to be incorrect**:
   Under these circumstances it is the surgeon's responsibility to take all steps to locate any missing item. If the item is not located and is retained, the surgeon will be held liable.
2. **Failure to investigate postoperative complaints in a timely manner**:
   There may be a situation when there is a delay in making the diagnosis of a retained foreign body. If the surgical count is represented by the nurse to be correct but a retained item is later found, the nurse will be responsible for erroneously reporting a 'correct count'. The main liability of the surgeon may be that there was a failure to promptly investigate the patient's unusual symptoms or pain, and also for any additional harm caused to the patient from the time the standard of care would have required an investigation of the patient's complaints.
3. **Surgeon's liability under the captain of the ship doctrine**:
   This doctrine makes the surgeon vicariously liable for negligence of all the operation team involved in the surgery of the patient. In retained surgical item cases, the plaintiff often alleges that the nurses and other staff follow the directions of the surgeon, thus under 'captain of the ship' doctrine, the surgeon is primarily responsible.

Sterilization/Family Planning Operation

Performing permanent female sterilization can be problematic for gynecologists due to failure of surgery, sometimes, even after many years have passed. The patient can demand compensation for such natural recanalization. *Failure of the procedure, i.e., conception may occur due to any of the following reasons*:
- Wrong structure such as round ligament occluded due to faulty identification.
- Client already being pregnant at the time of procedure, i.e., luteal phase pregnancy when proper selection of case cannot be done due to over-burden of cases especially in camp set-up. This cannot be treated as failure but as continuation of pregnancy.
- Pregnancy occurring due to tuboperitoneal fistula.
- Spontaneous recanalization of the fallopian tube.
- Improper, incomplete or partial application of rings over the fallopian tubes resulting in partial occlusion of the tube (*faulty surgical technique*)
- Auto-breakage of rings due to poor quality.

Safety Measures in Cases of Sterilization Operation
- Proper selection of case, i.e., performing the procedure in proliferative phase only.
- Counseling regarding failure rate should be documented and signed.
- Always give written instructions to the lady to report immediately in case of missed period. MTP should be offered to such cases when they report in time.
- Follow the national program guidelines strictly
- In case of malpractice lawsuits due to pregnancy even after sterilization procedure (*ring application*), histological proof of fibrosis at the site of ring application must be presented as a defence.

SURGICAL COMPLICATIONS: MEDICAL AND LEGAL IMPLICATIONS

During performance of major or minor surgical procedures an obstetrician-gynecologist can encounter various complications like drug reactions, anesthetic complications, errors in surgery, injury to vital structures, death on operation table or immediately after surgery, postoperative collapse, surgical infections, etc. Awareness of specific complications related to each procedure is essential to implement safeguards and reduce risk of occurrence through appropriate precautions where feasible. Informed, written consent about the nature of surgery and associated risk of complications with their appropriate management as indicated is a must to reduce risk of litigation.

Role of Consent

The landmark Supreme Court Judgment in case of *Samira Kohli versus Prabha Manchanda*[20] that has defined consent, was itself based on the suit against a gynecologist who performed hysterectomy in a 40-year-old lady after a diagnosis of pelvic endometriosis during laparoscopic evaluation of dysmenorrhea and chronic pelvic pain without taking specific consent for hysterectomy. Though the doctor was not found negligent for the surgery itself she was penalized for not taking specific written informed consent for hysterectomy prior to the procedure. Hence, it is imperative to be aware of the importance of written, informed consent in every major as well as minor procedure. Proper documentation of consent with signatures of patient as well as a close relative can often be a deciding factor in favor of the doctor during future litigation.

SPECIALIST AS AN EXPERT WITNESS IN A COURT OF LAW

It is the duty of all the medical practitioners who testify as expert witnesses on behalf of defendants, the government, or plaintiffs to do so solely in accordance with their observation on the merits of the case.[21] The moral and legal duty of physicians who testify before a court of law is to do so in accordance with their expertise. This duty implies adherence to the professional ethics. Truthfulness is essential. Misrepresentation of one's personal clinical opinion as absolute right or wrong may be harmful to individual parties and to the profession at large. Obstetrician–gynecologists must limit testimony to their sphere of medical expertise and must be prepared adequately. Witnesses who testify as experts must have knowledge and experience that are relevant to obstetric and gynecologic practice at the time of the occurrence and to the specific areas of clinical medicine they are discussing. They must make a clear distinction between medical malpractice and medical maloccurrence. The acceptance of fees that is greatly disproportionate to those customary for professional services can be construed as influencing testimony given by the witness, and it is unethical to accept compensation that is contingent on the outcome of litigation.

Medical maloccurrence is defined as a bad or undesirable outcome that is unrelated to the quality of care provided. *Malpractice*, in contrast, requires a demonstration of negligence (i.e., substandard practice that causes harm).

The following principles are offered as guidelines for the physician who assumes the role of an expert witness:

- The physician must have experience and knowledge in the areas of clinical medicine that enables him or her to testify about the standards of care that applied at the time of the occurrence that is the subject of the legal action.
- The physician's review of medical facts must be thorough, fair, and impartial and must not exclude any relevant information. It must not be biased to create a view favoring the plaintiff, the government, or the defendant. The goal of a physician testifying in any judicial proceeding should be to provide testimony that is complete, objective, and helpful to a just resolution of the proceeding.
- The physician's testimony must reflect an evaluation of performance in light of generally accepted standards, neither condemning performance that falls within generally accepted practice standards nor endorsing or condoning performance that falls below these standards. Experts and their testimony should recognize that medical decisions often must be made in the absence of diagnostic and prognostic certainty.
- The physician must make a clear distinction between medical malpractice and medical maloccurrence.
- The physician must make every effort to assess the relationship of the alleged substandard practice to the outcome. Deviation from a practice standard is not always substandard care or causally related to a bad outcome.
- The physician must be prepared to have testimony given in any judicial proceeding subjected to peer review by an institution or professional organization to which he or she belongs.

Questions that may be asked to the expert witness:
1. Has the standard of care been followed in the particular case?
2. What other treatment options could have been suggested?
3. Have necessary investigations been carried out?
4. Is there any negligence?
5. Is the poor outcome a result of substandard care?
6. What are the guidelines of professional bodies in dealing with such cases?

■ GENERAL PRECAUTIONS DURING DAY-TO-DAY PRACTICE: AVOIDING MALPRACTICE LAWSUITS

- *Be concerned and communicative*: Doctors who are hurried, uninterested, or unwilling to listen to and answer the queries are at risk of suit, even if they practice quality medicine. Conversely, those who are perceived as concerned, accessible, and willing to communicate are sued far less.

- *Educate and counsel*: Educate antenatal patients about few common conditions tackled during pregnancy and give printed material for discussion at next visit. Counsel the patient as well as her relatives about disease, potential complications and available options for management.
- *Informed consent*: Take written informed consent for surgical procedures whether major or minor.
- *Document refusal for treatment*: Do not forget to take documented negative consent of refusal for treatment, e.g., refusal for cesarean section, refusal for blood transfusion, refusal for second opinion, etc.
- Do not combine two surgeries as far as possible.
- Counsel if any perceived need for blood transfusion and keep rare blood group donors or blood ready in emergency.
- Take separate consent for blood transfusions when required with explanation of specific adverse effects.
- Advise necessary investigations with proper documentation of the medical indications for such investigations.
- In case prescribed medicines are substituted by patient or not taken as advised, make a note in prescription on next visit.
- Do not give false/unrealistic assurances of complete cure.
- Document noncompliance of the patient related to diet, medication or any other precaution.
- Inform well in time about the alternative specialist to be contacted in case of non availability of oneself due to any reasons.
- Suggest second opinion/consultation in complicated cases or when patient/relatives have unrealistic doubts. Document the suggestion of second opinion/consultation along with patient's signatures.
- Keep all records and registers updated as required by law of the country and submit regular reports to authorities as needed.

CONCLUSION

It is essential for every practicing obstetrician and gynecologist to be aware about law in general and specifically law relevant to their specialty. Fulfilment of legal requirements under various legislations is mandatory and must be followed diligently to avoid potential medicolegal problems. Developing a good doctor-patient relationship, adhering to acceptable standard of care, prompt response to emergencies, dealing with high-risk areas of potential litigation with good documentation and counseling alongwith high quality training, decision-making and timely intervention are the basis for a good practice and certainly a sound basis for avoiding litigation in obstetric and gynecology practice.

REFERENCES

1. UNFPA (United Nations Population Fund) is an international development agency that promotes the right of every woman, man and child. Available:http://esaro.unfpa.org/public/public/site/africa/cache/offonce/news/pid/10529%3Bjsessionid=1D9DC69 CFC6BAF73FFE558EF7BA5FC89.jahia01.
2. Prabuddh S Mittal. Medicolegal aspects in Obstetrics and Gynecology Practice. In: Tiwari S, Baldwa M et al. Textbook on Medicolegal issues related to various specialties. (Eds) 1st edn, Jaypee, New Delhi. 2012.pp. 186-97.
3. Richard B, Soders R. Chicken soup for the defendant physician-OBG management. 2003.p.52.

4. Princeton NJ: Princeton Survey Research Associate. Professional liability and its effect–report of a 1999 survey of ACOG's Membership.
5. John Patrick O'Grady, Dennis RA, Despina EH. The Borderland between law and medicine in current Obstet and Gynec-diagnosis and treatment. Ed Alan HD Cherney, Lauren Nathan, pp.1117-24.
6. Wilson N, Strunk AL. Survey on professional liability. ACOG Clin Rev. 2006;12(2):I,13-6.
7. http://www.bormanviolins.com/SC/keel.htmKeel vs. Banach. So. 2d. Ala. 1993;624:1022.
8. Kimble. Ala. Law. Ala. 1994;55:84.
9. Lollar vs. Tankersley So. 2d. Ala. 1993;613:1249.Available: http://www.leagle.com/decision/19931862613So2d1249_11822.xml.
10. American College of Obstetricians and Gynecologists. Screening for fetal chromosomal abnormalities. ACOG Practice Bulletin No. 77. Obstet Gynecol. 2007;109:217-27.
11. Callen PW. Obstetric ultrasound examination Available: http://www.radiology.ucsf.edu/sites/all/files/filemanager/Chapter_1_Callen_Textbook.pdf.
12. AIUM practice guideline for the performance of obstetric ultrasound examinations. Laurel (MD): AIUM; 2007. Available: http://www.aium.org/resources/guidelines/obstetric.pdf.
13. Kuczkowski KM. Medico-legal issues in obstetric anesthesia: what does an obstetrician need to know? Arch Gynecol Obstet. 2008;278(6):503-5.
14. Ashok Jadon. Complications of obstetric anesthesia. Indian J Anaesth. 2010;54(5):415-20.
15. http://ncdrc.nic.in/Consumer complaint no. 54 of 2013. Mr C Jayapal Reddy vs Shri GS Rao, Managing Director, Yashoda Group of Hospitals and Dr Padmini Valluri (Gynecologist), Yashoda Hospitals. 2013.
16. Lauwers PR, Van Hee RH. Intra-peritoneal gossypibomas: The need to count sponges. World J Surg. 2000;24:521-7.
17. Kaiser CW, Friedman S, Spurling KP, Slowick T, Kaiser HA. The retained surgical sponge. Ann Surg. 1996;224:79-84.
18. Emergencies, procedure changes contribute to left-behind surgical instruments. Patient Safety Monitor Insider, Jan 17, 2003. Available: http://www.hcpro.com/QPS-25552-873/Emergencies-procedure-changes-contribute-to-leftbehind-surgical-instrumentsPfizer-slaps-bar-codes-on-unit-dose-medicationsSenators-balk-at-Bushs-stance-on-malpractice-reform.html.
19. Gawande AA, et al. Risk Factors for Retained Instruments and Sponges After Surgery. N Engl J Med. 2003;348:229-35.
20. Samira Kohli vs. Dr. Prabha Manchanda and Anr. Available: http://www.indiankanoon.org/doc/438423.
21. Available:http://www.acog.org/Resources_And_Publications/Committee_Opinions/Committee_on_Ethics/Expert_Testimony.

CHAPTER 22

Medicolegal Issues in Surgery

Manu Shankar

> *"Science does not have a moral dimension. It is like a Knife. If you give it to a Surgeon or a Murderer, each will use it differently."*
> —**Wernher Von Braun**[1]

■ INTRODUCTION

Surgery originates from Chirurgery (Latin: *chirurgia*), which further has its origin from Greek words, *cheir* (hands) and *ergon* (work). Historically surgery was the branch of medicine that involved working with hands to remove the disease. During 16th century, Ambroise Pare a French surgeon, and *Surgeon in chief* to Napoleon's army stated that:

> *"To perform surgery is to eliminate that which is superfluous, restore that which has been dislocated, separate that which has been united, join that which has been divided and repair the defects of nature."*[2]

The past decade has seen dramatic improvement in the patient care provided by the surgeons. Many of these improvements may be traced to the improved understanding of disease, better diagnostic technologies, improved surgical techniques and tools, and above all the commitment of surgeons to provide the quality care. In spite of providing the best possible care, complications do occur. The very idea that complications can occur has always disheartened the surgeons, more so in the current scenario where complications engender litigation. A patient may resent a prolonged hospital stay, or a lifelong disability, which can have disastrous consequences on surgeon-patient relationship.

There are numerous medicolegal risk factors related to surgery. Most of them are overlapping, and if not managed properly, may interlink with each other to ultimately culminate into malpractice lawsuits. Some of these medicolegal issues may arise due to: unexpected/poor outcome, surgical complications, retained foreign objects, wrong site surgery, uninformed alteration in major surgery, sudden and irresponsibly referring a patient to other consultant/higher center, unexpected high cost of care, prolonged hospital stay, improper communication. There are certain risk factors, innate to the specialty of surgery which may not be avoidable, even in the best hands and care. However effective management of these innate risk factors is essential for patient safety as well as for legally safe practice.

PREOPERATIVE PERIOD IN SURGERY

A surgical patient may have multiple co-morbidities. In an elective setting, it is essential to optimize the medical comorbidities as much as possible, even if it means deferring the surgery by a few days/weeks. Failure to do so or lack of documentation may amount to negligence. In an emergency setting, when it is not possible to wait for comorbidities to become normal, document all such conditions, and have a base line values for the current status of the comorbidities. It is a good practice to have a consultation from relevant specialists and document all the verbal discussions with them. Documented informed consent with detailed discussion with the patient and one surrogate decision maker, and giving adequate time would keep most of the medicolegal implications away.

Document Preoperative Status

It is essential to document all the preoperative issues, comorbidities, addictions, allergies, co-existing medical problems or any other issue that is expected to affect the outcome of the current surgery to be performed. If the patient fails to reveal these conditions or hides any of the facts, then he has coliability. For illustration, a patient fails to inform his concurrent medicines, and has history of allergic reaction to one of the prescribed medicines. He would be considered negligent in not revealing his medical history to the doctor. Hence, it becomes very important to document that a medical and treatment history has been obtained. Such a routine of documenting the patient's preoperative status is not only a good clinical practice but also has a significant role in defending an allegation of medical negligence against a surgeon in a Court of law.

Document the Shared Decision Making Process

All communications with the patient and his family has to be documented, including plan of management, and the possible outcome. This becomes more important in critical patients, in which the commonest complaint is that: *surgeon did not explain the prognosis, else we would have taken a second opinion/thought of alternative management.* To avoid legal hassles, it is prudent to give a summary of the case to the patient/attendant and tell them that they are free to take a second opinion before giving consent for the surgery. This should obviously be documented in the case sheets. In case the patient/family refuses the treatment or intervention, it is recommended that the surgeon should document the communication, including the expected adverse outcomes of refusal. Failure to do so may amount to flouting the rules of an informed consent.

Involve Other Specialties

It is always better to recheck deranged lab results, especially when these are likely to affect the current surgery. A patient with borderline high serum creatinine, planned for a Contrast Computerized Tomography (CECT) may land up in contrast nephropathy, leading to high risk of malpractice lawsuit. However, timely consultation with a nephrologist, along with necessary precautions like hydration and n-acetylcysteine, and documentation of the fact that the benefits of CECT would outweigh the risks of contrast nephropathy, will be helpful in avoiding medicolegal issues later on, in case an unavoidable harm occurs. In case consultation from other specialists is taken, the operating surgeon must ensure that the specialist writes down his advice/medication orders in the case sheets. All the verbal discussions should also be written in chronological order.

Give Sufficient Time to Patient

A good informed consent allows sufficient time to the patient to decide before surgery and mentions all the pros and cons of the procedure. For elective surgeries, it is advisable to provide complete information to the patient and give him sufficient time to decide. Once all the information necessary for informed consent has been provided and the patient is taking time to decide, it is advisable to document the same and authenticate by taking patient's signatures. The window period when surgeon has provided all the information and is still waiting for the consent is extremely critical as during this period the patient's condition may deteriorate and later on may complain in a Court that he suffered harm due to surgeon's delay in treating the patient. To avoid such untoward complaint it is advisable to keep in safe custody a written statement from the patient:

> I have received from my doctor, all the information necessary to decide whether to allow/deny the consent for recommended surgery. I have no further queries from the doctor but I need some time to decide.
> Date:
> Time: Patient's/Relative's sign

The best time for obtaining consent is in the outpatient clinic before the patient is admitted as it gives adequate time to the patient to discuss the issues related to surgery and the outcome. If the patient is in critical condition, and it is not possible to take consent before performing the lifesaving surgery, then the operating surgeon along with a hospital administrator should take decision to perform the surgery without consent. Such a situation may arise more commonly in unattended patients who are not accompanied by any relative/attendant.

■ PEROPERATIVE PERIOD

Unexpected Peroperative Findings

In spite of thorough preoperative assessment and lab investigations, the surgeon may encounter certain unexpected findings, regarding which he has to take the best possible decisions while performing the surgery. He may be tempted to extend/modify the surgery for which no informed consent was taken. It is advised that the surgeon should limit the extended surgery to the extent of life saving procedure, as he cannot presume the patient's consent to the surgery that goes beyond lifesaving procedure. For illustration, a surgeon may find an ovarian cyst or endometriosis during surgery for acute appendicitis. The surgeon should not perform oophorectomy at the same go as it is not an acute emergency. Let the patient come out of anesthesia, and do the second surgery after the patient gives the consent. However, if the findings in the above case is tubal ectopic with bleed, further surgery as deemed necessary can be carried out after getting the consent from patient's husband/any other relative immediately available outside the operation theater.

Deviation from Planned Surgery

In the event of a major deviation from the planned procedure which would warrant removal of an organ, if the condition permits, it is better to let the patient come out of anesthesia, and do the second surgery after the patient gives the consent. If the condition of the patient is so critical that it is not possible to postpone the altogether new surgery for which there is no prior consent of the patient, it is better to take informed consent of two family members during the procedure. The reason for deviation from the planned surgery, and all the communication with relatives must be thoroughly documented in case sheets in chronological manner.

Need to Call Other Specialists During Surgery

While performing the procedure, surgeon may need to call upon another specialist due to some unexpected finding or any complication. For illustration, a gynecologist may need to call upon a surgeon to separate dense pelvic bowel adhesions during hysterectomy, or an oncosurgeon calling upon a vascular surgeon to repair a blood vessel during a cancer surgery. Many a times, such need to call upon another specialist may not be anticipated before starting the surgery. The unexpected findings, any injury/complication and the remedial measures taken should be documented in the case sheets. Any concealment of facts, due to apprehension of malpractice litigation may further worsen the situation. Taking help of another specialist in the course of a surgery for dealing with unexpected findings or a complication, and documenting the same, is always a safe-guard, rather than hiding such a fact.

■ POSTOPERATIVE PERIOD

Postoperative Complications

Postoperative complications after any surgery are well documented in the scientific literature. It is important to differentiate whether the complication that occurred was unavoidable or due to some negligence. A postoperative abscess/wound infection is a known complication. However, if it occurs because of retained surgical gauze, it is negligence. If operative notes mention that a thorough lavage was given at the wound site to remove all physical debris, it will be indicative of due care provided by the surgeon and his team. Similarly, if a pack is left inside the peritoneal cavity for securing hemostasis and a planned procedure after 48 hours, it is advisable to inform the same to the patient/attendant and also document the same in the case sheets. Lack of documentation may result in avoidable blames against the operating surgeon.

Repeat Surgery

Almost all surgical procedures can have a complication which can lead to a second procedure, or some findings might make the surgeon perceive the need for a second look procedure. Patients/relatives are aggressive if this includes a lot of financial burden. Appropriate counseling of the patient, discussing the possible outcomes and the plan for managing each outcome is a clinical practice that fulfils the requirement of informed consent as well as acts as a litigation prevention strategy. A second look surgery after finding mesenteric ischemia is a planned procedure. A patient not settling after a bowel surgery, having possibility of adhesions/anastomotic leak, necessitating a second look procedure is a complication. Discussing out the issues with the patient and relatives is essential. Educate the patient that, a relook will never kill a patient, but missing out on these signs may be detrimental. Having a second opinion helps in restoring your as well as the patient's confidence. If you have the privilege of having a senior colleague around, discuss the case with him/her. Sincere concern shows that the patient is being cared for and the surgeon is aware and trying to solve the unexpected outcome.

CONSENT IN SURGERY[3]

Informed consent is an integral part of the practice of surgery. All over India, there are diversities in the way consent is taken. The ambiguity in the documentation of consent leads to variable interpretations in court of law, which have resulted in damages to many Surgeons. The Supreme Court of India in a landmark judgment of Samira Kohli versus Prabha Manchanda[3] elaborated on various aspects of taking consent. It further laid down various guidelines for taking a valid consent. The Apex Court opined that any additional surgery however beneficial to the patient in saving time, expenses, pain and suffering are no ground for defence.

A well drafted consent should include the patient's details, diagnosis, planned surgery, name of surgeon/surgical team, anesthetists' name. It should also mention the common complications, anticipated outcome, need for any special procedures as needed. It should also have documentation of comorbidities with mention of any added risks associated with them. The consent should be written in a language that the patient can understand. Adequate time should be given to the patient/relatives to understand the disease, plan of management and ask questions. Consent should be preferably signed by the patient himself. In case of valid reasons only, the consent may be signed by patient's relative/representative. It should also be countersigned by the doctor explaining the consent and witnessed by a third person. Failure to communicate peroperative findings, any deviation from the expected course in recovery and not documenting the same may give rise to postoperative medicolegal issues. A consent for surgery has to be different from the consent for anesthesia as both are dealt with by separate teams, and complications related to surgery and anesthesia are different.

ROLE OF ANESTHESIA

It is said that, *a surgeon is as good as his anesthetist will let him be*. Gone is the era when the skill of a surgeon was determined by the speed of surgery in the operation theater. With the advent of safer anesthetic drugs, and excellent monitoring, the efficacy is now judged by the safe outcomes and uneventful recovery. Paramount to the above fact is the competence of the anesthetist in dealing with the perioperative period, ensuring a smooth recovery. If the anesthetist is able to anticipate the surgical procedure and steps, it helps to have a better outcome. Giving deeper plane of anesthesia during anal procedure and keeping the patient on spontaneous respiration during superficial procedures is in the hands of the anesthetist. Anesthesia needs to be tailored according to the medical comorbidities of the patient and the surgery planned. If the patient is high-risk for anesthesia for a planned surgery, it is better to defer the operation till the patient is stabilized rather than to indulge into hurried surgery. In a patient with myasthenia gravis, muscle relaxant is contraindicated as it potentiates the myasthenic crisis. Regional anesthesia in such a patient would be preferable. Anticipating blood loss, maintaining normothermia, euglycemia, adequate fluid replacement during prolonged or difficult surgeries, maintaining a sufficiently deep plane of anesthesia goes a long way in ensuring uneventful postoperative outcome. Anesthetists have a critical role in outcome of the surgery and may be held liable in case the patient suffers any harm due to surgery.[4]

SURGICAL COMPLICATIONS

Narrow demarcation exists between what is perceived as a surgical complication, and a poor outcome due to negligence. There is no standard definition of complication. A complication may be described as an adverse event caused by pre-existing factors that were outside the doctor's control.[5,6] All patients are not similar in health, habits, immunity or healing power, and have varying susceptibility to complications. A mistake, however, assumes there was a lapse of either quality or control by the surgeon out of keeping with normal expectation.

The concept of surgical complication, mistake and a negligent act may have a varied interpretation by the experts. For illustration, *recurrent laryngeal nerve* injury during thyroidectomy may be either of the three. If the surgeon identifies and preserves the nerve, and lands up in a postoperative hoarseness of voice, it is a complication. If he does not attempt to identify it, it may be labeled as a medical mistake, but if he tries to control bleeding in that area with haphazard application of hemostats or unipolar electrocautery, and lands with hoarseness of voice, it would be labeled as negligence.[7]

There is a common misconception among the surgeons that a known complication occurring due to specific surgery is an acceptable legal immunity against the claims for negligence. However, the real scenario is that courts are well aware that a known complication due to surgery can also occur due to negligent act or omission. In such cases, courts apply *bolam's rule* and look whether standard care was provided or not. For illustration, obstructive jaundice may occur as a complication of laparoscopic cholecystectomy. Such a complication may occur due to a slipped stone in common bile duct (CBD), but if a surgeon clips and divides the CBD, it may be labeled as negligent act, especially if the surgeon fails to detect and manage the problem in postoperative period. It may be extremely challenging to prove that the complication was because of surgical mistake, negligence or due to patient's comorbid conditions. It is advised to describe all the operative steps in detail, what all was done to avert the known complications. It is advisable that the case sheets must mention that the surgeon has ensured a safe clinical practice and all precautions were taken.

Definition of complication has been changing and till now, no standard definition is in place. What is considered a complication now may have been an acceptable outcome few decades ago. Similarly a known complication today may be an unacceptable event in a decade. Wound infection was a desired thing in the preantibiotic era (laudable pus) but now wound infection in a clean surgery is not acceptable and is considered as complication in a joint replacement or organ transplant surgery.

Complications related to anesthesia may occur due to failure of equipment or failure to identify warning signs. These complications may vary from delayed recovery, bronchospasm, aspiration to even death during procedure. It is important for anesthetist to document all these relevant findings in their preanesthetic check-up charts and take relevant informed consent from the patient and the relatives. Some of the complications can be avoided if proper preoperative planning is done.

Error of judgment can occur with any surgeon during a procedure. Different surgeons may behave differently during a similar situation. What a surgeon is thinking during the surgery, and what made him take that particular step is best understood by him only. For illustration, removal of a segment of bowel during surgery which was perceived to be diseased, but the biopsy showed it to be a normal segment might be considered as a right approach by one group of surgeons while the other group may consider it to be error of judgment. In case of doubt, it is better to take consultation of another colleague during the procedure (if available). Document your peroperative findings in detail, and if possible, mention the reason for adopting the particular approach during surgery. If at the end of the procedure, or in postoperative period, anything is found amiss, it is better to discuss the concerns with patient and the family, ask for relevant investigations, manage the case accordingly and keep the patient and family well informed.

Death during surgery or immediately thereafter creates an almost irrevocable suspicion in the minds of deceased's relatives about criminal negligence. Such deaths constitute a medicolegal case, and even if it was anticipated and documented in preoperative consent, it is essential to inform the police and get the medicolegal autopsy done. There are a few clear cut criminal negligence cases, like leaving a foreign body (mop/instrument), operating on a wrong patient, operating on the wrong site, of carrying out the wrong procedure. The World Health Organization (WHO) safe surgery checklist is a simple tool to reduce the risk of surgical errors.[8]

■ 'NEVER EVENTS' IN SURGERY

A never event is defined as a serious, preventable incident that should not occur if the available preventive measures have been implemented.[9] A retained surgical item and wrong-site surgery are the two avoidable events in surgery that may have devastating consequences both on patient as well as healthcare team. Mere fact that wrong site surgery was performed shows that due care and skill was not practised.

Retained Surgical Items

A retained surgical item refers to an unintentional retention of any surgical item, which is found to be inside the patient after he/she has left the operation theater. A surgical sponge is the most common retained surgical item but other items, such as needles and surgical instruments, can also be inadvertently left inside a patient. The foreign body can cause an acute injury leading to early detection or it may take weeks, months or years to be discovered. Such patients may present with complications such as infection, bowel obstruction, development of a tumor like lesion erosions through skin or fistula formation.

The risk of retained surgical item increases in patients who have emergency surgery, an unexpected change in surgical procedure and higher mean body mass index. Bypassing the surgical count, incorrect count or falsely correct count results in breach of line of defence to prevent surgical errors and increases the likelihood of retained surgical items.[10] Adhering to strict surgical safety protocols can help in reducing the incidence of this never event. The American College of Surgeons and the Association of Perioperative Registered Nurses have issued guidelines to prevent the occurrence of retained surgical items. These guidelines include the use of standard counting procedures, performing a thorough wound inspection before closing a surgical site, and using only X-ray detectable items in the surgical wound. An X-ray at the completion of an operation is recommended if there is any confusion regarding the counts even by a single member of the operation room team, or in the presence of risk factor.[11]

When a surgical item is erroneously left inside a patient, the doctrine of *Res ipsa loquitor* (*things speak for itself*) applies which presumes that mere presence of the foreign object in the patient indicates that the patient did not receive proper surgical care and that the surgeon was negligent in providing the standard care. The proof of negligence by the patient is not required, rather the burden of proof shifts to surgeon and his/her team.

Wrong Site Surgery

Wrong site surgery refers to any surgical procedure performed on the wrong patient, wrong body part, wrong side of the body, or wrong level of a correctly identified anatomic site.

The likelihood of wrong site surgery is more when there are multiple surgeons involved in the same surgery or multiple procedures are performed on the same patient, emergency surgery, abnormal patient anatomy, and morbid obesity.[12] Incomplete preoperative information (medical records are nonavailable or not reviewed), inadequate system in place to verify the correct surgical site, or lack of team work are some of the risk factors for wrong site surgeries.[13] The legal standing of *wrong site surgery* is similar to that of erroneously *retained surgical items*. Mere fact that wrong site surgery occurred shows that due care and skill was not provided to the patient. The doctrine of *Res ipsa loquitur* applies. Proof of negligence is not required from the plaintiff, rather the burden of proof shifts to the surgeon.

■ TAKE HOME MESSAGE FOR THE SURGEONS

- Legible documentation of the whole process of patient care in chronological is extremely important.
- Take written informed consent from the patient and get it countersigned by patient's relative and a staff member.
- For emergency, lifesaving or unplanned procedures, take consent from the patient, if possible, and if the patient is not able to give consent due to his critical condition/unconsciousness/altered sensorium take consent from patient's relative, and document the indication of surgery, possible outcome, risk factors and complications.
- If any additional procedure is to be performed during surgery which was not anticipated earlier, and is not a lifesaving procedure and can be afforded to be postponed, it is better to postpone the same till the patient gives consent for that additional procedure. Let the patient recover from the first surgery, and then go ahead with the additional procedure after getting a fresh consent.
- In cases where chances of good outcome after the surgery are low, and in cases of anticipated complications, get the opinion of another colleague and document the same. Also educate the patient's relatives about the nature of surgery and expected outcome.
- Follow the WHO safe surgical checklist.
- Always recheck the counts before and after the closure.
- Use gauze or mops with radio-opaque markers, so that they can be screened by C-arm if counts are incorrect.
- In case of complications or any deviation from expected postoperative course, be vigilant to detect and manage the complications. Document your findings and relevant investigations. Also document in detail further management of the case and keep the patient well informed.
- Involve other colleagues if any doubt arises and also involve the patient/relatives in shared decision making.

■ CONCLUSION

Although the quality of care being provided by the surgeons has improved dramatically, every surgical procedure has a risk of complications. In spite of providing the best care, complications still dismay the surgeons. There are numerous medicolegal issues related to surgery. There are certain risk factors, innate to the specialty of surgery which may not be avoidable, even in the best hands and care. However effective management of these innate risk factors is essential for patient safety, nurturing into healthy surgeon-patient relationship. Regularly updating the recent trends in surgery as well as current medicolegal trends is a must for every surgeon.

REFERENCES

1. Bob Seidensticker. Future Hype: The Myths of Technology Change. 2006.
2. Available: http://www.historyofsurgery.co.uk/Web%20Pages/0419_1.htm.
3. Samira Kohli vs. Dr. Prabha Manchanda and Anr. Available: http://www.indiankanoon.org/doc/438423.
4. C Parakh. Legal aspects of anesthesia practice. Indian Journal of Anesthesia. 2008;52 (3):247-57.
5. Daniel K Sokol, James Wilson. What is a Surgical Complication? World J Surg. 2008;32:942-4.
6. Adedeji S, Sokol DK, Palser T, McKneally M. Ethics of surgical complications. World J Surg. 2009;33(4):732-7.
7. Available:http://www.kevinmd.com blog/2011/03/surgical-error-difference mistake-complication.html.
8. Available:http://www.who.int/patientsafety/safesurgery/tools_resources/SSSL_Checklist_finalJun08.pdf.
9. Hadjipavlou AG, Marshall RW. Wrong site surgery the maze of potential errors. Editorial Bone Joint J. 2013;95-B:434-5.
10. Gawande AA. "Risk factors for retained instruments and sponges after surgery". N Engl J Med. 2003;348:229-35.
11. Gibbs VC, Coakley FD, Reines HD. Preventable errors in the operating room: retained foreign bodies after surgery-part1. Curr Probl Surg. 2007;44:281.
12. Clarke JR, Johncton J, Finley ED. Getting surgery right. Ann Surg. 2007;246:395.
13. Charles H. Chodrof Doing the right things to correct wrong-site surgery. Pennsylvania Patient Safety Reporting System (PA-PSRS) Patient Safety Advisory. 2007;4(2):29-68.

CHAPTER 23

Medicolegal Issues in Orthopedics

VJ Purushotham

> *"A good surgeon doesn't just concentrate on technical ability, but also on the appropriateness of what you're doing."*
> — Benjamin Carson

■ INTRODUCTION

Orthopedic surgery is a branch of medicine dealing with musculoskeletal system which is responsible for the locomotion of our body. The term "orthopedia" was coined by French physician, Nicolas Andry in 1741 meaning "straightening the child" as correction of deformity was becoming increasingly common those days. Nicholas Andry published a book, titled "Orthopaedia: The Art of Correcting and Preventing Deformities in Children."[1] The book has depicted a crooked tree tied to a strong post (**Fig. 1**). This depiction reflects the basis

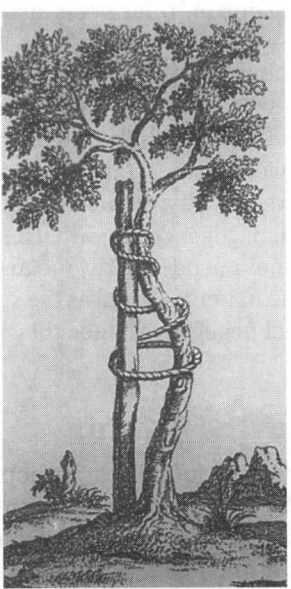

FIG. 1: Famous engraving of the "Crooked Tree".

of orthopedic surgery, i.e., to correct deformities. Many developments in orthopedics have resulted from experiences in wartime. Though the initial progression was slow, rapid developments took place in the 19th and 20th century. Dr Hugh Owen Thomas and his nephew Dr Robert Jones contributed to the growth of innovations in orthopedics in the 19th century.[2,3]

Jones founded British Orthopaedic Society in 1894, which propelled the advances in surgical section of orthopedics.[4] The intramedullary rods and plates were invented and the association for study of internal fixation (AO) was founded in Switzerland in 1958.[5] The modern hip replacement was pioneered by John Charnley in 1960, at Wrightington, UK.[6] Thus, what started as the field of deformity corrections in early 18th century led to the present era of replacement of most of the joints and fixing all the fractures. Perhaps, orthopedic field's advancement from nonoperative treatment to operative treatment, has led it to being one of the most often dragged fields to consumer courts! In addition to clinical challenges, it is expected from the orthopedic surgeons to fulfill legal requirements associated with medical practice.

MEDICOLEGAL RISKS IN ORTHOPEDICS

Morbid Results are Easily Noticeable

One of the biggest risks in orthopedics, in terms of lawsuits, is that the radiological findings are quite obvious, sometimes even to laymen, thus what normally is a slight deviation from the standard protocols of fracture fixation, reconstruction or deformity correction, may present as a glaring mistake. The rising trend of patients seeking second opinion due to lack of faith in healthcare system further magnifies the conflict, ultimately ending up as medical negligence lawsuit. Similar to other medical specialties, in case of orthopedics, different treatment modalities under different schools of thoughts exist and are routinely practiced, thus identifying a clear and definitive standard protocol for treating any specific disease is not possible. So, when there is a difference of opinion in any given treatment modality, criticism, or vague comments against the treating doctor by his peers gives way to the suspicion ultimately ending up as malpractice lawsuit.

In orthopedic patients, often, the complications are easily noticeable in the form of persisting deformities, discharging sinuses, etc. In spite of providing reasonable care, when a petitioner in the form of patient with walking aids, wheel chairs, and deformities, enters the Court, there is a possibility that he would gain sympathy of the Court. Often, on the very face of it, the complications are still viewed as a byproduct of negligence. However, it is now clear through many judgments in medical negligence cases that a patient suffering from an ailment or complication even after surgery does not necessarily mean negligence on the part of treating doctor. There is a need to educate the patients as well as the society at large that complications do not necessarily represent medical negligence, since they are not always preventable even with best possible care.

Lack of Proper Rapport with the Patients

It may sound awkward, but studies have found that orthopedic surgeons are known to be relatively arrogant, and thus may be misinterpreted to be unsympathetic to the patients. A survey done by American Association of Orthopedic Surgeons (AAOS) revealed that patients feel that orthopedic surgeons are not friendly and are not sympathetic.[7] The opportunity of building doctor–patient rapport before the start of treatment is very less especially in trauma and emergency cases. Often, the orthopedic cases assessed in emergency room are in critical condition, and thus chances of uncertain decisions are more. Unlike other fields where the patient has an existing relationship before any complications occur, this may be absent in orthopedic practice especially when dealing with trauma and other emergency situations.

Scope of Consent in Orthopedics

In multiple trauma and other emergency cases, optimal management of the injured requires rapid decision making and procedural skills often without getting time for informed consent of the patient. The patient may not be in a sound state of mind to give a valid consent, and treatment is often required to be life-saving. Because of these circumstances, the risk of liability always hangs over the orthopedic surgeon like the "sword of Damocles."

Given the current scenario of rising trend of malpractice litigation, every orthopedic surgeon must have a thorough understanding of the informed consent. Informed consent has a significant role in medical practice. A well-informed patient, participating in the decisions related to his/her treatment is a must for validity of the consent. A surgeon should provide all the information to the patient in a complete and understandable manner and then obtain his/her consent. The key components of this process include explanation of the diagnosis, description of the proposed surgery with its benefits and risks, any alternative treatment available, and probability of success of the proposed surgery. While taking consent in orthopedic cases, it may be required to provide additional information:

- Chances of repeat surgeries,
- Statement of no guarantee,
- Need for bone grafts and blood products,
- Potential complications,
- Possibility of unforeseen problems and even the risk of death in some cases.

Documentation in several formats, such as patient-signed consent form, case sheets, teaching videos, and patient information pamphlets, are helpful to ensure that the patient was well informed and played active role in the decision to proceed with the surgery.

Reasons of Litigation Against Orthopedic Surgeons

Poor outcome due to nonunions, malunions, limb length discrepancies, loss of movement, and residual deformities are some of the common cases that are being dragged in to Consumer Courts. Nowadays life style surgeries such as total hip replacement (THR), total knee replacement (TKR), limb lengthening surgeries by Ilizarov surgeries, and arthroscopic surgeries are becoming more common. Perhaps here the aggressive marketing by some corporate hospitals, influencing the patient to undergo such surgeries are the source of such conflicts. In the opinion of author, the patient should seek for surgeries rather than the surgeons pushing for it! It is advisable that the decision to perform surgery should be a shared decision in which the patient should be actively involved. Common causes of litigation against orthopedic surgeons are depicted in **Box 1**.

Recently, postoperative infections are also being drawn to courts in the name of negligence. It is commonly claimed that hospital conditions and operation theater set up are causative factors resulting in postoperative infection. So, it is of paramount importance to uphold the standard operating setup. Often, the orthopedic surgeons are dragged into the lawsuit for anesthesia-associated complications. It is advisable that the surgeon should know about the type of anesthesia to be administered by the anesthesiologist and possible

> **BOX 1** **Common causes of litigation in orthopedics.[8]**
> - Poor outcome of the treatment
> - Improper treatment
> - Improper communication/documentation
> - Hospital acquired infection
> - Diagnostic errors
> - Wrong side/level surgeries
> - Nerve/vessel injuries and compartment syndrome

> **BOX 2** **Top 10 conditions commonly resulting in medicolegal conflicts in orthopedics.[8]**
> 1. Fracture of femur
> 2. Fracture of tibia
> 3. Disc lesions
> 4. Osteoarthritis (arthroplasty)
> 5. Fractures of radius and ulna
> 6. Ankle injuries
> 7. Back disorders: Lumbago, sciatica
> 8. Knee ligament/meniscal injuries
> 9. Humerus fracture
> 10. Hand injuries

complications in the chosen type of anesthesia. Another increasingly common medicolegal issue is the arrangement of ICU backup for surgeries and even for some procedures. Any procedure under anesthesia should have an ICU backup, in case anything goes wrong. Top 10 conditions in orthopedics in which chances of medicolegal conflicts are higher are shown in **Box 2**.

Wrong-site Surgery

Wrong-site surgeries can be devastating events for patients as well as the healthcare providers. Wrong-site surgery has been listed as "never events" by the NHS's National Patient Safety Agency. A "never event" is defined as a serious and largely preventable incident that should not occur if the available preventive measures have been implemented.[9] The Joint Commission identified a number of factors contributing to an increased risk of wrong-site surgeries (**Table 1**).[10] The majority of cases involved a failure in communication between surgical team members and the patient and family. Other contributing factors included: (a) Policy issues, such as marking of the surgical site not being required; (b) Absence of verification in the operating theater and of a verification checklist; (c) Incomplete preoperative assessment; (d) Staffing issues; and (e) Distracting factors. The Joint Commission also described negative factors such as:
- Exclusion of certain surgical team members from the patient assessment;
- Failure to include the patient or family when identifying the correct site;
- Lack of policies, procedures, and controls;
- Miscommunication;

TABLE 1: Factors contributing to an increased risk for wrong-site, wrong-person or wrong-procedure surgery.[10]

Contributing factors	Proportion of cases (%)
Emergency cases	19
Unusual physical characteristics, including morbid obesity or physical deformity	16
Unusual time pressures to start or complete the procedure	13
Unusual equipment or setup in the operating room	13
Multiple surgeons being involved in the case	13
Multiple procedures being performed during a single visit to the operating theater	10

- Pressure to reduce preoperative time;
- Illegible handwriting;
- Reliance solely on the operating surgeon to determine the correct site and use of abbreviations to explain the operation site or side.

TIPS ON PREVENTING MEDICOLEGAL CONFLICTS

Good Communication and Rapport

Good communication and rapport are the most important aspects that can nurture a warm doctor–patient relationship. Even though the concept of considering medicine as a noble profession and the doctors as equivalent to God is rapidly fading away, patients still look upon at their doctor as a savior of their problems. Patients go to their doctors with faith and trust, though sometimes they may have some suspicious thoughts and apprehensions. To build a healthy and warm doctor–patient relationship, proper communication is a must. Clear and complete communication is very crucial to win over patient's confidence. Communication also helps the patient to understand most of the matters related to his illness and the proposed treatment. Good communication and excellent rapport are helpful in educating the patient during the process of taking the "informed written consent" and thus preventing possible litigations.

Documentation and Informed Consent

Having established a good communication and rapport with the patient, next very important step is documentation. Most of our lawsuits are lost for want of proper documentation, including consent. Each event of the patient's interaction related to the illness and treatment has to be recorded. The consent to be documented has to be comprehensive one, with details of the proposed surgery/procedure, risks, benefits, and alternatives (if any) available. It is very important to ensure that the consent is signed by the patient, the treating doctor, impartial witness, and preferably by the attendant. Counseling of the patient and attendants in the language they understand is important.

Another important aspect of documentation is "discharge summary." The postoperative advice has to be clearly written especially with regard to wound care, ambulation, and follow-ups. The documentation has to be clear, legible, and devoid of abbreviations.

Advocating Treatment Options

Orthopedics has evolved tremendously in terms of management of both trauma as well as nontrauma conditions. While operative treatment has replaced nonoperative treatment in almost all situations, the scope for nonoperative option still exists, and the patient must be educated about both the options including their advantages and disadvantages, and a shared decision making should be done. In lifestyle surgeries, like joint replacements, the patient should ask for surgery rather than the surgeon pushing for it.

Avoid Medical Jousting Please!

Medical jousting is the uninformed criticism of a healthcare colleague. It means criticizing the treatment that a patient has already undergone so far before consulting the other doctor. Usually the jousting is unintentional, however, it can also be intentional. Intentional jousting may occur in privatized healthcare systems where colleagues can become competitors. Negatively commenting about a competing doctor's decisions might be seen as a way to boost one's own business. The scope of jousting can vary widely. Some of the examples are:[11]

- Oh! What has been done.
- I would not have treated like this.
- Who gave you this complication? This could've been avoided.
- Oh! you should not have been put on that medication.
- Body language such as a look of surprise or horror when a patient mentions something about their previous care.

The implication of medical jousting is that patients get disheartened about the treatment and lose faith in doctors. The patients get confused as to which doctor's advice should be followed, when they keep on getting conflicting opinions about the treatment already received so far. It leads to loss of trust in healthcare professionals, and it risks malpractice litigation against the professionals involved. However, this does not mean that bad healthcare should be concealed. All doctors have an obligation to highlight when things have gone wrong. Jousting, however, is different, since the criticism in jousting is unsupported by the full facts. It is advisable that doctors should take a resolution not to pass any negative comments against their colleagues and the treatment offered so far. Remember that what you are doing to others, others may do to you!

Practice Evidence-based Orthopedics[12]

Evidence-based medicine (EBM) means judicious use of current best evidence in deciding to offer the best healthcare services. Always adopt a standard and universally accepted protocol during the management of the condition. While treating a patient, due attention should be given to evidence-based orthopedics. This, however, has to be combined with doctor's own experience and expertise in orthopedics. It is advisable to use both individual clinical expertise and best available evidence since neither alone will be adequate. Update your knowledge periodically through regular participation in CMEs, conferences, workshops, etc., as and when required.

Safe Operation Theater Setup

An operating theater is a complex system which has several risk factors, associated not only with the structure and its equipment, but also the performance of healthcare workers. A safe operating theater setup is an environment in which all risk factors are kept strictly under control. This can be achieved through careful planning, implementation, and maintenance of OT standards along with periodic audits as well as proper ongoing training of every member of the OT team. Never compromise on the standards of the operation theatre. No surgery or procedure should be allowed without maintenance of high standards of the operation theater.

■ ORTHOPEDIST IN THE COURT OF LAW

Having known the common situations in orthopedics that can have legal implications, it is better to be acquainted with the common questions that may arise in the Court. Usually, the technical aspects of the case are very difficult for the lawyers to understand. Thus, in a Court of law the doctor should try to provide the details in the most understandable way.

Common questions asked in the Court
- Have you treated this case?
- Are you qualified and skilled to execute this treatment?
- Did you explain the details of the treatment to the patient and his/her attendants?
- How did this "complication" occur? (nonunion, malunion, infection, etc.)
- Does your hospital have standard setup of ICU?
- How do you say this is not negligence?

If looked into the above questionnaire there is enough scope for the answering doctor to defend the case (if there are some grounds). Essentially it is required to prove that you are qualified and you have reasonable skill to treat the patient, and followed a standard protocol of treatment. The defending doctor has to educate his advocate with required content so that it can be defended effectively. The national and state associations can work on bringing standard treatment guidelines and protocols, which will define the actual standard protocol, which is very subjective at present.

■ CONCLUSION

In the era of decreased tolerance and general attitude of "consumer is the king", the service provider in all walks of life is at the receiving end. The medical profession is no exception to this. Our profession which was "once upon a time", considered as noble is now being labeled as a "heartless profession" both by the society as well as by the media. Unfortunately, what has not been understood by them is that medical science is not an exact science and often, the results are unpredictable and not reproducible all the time. At this point, it is very important for us to be more cautious and careful. It is imperative for us to be aware of the legal implications of our profession. As accidents and trauma are increasingly common in the modern lifestyle, cases from specialty of orthopedics are now more often dragged in to the consumer courts. So, not just the methodology of the treatment, but the legal aspects of such treatment have to be inculcated in our practice. Equally important is to have a good patient- doctor relationship, which will be helpful, especially when things go wrong! The associations of all specialties should focus on educating its members on medicolegal aspects of their field.

"Here's wishing all the readers a very safe and fulfilling practice!"

REFERENCES

1. Wikipedia. Nicolas Andry. [online] Available from http://en.wikipedia.org/wiki/Nicolas_Andry. [Last Accessed on August, 2019].
2. Cope R. Hugh Owen Thomas: bone-setter and pioneer orthopaedist. Bull Hosp Jt Dis.1995;54(1):54-60.
3. Tham W, Sng S, Lum YM. A Look Back in Time: Sir Robert Jones, "Father of Modern Orthopaedics". Malays Orthop J. 2014;8(3):37-41.
4. Platt H. British Orthopedic Association: first Founders' lecture. J Bone Joint Surg Br. 1959;41-B(2):231-6.
5. Matter P. History of the AO and its global effect on operative fracture treatment. Clin Orthop Relat Res. 1998;(347):11-8.
6. Wikipedia. John Charnley. [online] Available from https://en.wikipedia.org/wiki/John_Charnley. [Last Accessed on August, 2019].
7. Committee on Professional Liability. Managing Orthopaedic Malpractice Risk, 2nd edition. Illinois: American Academy of Orthopedic Surgeons. 2000.
8. Klimo GF, Daum WJ, Brinker MR, et al. Orthopaedic malpractice: an attorney's prospective. Am J Orthop (Belle Mead NJ). 2000;29(2):93-7.
9. Hadjipavlou AG, Marshall RW. Wrong site surgery: the maze of potential errors. Bone Joint J. 2013;95-B(4):434-5.
10. Joint Commission on Accreditation of Health Care Organizations. Sentinel Event Alert: Follow-up Review of Wrong Site Surgery. [online] Available from http://www.jointcommission.org/SentinelEvents/SentinelEventAlert/sea_24.htm. [Last accessed Aug., 2019].
11. Capson. Doctor Jousting: What It Means and the Dangers. [online] Available from https://www.capson.com/blog/doctor-jousting. [Last Accessed on August, 2019].
12. Sprague S, Smith C, Bhandari M. OrthoEvidenceTM: A clinical resource for evidence-based orthopedics. Orthop Rev (Pavia). 2015;7(2):57-62.

CHAPTER 24

Medicolegal Issues in Ophthalmology

Dinesh Verma, Amandeep Singh

"He that is stricken blind cannot forget the precious treasure of his eyesight lost."
—**William Shakespeare**[1]

■ INTRODUCTION

Description of ocular diseases and their treatment form a part of the oldest medical treatises, *the Sushruta Samhita*. The Indian surgeon *Sushruta*, described the technique of cataract surgery in 800 BC India. For next 2,000 years there were no major breakthroughs until the invention of *ophthalmoscope* that enabled direct visualization of retina. Introduction of *intraocular lens implants* in 1940s, *lasers* in 60s and *phacoemulsification* in 70's transformed the practice of ophthalmology dramatically.[2-4]

Ophthalmology has since evolved into a very 'high-tech' specialty involving highly complex surgical procedures. While many retinal conditions like macular holes which were considered untreatable can now be cured with surgery, several types of Lasers have been used to burn unwanted tissues/blood vessels, to make holes in the soft eye structures to clear the path of vision and to reshape cornea to change the refractive power of the eye aiming to remove the need for glasses, last one involving the most popular technique called LASIK. The other significant developments have been on pharmaceutical area, where an array of therapeutic options has become available for glaucoma, macular degeneration and retinal vascular disorders like diabetic retinopathy. These have brought new problems to the fore as updated knowledge about suitability or otherwise of all available options become imperative for practicing ophthalmologists.

Why Ophthalmology is Vulnerable to Malpractice Litigation?

In addition to the already proven, highly effective therapies, recently there have been a series of reports about emerging treatments of yet incurable eye conditions involving stem cells, artificial retina (micro-chip implants) and gene therapies making this field one of the most rapidly advancing ones in whole of medicine. Latest technology addition to this armamentarium has been Laser assisted cataract surgery that seems to be raking up a storm of controversy. This rapid advance and high-tech status brings its own challenges to the practicing ophthalmologists. Patient expectations have become very high due to the media hype as well as very high cost of these new procedures. When complications occur or just the result is suboptimal, the risk of medical negligence litigation in a consumer court rises sharply. This chapter will help the readers to become aware of the specific risks and to reduce them significantly by following the guidelines and suggestions. There have been studies done to determine the relative percentage of medical negligence cases in various ophthalmic subspecialties.

Medicolegal Issues in Ophthalmology

Medicolegal awareness is a must for ophthalmologists. They may be commonly involved in medicolegal cases in following three circumstances:
1. As treating doctor where legal proceeding has been started against him/her for negligence or malpractice which could be civil or criminal depending on the seriousness of the allegations.
2. When the ophthalmologist has examined or treated a patient as an expert in civil or criminal matters unrelated to their own involvement in that patient's care.
3. As a third party expert witness in a Government inquiry, investigating committee, police or court of law for giving evidence in cases of mishaps like cluster infections, camp surgery complications or complex medical conditions treated by other ophthalmologists.

■ VULNERABLE DOMAINS IN OPHTHALMIC PRACTICE

Laser Assisted In Situ Keratomileusis Complications (Suboptimal Visual Outcome)

Laser Assisted In Situ Keratomileusis (LASIK), a type of refractive surgery for the correction of myopia, hypermetropia, and astigmatism. The surgery is performed with the help of a laser or microkeratome to reshape the cornea in order to improve visual acuity. The popularity of refractive surgery has been rising rapidly, especially in India where a large number of young girls and some boys want to get their glasses removed, apparently to improve their matrimonial prospects. This popularity has also increased the expectations to a very high level. Furthermore, since LASIK is a cosmetic surgery, any complication as a result of the procedure is totally unacceptable since the visual result would have been better if no surgery was done. These factors have made refractive surgeons much more vulnerable to malpractice claims. This is reflected in the Medical Protection Society or Medical Defense Union subscriptions in UK which are highest for refractive surgeons.[5]

As any surgery has intrinsic risks, LASIK is also associated with certain risks and complications which however are much smaller compared to other types of eye surgeries. Infection, inflammation, dryness and ectasia (corneal thinning) may occur. Complications with the corneal flap may occur. Permanent damage to a patient's vision, including blindness, is possible. Diffuse lamellar keratitis, also called the "Sands of Sahara" syndrome, may occur which is an inflammatory reaction and not an infection. This occurs when the tissue under the flap reacts to minute traces of microorganism toxins. Likelihood of its occurrence is based on each patient's sensitivity and/or the amount of exposure. It can usually be well controlled with steroid drops, although in extreme situations it may be better to lift the flap, wash out the inflammation and place steroids directly on the affected tissue. Quick recognition and treatment can mean the difference between a good outcome and an eye with a refractive error.[6,7]

Some patients with poor outcomes from LASIK surgical procedures may complain of reduced quality of life because of vision problems. A small percentage of patients may need to have another surgery because their condition is over-corrected or under-corrected. Some patients may need to wear contact lenses or glasses even after treatment.

The risks of LASIK surgery should be discussed during the process of taking informed consent. The majority of LASIK malpractice claims involve missed contraindications rather than errors during the procedure. Contraindications are pre-existing conditions in a patient that reduces the chances of success and increases the probability of complications. If an ophthalmologist who knows that contraindications are present and still proceeds with the LASIK procedure anyway, and unfortunately that resulted in injury to the patient, the chances of surgeon's losing the malpractice lawsuit are very high.[8]

The key to avoiding a negligence or malpractice claim for refractive surgery is an informed consent which clearly describes the expected results and potential complications. This is the effective way to manage patient expectations and avoid litigation. It is false economy to try and get more customers by painting a very rosy picture and then ending up with a law suit which will destroy your reputation. A professional counseling is essential in a LASIK set-up. Only well motivated clients who understand the risks (howsoever small) should be taken for LASIK surgery.

Cataract Surgery

Cataract surgery is one of the safest and most rewarding surgical procedures ever devised in ophthalmology. Often, the surgery is usually performed in an ambulatory setting under local anesthesia, causing little or no discomfort to the patient. Current success rate in experienced hands is close to 97% but that also means that 3% of patients do suffer from untoward complications, which does not allow their vision to improve or even deteriorate further.[9]

One of the most controversial and medicolegally challenging issues is the recently introduced *femtosecond laser assisted* cataract surgery. The surgery is being promoted as the *best and safest*, and charging two to three times more for the procedure as compared to well established *phacoemulsification*. However there is no firm evidence in literature till date that the results are any better or the complications are any less. In fact there is a steep learning curve which may result in more complications.[10,11] Surgeons should be careful in making those claims of superiority without evidence from peer reviewed literature; otherwise they are liable to medical negligence claims.

The medical negligence claims in cataract surgery mainly revolve around infection, mismanagement of known complications and operating on wrong eye or putting in wrong power of intraocular lens (IOL). Another area of potential litigation is nonimprovement of vision due to co-morbidity like glaucoma or retinal pathology, if these were not diagnosed prior to surgery.[12] It is very important to check intra ocular pressure (IOP) and do a fully dilated pupil fundus examination in every patient undergoing cataract surgery. A proper informed consent before surgery explaining the prognosis, complication rates in a written information sheet is an advantageous approach to prevent the litigation later in event of less than expected result. If a surgical complication occurs, an honest explanation must be given to the patient and relatives. Most litigation cases in consumer courts or criminal cases occur because patients lose trust as they find out about a surgical complication from another doctor after second opinion. Keeping patients informed all the time of the progress and being honest about genuine complications is beneficial in satisfying the patient and thus avoiding legal action. Prompt referral to a vitreoretinal surgeon for complications such as dropped nucleus and severe endophthalmitis are again conducive to enhancing trust between patient and surgeon. Eventual outcome of surgery may affect the patient's satisfaction but the role of confidence and trust in the surgeon cannot be overemphasized.

Ocular Trauma

Ocular trauma (accidental or intentional) often has medicolegal implications in ophthalmic practice. Globally more than half a million blinding injuries occur every year. Approximately 50% of all patients visiting an eye casualty department do so because of ocular trauma.[13] The ocular injuries may range from mild and nonsight threatening to extremely serious with potentially blinding consequences. Serious ocular injuries may be classified into those caused by blunt objects, sharp objects, flying particles or burns. Blunt or contusion injury may result in a simple black eye to severe intraocular disruption, including rupture of the globe, raised intraocular pressure and/or secondary hemorrhage 4–5 days later may complicate the bleed and result in corneal or optic nerve damage. Thorough ocular assessment, paying particular attention to the intraocular pressure, structures within the drainage angle, clarity and stability of the lens, the posterior pole and the peripheral retina is extremely important. Penetrating injuries, generally, carry a poorer prognosis in comparison to blunt injuries, although the extent of damage will depend on where and how far the object enters the eye. Foreign bodies that enter the eye may cause structural damage to the intraocular contents and may cause toxicity to tissues as they degrade or oxidie, if not removed rapidly, small foreign particles may be missed, even with the assistance of slit lamp magnification. Intraocular structural damage may be undetectable at the time of injury, leading to potential medicolegal hazard for the ophthalmologist. In case of slightest suspicion of ocular injury due to penetrating foreign body, the patient must be fully examined and managed by an ophthalmologist.[14]

Retinal Conditions

Retina being the light sensitive part of the eye that takes the vision to the brain is vulnerable to various serious disorders. Only 40 years ago, most of the retinal conditions were untreatable but now with major advances in technology we can cure, control or at the least slow down the progress of most retinal conditions. This is good news for patients but unfortunately these advances often give rise to unrealistic expectations of perfect visual results. From Ophthalmologists' perspectives, it is their duty to manage these expectations by educating the patients and their relatives. This is more so while treating retinal disorders, viz. like late stage proliferative diabetic retinopathy, complex retinal detachments with proliferative vitreo-retinopathy (PVR), macular whole surgeries and newer therapeutic options for age-related macular degeneration (AMD). Proper informed consent detailing the potential outcomes, and known complications is must in these circumstances. In retinal surgery, patients must be warned about serious complications like losing all vision or even the eye as long as the benefits of surgery outweigh the risks, the surgery is justified.

Vitreoretinal surgeons are at much higher risk of malpractice claims because of significant potential for severe visual impairment or blindness and more complex nature of most vitreoretinal surgeries than general ophthalmic surgery. In a study the members of the macula, retina, and vitreous societies were mailed questionnaires regarding their malpractice litigation experience, and the responses were analyzed. Rhegmatogenous retinal detachments were the most common presenting diagnosis in ophthalmic malpractice litigation, and most of these patients are treated by vitreoretinal specialists. Negligent treatment (surgical or medical) (63%) was alleged more than negligent diagnosis (10%).[15] These risks strongly indicate for a thorough discussion of informed consent and the development of a good physician-patient relationship.

Missing Serious Systemic Diseases

Eyes are like windows to the body. The blood vessels in the retina reflect what is happening in rest of vascular system of the body. The state of optic nerve is a clear indication of brain functions. In conditions like diabetes and hypertension, the detailed retinal examination reveals a lot about the condition of heart, kidneys and nervous system. Often, ophthalmologist may be asked to do a routine eye checkup on a patient. If there are changes which indicate serious systemic illnesses, these must be picked-up and appropriate referral must be made. Many patients with brain tumor, minor stroke, systemic vasculitis, *systemic lupus erythematosus,* HIV, etc., may present first to the ophthalmologist with a visual symptom. Missing any of the signs in such situation may render the ophthalmologist liable to negligence claim. The only remedy to prevent such allegations is to do a thorough examination, listen carefully to all the complaints and refer the patients for further investigations if no ocular cause is found for the visual symptoms rather than saying *go home, there is nothing wrong with you.* It goes without saying that proper management should also be accompanied by proper documentation in the medical records of the patient.

Organ Donation

Last bastion in the medicolegal quagmire is the issue of organ donation. Since eye donation is very important source for corneas for transplant, we should be aware of the medicolegal implications of the rights of the relatives and the legal status of organ donor cards that people fill prior to their death.

The law for organ donation in India is available as a specific legislation, namely, *The Transplantation of Human Organ Act, 1994.*[16] This Act regulates removal, storage and transplantation of human organs for therapeutic purpose and for the prevention of commercial dealings in human organs. All the eye banking and collection of eyes must be done as per this Act. The eye donation of the deceased can be authorized by the next of kin even if the deceased did not pledge to donate his/her eyes before death. If any person in writing at any time or orally in the presence of two or more witnesses has expressed a request for donating after his death, then the person in lawful possession of his body after his death may do so unless he has reason to believe that the request was subsequently withdrawn or there is an objection by near relative which are defined in Sec 2 (i) as spouse, son, daughter, father, mother, brother or sister.

There are circumstances when removal of eyes authority cannot be given:
- If inquest is required by a person empowered to give such authority or by police.
- No authority for removal of eyes if the body is entrusted to another only for cremation.
- In brain stem cell death, eyes cannot be removed unless such death is certified by a Board of Medical experts.
- Removal cannot be done from unclaimed bodies in the prison and in hospitals.
- In the case of medicolegal autopsy no organ should be removed without legal permission from the investigating officer.

- Section 10 (1) (a) provides that, "No hospital, unless registered under this Act shall conduct or associate with or help in the removal, storage, or transplantation of any human organ."

Offences and Penalties:
- Punishment for removal of human organs without authority is imprisonment for a term which may extend to 5 years and with fine which may extend to ₹10,000. The doctor's name shall be reported to state Medical Council for suspension for 2 years for first offence and permanently for subsequent offence.
- Punishment for Commercial dealings in human organs is with imprisonment for a term which shall not be <2 years but which may extend to 7 years and with fine which shall not be <10,000, may extend to 20,000.
- Eye Bank is a nonprofit organization affiliated to Eye Bank association of India which is entitled to procure, medically evaluate, and distribute eyes. The recipient information is always kept confidential and anonymous. It should not be revealed to the donor's family on whatever grounds. There are severe penalties in law for breach of such confidentiality.

MANAGING THE RISK OF LAWSUITS

Ophthalmologists who are sued are prone to the emotional feelings of anger, guilt and depression. Even if they win the case, it costs them waste of time, money, and emotional distraction of defending a lawsuit. With emotional and financial stakes being high, it is strongly recommended to incorporate risk management strategies in daily ophthalmic practice. Following protocols and checklists, legible and comprehensive medical records, good quality informed consent supplemented by documentation of the communication with the patient, attentiveness to the patient's concerns are some of the general risk management modalities that may help to prevent the lawsuits or at least provide a good defence later on in the court.

The Informed Consent

The purpose of informed consent is to enable the patients to make decisions about their healthcare by providing them all the relevant information and also helping them in understanding the intricate concepts of the disease and the proposed treatment. Other than the medical indication, the process of informed consent is also a legal requirement that makes it mandatory for the healthcare providers to take patient's consent before providing the proposed treatment (although exceptions to informed consent do occur).

Good quality informed consent form is a critical defence against medical negligence lawsuits. It is one of the areas of ophthalmic practice that can be easily improved and at the same time, it is one of the strongest risk management strategies. Ophthalmologists must be aware that a good quality informed consent has to stand to the challenge of denial by the patient who although was thoroughly informed says in a court of law: *The surgeon just asked me to sign the consent form and I was not given the opportunity to discuss my queries.* Keeping in mind such denial by the patient all the communication related to the process of informed consent must be documented in the medical records and preferably signed by the patient/relatives. In current scenario of degrading physician—patient relationship and advanced information technology, the concept of video recorded informed consent must be considered.

The Documentation

Gaps in documentation are one of the primary targets in medical negligence litigation. Any cutting, overwriting or alteration may raise suspicion in court of law, and if not suitably justified may put the defending doctor in severe jeopardy. Ophthalmologists should be cautious in glaucoma patients, where non compliance is more common. Glaucoma patients may skip medication particularly when they are experiencing loss of vision. Any incident of non compliance with medication, and missed appointments, refusal of testing, treatment, or referral, and leaving against medical advice must be duly documented in the medical records. It is preferable to get such documentation authenticated by countersigns of patient/relatives. In case the patient/relatives refuse to sign, the same should also be documented.

The Protocols and Checklists

Enforcement of mandatory surgical checklist is the most effective way of eliminating the surgical errors. Following protocols and checklists are essential for patient safety. The indispensable role of final check to ensure right patient, right procedure and right site cannot be overemphasized. In case of cataract surgery, a final check of the intraocular lens to be implanted is extremely risk prevention strategy. In a 'perfect surgery' case a wrong power lens was implanted due to cascade of preventable mistakes leading to medical liability consequences. The ophthalmologist was too busy with the surgical concerns to be sure that the power of the lens was correct. This is an illustration of risk management failure due to lack of system in place.

The Communication

Appropriate communication with a patient especially when complications develop is extremely critical. Patient must be explained about the complication and how it was dealt. Such revelation is not an admission of mistake. All communications including the patient's queries and the replies should be documented in the medical records. Postoperative instructions to the patient should be clear, easily understandable, and written. Use language that patient can understand.

In case harm occurs to the patient due to medical error, disclosure about the same to the patients (in a structured manner) is the right thing to do. If the medical error is concealed and the patient comes to know about the mistake from some other source, the medical practitioner will be at a greater risk of law suit.[17]

■ CONCLUSION

Most of the complaints against the ophthalmologists are driven by unfavorable outcomes. Ophthalmologists must explain to their patients that poor outcomes may occur unavoidably without negligence. Risk management strategies must be followed to improve the patient safety as well as professional safety. Good communication along with appropriate documentation, maintenance of high standards in daily practice, and keeping oneself abreast with the latest trends in ophthalmic practice can go a long way in improving the professional safety of the ophthalmologists.

REFERENCES

1. Quote by William Shakespeare. Available: http://izquotes.com/quote/383068.
2. Roy PN, Mehra KS, Deshpande PJ. Cataract surgery performed before 800 BC. Br J Ophthalmol. 1975;59:171.
3. A historical tour of ophthalmology. Available: http://www.mrcophth.com/Historyofophthalmology/introduction.htm).
4. Mark L. Dlugoss. Editor's Blog: How 'strange' is evolution in ophthalmology?–Ophthalmology Times. APR 19, 2013 Available: http://ophthalmologytimes.modernmedicine.com/ophthalmologytimes/news/editor%E2%80%99s-blog-how-%E2%80%98strange%E2%80%99-evolution-ophthalmology?page=full.
5. Tomkins C. Over 120 years of defending ophthalmologists. Br J Ophthalmol. 2006;90(9):1084-5.
6. Bethke W. Don't Get Lost in the Shifting Sands. 10/4/2012. Available: www.revophth.com/content/d/refractive_surgery/c/36933.
7. LASIK Laser Complications available: www.lasik1.com/LASIK_Risk_Complications.html.
8. Lasik Surgery Risks and Malpractice. Available: http://www.medicalmalpractice.com/lasik-surgery.cfm.
9. American Academy of Ophthalmology Cataract and Anterior Segmental Pannel Guidelines. Preferred Practice Pattern. Cataract in the adult eye. San Francisco, CA: American Academy of Ophthalmology; 2011. Available: www.aao.org/ppp.
10. Sutton G, Bali SJ, Hodge C. Femtosecond cataract surgery: transitioning to laser cataract. Current Opin Ophthalmol. 2013; 24:3-8.
11. Bali SJ, Hodge C, Lawless M, Roberts TV, Sutton G. Early experience with the femtosecond laser for cataract surgery. Ophthalmology. 2012;119:891-9.
12. Bettman JW. Seven hundred medicolegal cases in ophthalmology. Ophthalmology. 1990;97:1379-84.
13. Negrel AD, Thylefors B. The global impact of eye injuries. Ophthalmic Epidemiol. 1998;5(3):143-69.
14. Macewen CJ. Ocular injuries. J R Coll Surg Edinb. 1999;44:317-23.
15. Kraushar MF. Medical malpractice experiences of vitreoretinal specialists: risk prevention strategies. Retina. 2003;23(4): 523-9.
16. The Transplantation of Human Organ Act, 42 of 1994.
17. Robertson G. Fraudulent concealment and the duty to disclose medical mistakes. Alberta Law Rev. 1986;25:215-23.

CHAPTER 25

Medicolegal Issues in Pediatrics

Yogesh dave

"Children don't care how much you know, until they know how much you care."
—**John Maxwell**[1]

■ INTRODUCTION

Pediatrics as a specialty of medicine has advanced a lot from the time when children were treated by physicians primarily responsible for adult medical service, to the current times when super specialties exist within the field of pediatrics.[2] Pediatricians provide medical care to infants, children, and adolescents, and the age limit usually ranges from birth up to 18 years. Often the diseases and disorders of children are unique, and require a significantly different approach to management as compared to adult patients. Children are not miniature adults. The smaller body of an infant or neonates is substantially different physiologically from that of an adult. The common clinical pitfalls in pediatric practice, stemming from failure to appreciate the age-related physiological and developmental distinctions, provide the grounds for medical malpractice actions. In case of allegation of negligence in providing healthcare to the children, the standards laid down for pediatric age group are considered by the courts. Before discussing various medicolegal issues related to pediatrics, it is important to be know: who is child and who is a pediatrician?

Who is a Child?

As per the Indian Academy of Pediatrics, age limit up to and including 18 years come within the purview of pediatrics for the purpose of providing healthcare. This policy has been adopted by the Academy during the annual conference at Jaipur, in 1999.

Policy on Age of Children for Pediatric Care (1999)

For fulfilling the professional obligations of pediatricians to the society at large, the purview of pediatrics commences with the fetus and continues through newborn, infancy, preschool and school age including adolescence up to and including 18 years of age.

The explanatory note of the said policy further mentioned that, children with chronic illnesses and who are under the continuous care of a pediatrician will continue to be cared for by the same doctor for a while longer, and not just up to the age defined here.[3]

Who is a Pediatrician?

A Pediatrician or 'Child Specialist' is a doctor who has specialized in treating a child. He/she may have postgraduate degree (MD) or diploma (DCh) in Pediatrics. As per the Indian Medical Council (Professional conduct, Etiquette and Ethics) Regulation, 2002 Clause 7.20, *A Physician shall not claim to be specialist unless he has a special qualification in that branch.* The medical practitioners should practice within the scope of one's qualifications and skills. The Apex Court has ruled against any crosspathy and explained that if a doctor is practicing any other system it is *negligence per se.*[4] National Consumer Dispute Redressal Commission also reiterates the same principle that, 'when a patient is admitted in a hospital, it is done with the belief that the treatment given in the hospital is being given by qualified doctors under the Indian Medical Council Act, 1956.[5]

An MBBS graduate who has attained experience in Pediatrics (worked as houseman in pediatrics) cannot practice as a pediatrician because of nonattainment of qualification (degree or diploma) in Pediatrics.[6]

Why Study Medicolegal Issues in Pediatrics?

Most of the medical practitioners feel anxious while dealing with medicolegal cases. For them *medicolegal* means entangling oneself into police cases, indefinite hours to be spent in the court, facing unrelenting defense counsels, etc. Many practitioners realize the importance of medicolegal domain once they are entrapped in a malpractice lawsuit. The best approach for a pediatrician to avoid malpractice litigation is to have a basic knowledge of legal principles related to medical practice and implement the medicolegal knowledge into the medical practice.

The increasing cost of investment for medical practice, fierce competition amongst the specialists, corporate culture in healthcare are some of the factors responsible for a commercial approach in patient care. The patients are also attracted by the star facilities and assurance by the corporate hospitals. In such a scenario, patient's expectation from his/her physician rises to unrealistically high level. Allegations of rashness or negligence are often raised against doctors by persons with no medical knowledge, to extract unjust compensation. Pediatricians need to acknowledge the current scenario where the risk of malpractice lawsuits is manifold as compared to earlier days.

Parents are not willing to accept any complication occurring to their children due to negligence or deficiency in service. Once the physician-patient relationship has been established, the physician is obligated to diagnose and treat the patient's illness with *due care* and *diligence*. Failure to use due care constitutes negligence, for which the patient may recover monetary damages. Error of judgment or poor outcome, is by no means assumed to be negligence if due care is diligently provided. It is important to understand the legal principles applied to evaluate medical negligence cases.

Informed Consent in Pediatrics

The issue of informed consent is often viewed by medical practitioners as a baffling imposition on them by the plaintiffs. A common misconception of physicians is that, getting signatures of the patient on a consent form is sufficient. The reality is that 'signed consent forms' is not a complete remedy. Adequate communication between the physician and the patient goes a long way in preventing malpractice suits.

The concept of informed consent is not only a legal requirement, but also has an indispensable role in *shared decision making* as a part of good clinical practice. Inadequate discussion with the patient, followed by asking for a signature is regarded as improper consent by the law. The best approach to avoid a medical negligence lawsuit is to have a thorough discussion with the patient followed by documentation in medical records, the details of the information given to the patient, such as risks of the procedure, expected success rate as well as failure rate, alternatives available, risks of refusal to treatment, etc. Thus, when the patient has any untoward outcome and claims that he was not informed of the risk then medical records will support the medical practitioner in defending the lawsuits successfully.

A major difference between *pediatrics* and adult medicine is that children being minors, are generally considered incompetent to give legally binding decisions regarding their healthcare. The issues of guardianship, privacy, legal responsibility and informed consent must always be considered in every pediatric procedure. In general, parents or guardians are empowered to make healthcare decisions on behalf. However, parental empowerment is not absolute. In certain circumstances adolescents may insist on making their health related decisions independently. Pediatricians should carefully listen to the wishes of children and should strive to obtain their assent.[7]

Age for Consent in Pediatrics

A person who has capacity and competence to understand the necessary information can consent to his/her treatment. In India, majority is achieved at an age of 18 years and any person who is a major and of sound mind can give consent for his/her treatment. A child below 18 years of age cannot give consent. Parents/guardians can give consent for their medical/surgical treatment. A child between 12-18 years can give assent only for medical examination but not for any procedure. Pediatricians have legal obligation to take *parental permission* to undertake medical/surgical procedure in patients below 18 years (except in emergencies when parents cannot be contacted). Such a consent given by parent or guardian, on behalf of patient below 18 years is known as *consent by proxy*.

In an attempt to adapt to the concept of informed consent in *pediatrics*, authority has been given to child's parents or guardians to give *consent by proxy*. In India, proxy consent has seemed to work reasonably well. However, the concept of proxy consent may comprehend problems in adolescents. Rarely conflicts may arise in interests of minors and the parental desires or proxy consent. Adolescents may not be legally authorized to give consent for their treatment, but are in the process of developing competence to decide on the issues of their healthcare. Physicians should also solicit *patient assent* from adolescents on the proposed treatment.[8]

For medicolegal examination, the age for consent is 12 years and above. In 2014 Minsitry of Health and Family Welfare, Govt of India published 'Guidelines on medicolegal care for survivors/victims of sexual violence'. These guidelines have provided the age of consent for medicolegal examination of a survivor of sexual violence as follows:

"The consent form must be signed by the person him/herself if s/he is above 12 years of age. Consent must be taken from the guardian/parent if the survivor is under the age of 12 years."

Error in Diagnosis During Emergencies

Failure to diagnose the disease early enough to manage it properly may expose the pediatrician to increased risk of allegation of negligence. Lapse or delay in the diagnosis of surgical emergencies in children resulting in poor outcome, tend to end up in courts as malpractice lawsuits. In a child presenting with pain abdomen, appendicitis and intussusception should be seriously considered as differential diagnosis. Often, doctors wait for the classical symptoms and signs of the disease, not realizing that a crying child of 3 or 4 years of age can become desperately ill with appendicitis and show no other symptoms than anorexia, vomiting, and pyrexia. In a case of intussusception, the classical symptoms and signs have been so emphasized that in their absence, serious delay may lead to death of a child in spite of the treatment. For the diagnosis of intussusception, it is not necessary that a child must have spasmodic abdominal pain, vomiting, and passage of blood per rectum. Indeed, blood is passed per rectum in probably fewer than half of the cases before admission to hospital.

Similarly, torsion of testis during the age of 5 to 10 years is not uncommon. Unless treated early the effects can be disastrous. Most medical malpractice cases regarding testicular torsion injuries arise from the failure to timely diagnose and treat that injury. An immediate physical examination is a must. Once diagnosis is made, testicular torsion usually requires immediate surgery. If surgery is not performed, the testicle may atrophy and will need to be removed. Infection is also possible. The main concern associated with loss of a testicle is the potential inability to father children. Testicular torsion litigation mostly involves the urologist. However, the initial treating pediatrician must have a high index of suspicion for the diagnosis and refer promptly as a part of safe clinical practice.[9]

Avoidable Surgeries

Sometimes surgical conditions are self-limiting/self-correcting that the early surgery may be considered unnecessary. For illustration in case of umbilical hernia, if these patients are referred at an early age (1 or 2 years) directly to surgeons there will be a tendency to perform an avoidable surgery. Admittedly they will probably cure the child, but some may suffer complications related to the surgery performed. In such cases if surgical complications occur the surgeon will be vulnerable to criticism for doing unnecessary surgery.

Removal of large tonsils in children which otherwise, pass through a phase of their natural history, and resolve without surgery can also expose the surgeon to avoidable criticism. In cases where management of the disease by conservative approach vis-a-vis surgery is a gray area, it will be safe to have thorough discussions with the parents of the child as a team including both pediatrician and surgeon, so that parents are well informed and play vital role in *shared decision making* related to treatment option.

Patient Safety in Pediatrics

Patient safety is a major issue in pediatric practice. Special risk factors in this speciality are due to many factors like, wide variations in age, dosing range, formulations, etc. During the treatment process harm may occur to the child from the underlying medical condition, from the inherent risks of investigations and treatments, system failures, provider performance issues, adverse events or a combination of these. While analyzing the patient safety incident, the main focus should be on improving the healthcare system. After an unexpected clinical outcome occurs due to medical error, be prepared to acknowledge and deal with it. There should be uniform policy about medical error disclosure and especially it should be a corrective measure to prevent future repetition rather than blaming some body.

Neonatal Intensive Care: Vulnerable to Malpractice Lawsuits

Pediatricians need to manage a variety of potentially harmful conditions in the newborn nursery. Delay in initiation of neonatal resuscitation, missed or delayed diagnosis and improper management of hyperbilirubinemia, sepsis or meningitis, asphyxia, and congenital heart disease, neonatal hypoglycemia and neonatal seizures may give rise to medical malpractice liability against newborn healthcare providers. Other factors that contribute to potential liability include failure to perform appropriate screening evaluations, incomplete documentation, failure to recognise high-risk conditions that may contribute to a particular neonatal condition, and inadequate or delayed follow-up care.

In pediatric care, neonatal intensive care is a highrisk management priority. Risk prevention in neonatal care includes honest implementation of standard clinical guidelines into everyday practice. Certain zones of risk exist in each stage of neonatal care. Understanding and incorporating risk management strategies into practice will serve to reduce the risk of real or perceived complications.

Neonatal medicine, providing care to those in the most demanding age group requires well defined clinical guidelines for the best interest of the ill newborn. Providing care to the newborn requires trained professionals of many disciplines to create an effective team of providers who render neonatal intensive care; no single professional can do this alone. Although newborn is treated, but the whole family has to live with the long-term consequences of the care provided to the baby. Reasonable expectation from those providing care to the neonatal includes: a) steady improvement, b) absence of unnecessary pain and avoidable suffering. To determine the best interests of a neonate, the parents are considered to be the spokespersons; hence, it is imperative to seek their opinions.

Pediatricians must be vigilant enough to minimize the iatrogenic sequelae of neonatal intensive care. The potential for negative iatrogenic effects in neonatal practice must be recognized. To prevent the undesired iatrogenic effects, multiple factors as mentioned below must be standardized:
- Type, doses, and results of medications used
- Foreign bodies or devices used
- Environment in which the baby is managed (e.g., light, noise, temperature)
- Baby's nutritional needs (enteral nutrition vis-à-vis parenteral nutrition)
- Mode of ventilation (e.g., conventional, synchronized, high-frequency).

Practitioners might have rudimentary understanding of the basic concepts of law regulating the clinical practice. Principles of duty of care, breach and causation, doctrine of informed consent, are to be applied in patient care. Medicolegal issues may creep in the practice of neonatology due to multiple reasons. Recent developments in neonatal care has raised the parent's expectations of what a medical practitioner can offer and puts healthcare professionals under pressure to continue treatment, which may ultimately be futile. Doctors may refuse to continue futile treatments where it is felt that further continuing the treatment is not in the best interests of the child. On the contrary sometimes, the doctors feel that treatment options do exist but parents refuse to give consent for further treatment. Disagreement between the physician and parents may end up as unsatisfactory parents ready to sue the physician for negligence or deficiency in service. The best interests of the child are paramount and their welfare should always be the primary consideration. While the courts generally support the views of the healthcare professional, this cannot be guaranteed.

Parental Refusal to Medical Treatment

It is a basic principle of medical practice that physicians cannot treat a patient without valid consent unless the case falls within the category of 'exceptions to informed consent' (*discussed in chapter of informed consent*). Doctor cannot substitute his will for that of the patient despite the best of intentions or the reasonableness of the proposed treatment. It has also been generally accepted that a person of sound mind has the right to refuse treatment even though refusal may well lead to an avoidable death.

Children are generally considered incompetent to provide legally binding decisions regarding their healthcare, and parents or guardians are the decision makers on their behalf. In order to be able to make the correct decisions for their children, the parents must have the correct information. It is morally prohibited to disrespect a parental refusal of treatment, unless the refusal constitutes child abuse, child neglect, or violates a right of the child. However, there is no clear cut protocol for intervention. These are the gray areas and one should opt for legal advice. In situations when the parent or person having charge of the child refuses to give consent to medical treatment required to alleviate physical harm or suffering of the child, and the refusal is suspected to constitute child abuse, it is advisable to handle the case as a medicolegal case, keep the child in safe custody and inform the police and obtain authorization to the proposed treatment over the objections of the parents.

Communication Skills—Key Role in Pediatrics

Good communication skills are integral to a healthy professional-patient interaction. Effective communication may increase patient's understanding of treatment, improve compliance ultimately leading to improved healthcare. Better communication between the doctor and patient has a beneficial effect in terms of promoting better emotional health, resolution of symptoms and pain control.

A study found that doctors frequently interrupt patients so soon after they begin (after a mean time of only 18 seconds!) their opening statement, that patients fail to disclose significant concerns. Doctors often interrupt patients after the initial concern, apparently assuming that the first complaint is the chief one, yet the order in which patients present their problems may not be related to their clinical importance.[10] Interviews were particularly likely to become dysfunctional if there were shortcomings in that part of the consultation relating to "discovering the reason for the patient's attendance." Doctors often pursue a "doctor-centered", closed approach to information gathering that discourages patients from telling their story or voicing their concerns.[11] 800 patient visits to the Children's Hospital of Los Angeles were studied by means of tape recording the doctor-patient interaction and by follow-up interview. In 24% cases, there was dissatisfaction. A number of communication barriers between pediatrician and patient's mother contributed significantly to patient dissatisfaction. Mothers were confused by the terms used by doctors yet rarely asked for clarification of unfamiliar terms.[12]

To become a good practitioner, practice good communication. A physician must demonstrate respect, genuineness and empathy. These skills can be learned with practice! Developing strong communication skills is integral to becoming an effective health provider. Pediatricians need to improve the ability to elicit information from patients, interpersonal skills to respond to patients' feelings and concerns. The longer the doctor waits before interrupting at the beginning of the interview, the more likely he is to discover the full spread of issues that the patient wants to discuss and the less likely will it be that new complaints arise at the end of the interview.[10]

Legal Risks of Ineffective Communication

The medicolegal consequences of ineffective communication between physicians and patients are:
- Improper medical care
- Legal vulnerability for a lack of informed consent
- Breach of the duty to warn of risks associated with treatment methods and medications
- Breach of the patient's privacy rights.

Communicate Well with Children and Families

People don't sue the doctors they like. Excellent communication is an important factor in reducing medical legal risk. Communication with families is particularly critical. Parents are often anxious as they enter the healthcare establishment. Their perception, right or wrong, is that their child is sick or hurt enough to require immediate care. Parents will sense your level of concern and caring seconds after they arrive. "It is essential to explore how various methods help capture or impede capturing—clinical information." In fact, their opinion and bias towards the anticipated level of care was formed at the reception of the hospital. Does your healthcare establishment send out welcoming vibes *we are here to help you* when families arrive? It is essential that everyone providing clinical care take time to listen to the child's and/or parents' concerns, and reflect those concerns back in a way that makes it clear they are heard and understood. Communicating and demonstrating that you care is a great step forward that goes a long way in reducing potential medical legal problems that may arise much later.

■ CONCLUSION

Although pediatricians are not sued as frequently as other physicians, they have higher average malpractice indemnity. Most paediatricians are extremely concerned about the threat of malpractice litigation. It is important that pediatricians at all levels of experience enhance their knowledge of medicolegal principles. Training should begin with the development of a strong foundation in medicolegal education during medical school. Risk-management principles should be emphasized for at-risk scenarios. Problems with communication leading to medicolegal problems must be handled appropriately by training communication skills to the practitioners by the experts in the field of communication. The best way to deal with medicolegal problems is to prevent them with good communication, empathic attitude and practicing standard of care, timely referral service with avoidance of crosspathy and attention on *patient safety* and *quality healthcare*.

Ignorance of law is not an excuse. Pediatricians should have basic idea of malpractice lawsuits, how to cope with malpractice litigation stress, effective handling of suits, and professional indemnity insurance scheme, etc. Medicolegal issues related to emergency medical care, the vaccine injury, medication errors, newborn issues such as those related to the futility of care, etc., should be thoroughly discussed in CMEs. Policies on standard care and related medicolegal issues should be developed and regularly updated by the professional bodies of Paediatricians.

REFERENCES

1. John C. Maxwell, an internationally speaker and author. Available: http://quozio.com/quote/c4c5204e#!t=1003.
2. Bansal CP, Gupta S. The Past Half Century of Indian Academy of Pediatrics. Indian Pediatr. 2012;50:39-48.
3. John TJ. IAP policy on age of children for pediatric care. Indian Pediatrics. 1999;36:461-3.
4. Poonam Varma vs. Ashwin Patel AIR 2111,1996 SCC(4) 332.
5. Prof. P N Thakur vs. Hans Charitable Hospital III. 2007;CPJ 340.
6. Tiwari S, Baldwa M. Who is child specialist/pediatrician? Indian pediatrics. 2007;44(17): 527-8.
7. Committee on Bioethics, American Academy of Pediatrics. Informed Consent, Parental Permission, and Assent in Pediatric Practice. Committee on Bioethics. Pediatrics. 1995; 95(2):314-7.
8. Yadav M. Age of consent in medical profession: A food for thought. JIAFM 2007;29. Accessed: http://www.indianjournals.com/ijor.aspx?target=ijor:jiafmandvolume=29andissue=2andarticle=014.
9. Matteson JR, Stock JA, Hanna MK, Arnold TV, Nagler HM. Medicolegal aspects of testicular torsion. Urology. 2001;57(4):783-6.
10. Beckman HB, Frankel RM. The effect of physician behavior on the collection of data. Ann Intern Med. 1984;101(5):692-6.
11. Byrne P, Long B. Doctors talking to patients. Exeter: Royal College of General Practitioners, 1984.
12. Korsch BM, Gozzi EK, Francis V. Gaps in doctor-patient communication. Pediatrics. 1968;42:855-71.

CHAPTER 26

Medicolegal Issues in Radiology

Chandrashekhar A Sohoni

> "Great discoveries are made accidentally less often than the people like to think.
> ...Commenting on how an accident led to the discovery of X-rays."
> —**Sir William Cecil Dampier**[1]

■ INTRODUCTION

When Wilhelm Conrad Roentgen, the German physicist, accidentally discovered X-rays in 1895, hardly did he know that this *accident* was the foundation of a spectacular specialty in medical science—*Radiology*. The technological progress in the field of radiology has been amazing. With the scientific advancement in imaging, not only has the information related to medical disorders improved but the dependence upon imaging for the diagnosis has also amplified manifold. In the era of X-rays, the diagnosis was made clinically and only corroborated by imaging. Today, it would not be an exaggeration to say that in many situations, the diagnosis is made primarily by imaging. This paradigm shift has happened due to the following factors:
- Highly sensitive and specific diagnostic imaging modalities
- Practice of evidence based medicine
- Increased awareness regarding health issues in the society
- Raised legal accountability of medical practitioners.

Today, *medicine* is broadly divided into two categories—*diagnostic* and *therapeutic*. The burden of diagnosis is being increasingly put on radiology and pathology. Because of the possibility of medicolegal conflict, clinicians feel uncomfortable in treating the patients without documentary evidence of a disorder. Diagnosis has an extremely critical role in patient management and diagnostic modalities are inherently prone to controversies and criticism due to their vital status in the hierarchy of patient care.

Errors in Radiology

Missed radiological findings, radiological error reports or failure to communicate significant findings leading to delayed diagnosis ultimately resulting in harm to the patient are the common reasons for medicolegal conflicts in the practice of radiology. Whether a missed radiological finding constitutes an error or medical negligence is indeed a tough question, yet to be answered precisely and may vary from case to case. Non-compliance with the provisions of Preconception and Prenatal Diagnostic Techniques (PCPNDT) Act is also responsible for causing legal disputes for the radiologists.

Radiological errors can be classified as represented in (**Flowchart 1**):[2-4]
Salient features of the spectrum of errors in the practice of radiology are enlisted here:

- Perceptual or observation errors constitute 80% of the problem. Perceptual errors are related to multiple psychophysiological factors such as observer's alertness, fatigue, duration of the task, distracting factors, conspicuity of the abnormality, etc.[5]
- Scanning error is the result of failure to fixate in the area of abnormality.[4]
- Recognition error is the result of failure to recognize after fixation.[4]
- Decision-making error is the result of failure to interpret a seen lesion as an abnormal structure.[4]
- Satisfaction of search error is the result of being satisfied by finding one abnormality and thus failing to see another abnormality.[6]
- Intentional under-reading is the tendency to interpret an equivocal radiological finding as normal, most likely due to collegial pressure to reduce the rate of false positive readings and thus reduce unnecessary investigations.[7]
- Bias may be created due to previous normal reporting on radiological examination. If the first radiologist has missed a finding, and the next radiologist has read the report before scanning the patient, then there is a chance to miss the finding even during subsequent radiological study.
- A busy radiologist depends upon the typist to document the report. No matter how careful the specialist is, problem of typographical error is often encountered and is prone to emerge later on as an allegation of *omission* (breach of duty) against the radiologist. Many radiologists have ready-made formats for reporting imaging studies called as *normal formats*. These *normal formats* must be edited while reporting each case. The most common illustration of an error due to such a *normal format* is the reporting of a normal gallbladder in a post-cholecystectomy patient.

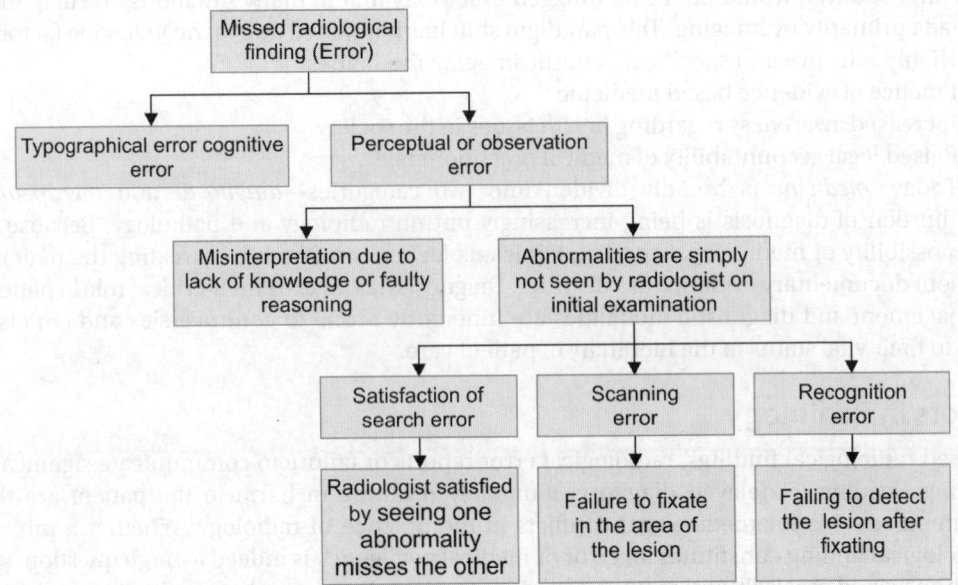

Flowchart 1: Types of radiological errors.

WHY RADIOLOGY IS VULNERABLE TO MEDICOLEGAL CONFLICTS?

Nature of the Specialty

Radiology differs from other medical specialties, in that it depends largely upon visual perception within a fixed time-frame. It is a unique specialty where mechanical, physiological and psychological factors create a complex interplay, and imbalance in any one of them can result in an error in radiological diagnosis.[2]

Radiological Opinion as 'Written and Signed' Document

Unlike clinical opinion, a radiological opinion is a written and signed document. It is a radiologist's opinion frozen in time and available for scrutiny. Despite knowing the liability that a written document brings, radiologists usually commit themselves to a diagnosis. Films from radiological studies are available for re-evaluation. This factor plays a crucial role in medicolegal cases where the court of law seeks an opinion from another expert in the field while deciding the standard of care. There is a lot of meaning in the saying *Hindsight is 20/20*, especially in case of missed radiological findings. The saying means that It is *easy to know the right thing to do after something has happened.Hindsight bias* is the tendency for the people with knowledge of the actual outcome of an event to believe falsely that they would have predicted the outcome correctly.[8] Although most people are not consciously aware that they are being influenced by hindsight bias, physicians, patients and other lay people remain susceptible to such bias in their judgments.[9] Nothing else can hurt a defending radiologist more than another radiologist appearing in the court of law, giving opinion under the influence of hindsight bias. The outcome of medicolegal cases can be influenced adversely by such biased opinions.

Commercialization of Healthcare

Like many other subspecialties of *medicine*, radiology has also been largely influenced by commercialization of healthcare. *Profits* depend on *increasing the volume* of services. Today every field is competitive and so is the case with radiology. In radiology practice, the word *efficacy* means generating more reports in less time. Hence, radiologists are increasingly under pressure to reduce the turn-around time for reports. Haste increases the chance of errors. The volume and complexity of work in radiology can potentially threaten the quality of care and patient safety. As the report is signed by the radiologist, he is often at the receiving end, whenever a patient complains about typographical or diagnostic error.

Unclear Baseline for Standard of Practice

In radiology, there is no formal documentation of the *process* of making a diagnosis. No matter how well the protocol of making a radiological diagnosis is followed, if the final report is erroneous any justification on the part of the radiologist usually fails to satisfy the patient or the referring clinician, especially if the wrong diagnosis resulted in harm to the patient. *Average diagnostic standard* in radiology is difficult to define, and it certainly cannot be based upon the ability to correctly diagnose every single time. Even an experienced radiologist can miss a finding, which in retrospect may seem obvious. The radiology infrastructure, working conditions and method of practice is not of uniform quality. The degree of experience and expertise amongst radiologists is also variable. Wood proposed the concept of *pseudodiagnostics*, wherein inexperienced radiologists make premature conclusions in the belief that a high true-positive rate of supportive evidence is diagnostic in itself.[10] Such bias has been described as anchoring bias, where one locks on to a diagnosis early in the work-up of a case and undervalues data that would support another diagnosis.

Expectation vis-à-vis Performance: A Mismatch

With increasing dependence upon radiology as a final step before decisive action, the focus is primarily on radiology reports. The general feeling among patients is that they pay more for imaging reports which are generated by high-end machines and therefore are entitled to 100% accurate diagnosis. The inherent nature of radiology practice, limitations of human perception and the inevitable element of human error negate any possibility of 100% accuracy every single time. Medical literature mentions that the general rate of missed radiological findings can be as much as 30% despite the improvement in imaging machinery.[11] This disparity in expectation vis-à-vis performance is the cause of discord between the patient and the radiologist, which may ultimately manifest as malpractice lawsuit.

Emotional Facet of the Disease

Disease and disability is often associated with a lot of emotional burden and the person at the crux of diagnostic process is likely to bear the brunt of misdiagnosis. This is especially true in cases where ultrasound scan misses a fetal anomaly at an earlier stage and detected at the later stage of pregnancy or after birth, creating an emotional turmoil in the family. Such emotional trauma, and many other similar sufferings of the patient are likely to get sympathy of the judiciary, resulting in penalization of the radiologist. Researchers have suggested that the attribution of blame satisfies the psychological need to find an object to punish, because by punishing another we annul the wrong and lessen the hurt.[12] A patient undergoing a wrong surgery or suffering a complication due to radiological error appears to be justified in claiming compensation. *Outcome bias* is a phenomenon characterized by a tendency to attribute blame more readily when the outcome is serious than the cases, where the outcome were comparatively trivial.[13] Brennan et al. summarized it and expressed, If the permanence of a disability, not the fact of negligence, is the reason for compensation, the determination of negligence may be an expensive sideshow.[14]

In two different surveys, two-thirds of the public were of the opinion that a physician should be sued for committing an error, if that error results in death or other serious injury to the patient.[9,15]

Ignorance About the 'Diagnostic' Limitations of Radiology

A sizeable number of medical practitioners are unaware of the capabilities and limitations of radiology. When it comes to patients, the situation is even worse. The patient's perception of an *image* is usually that of *a clear picture revealing all the abnormalities*, which actually is not the case with radiological images. Hence, patients and referring clinicians who are unaware of the limitations of medical imaging may find it difficult to understand and accept the diagnostic errors. Radiologist's rapport is largely affected on the way a referring physician counsels the patient about a radiological errror. If a clinician criticizes a radiological diagnosis, there is high probability that a patient may develop an adverse opinion against the radiologist.

Easy to Accept Cause-effect Relationship

Unlike complex clinical issues which are difficult for patients to comprehend, an error in a radiology report and the subsequent harmful effect can be easily accepted to have *cause-effect relationship*. According to the principles of law, to establish medical negligence, it must be shown by a preponderance of evidence that the injury caused to the patient was the result of act of commission that a reasonable physician would not have done under similar circumstances, or omission to do something that such a physician would have done under similar circumstances. Establishing the *cause-effect* relationship in a lawsuit is relatively easy in case of radiological errors. Whether the *error* is acceptable as per the *standards of practice* or not is a significant factor that helps to solve the issue related to negligence of a radiologist.

Judicial Decisions on Radiological Errors

According to the law, an error of judgment is not negligence. A physician is expected to exercise reasonable degree of care which is in accordance with the average level of competence.[16] A physician is required to exercise *reasonable care* and not necessarily perfect care.[11] Just the fact that a mistake has been made does not automatically make the physician negligent. The judgment given by Wisconsin appellate court is extremely important to understand the legal perspective on radiological negligence.[9] As stated by Berlin, in the case a Wisconsin radiologist had been sued for malpractice twice, once for missing a fracture of the proximal tibia and again for missing a carcinoma of the colon. Both lawsuits were settled with payment made to the plaintiff-patients. Soon thereafter, the Wisconsin Department of Regulation and Licensing instituted legal action to suspend or revoke the radiologist's medical license for medical negligence. A lower court exonerated the radiologist of charge of negligence and the department appealed to the State's appellate Court. The higher Court upheld the lower Court's decision in favor of the radiologist and expressed that:

> *"Radiologist may review an X-ray using the degree of care of a reasonable radiologist but fail to detect an abnormality that, on average, would have been found....Radiologists simply cannot detect all abnormalities on all X-rays...Errors in perception occur when a radiologist diligently reviews an X-ray, following all proper procedures and using all the proper techniques, and fails to perceive an abnormality which in retrospect, is apparent...*
> *Several reasons for errors in perception include:*
> - *Humans differ in the perceptions of a single item*
> - *The finding of one object may cause a physician to overlook another abnormality*
> - *The patient's body structure may make an abnormality more difficult to detect.*
>
> *Errors in perception by radiologists viewing X-rays occur in the absence of negligence. The medical literature states that, in controlled tests, radiologists miss a certain percentage of abnormalities despite using extraordinary efforts....There is no evidence in the record...to establish that (the defendant-radiologist's) errors in having failed to detect those defects came as a result of his failure to conform to the accepted standard care in the field of radiology....*
>
> *The judge went on to reason further that the average radiologist should be expected to see obvious lesions but may not see those that are subtle. To expect the average radiologist to diagnose all subtle lesions would be, to elevate the average physician to the perfect physician, and perfection is a standard to which no profession can possibly adhere."*

This judgment more or less summarizes the fundamental nature of radiology practice and radiological errors. However, the problem is the unclear definition of the words such as *reasonable, average* and *subtle*. Though one can easily find the dictionary meaning of these words, their exact connotation with respect to medical negligence concerning different medical specialties has never been spelled by courts.[9] The usual explanation offered for missing a radiological finding is the lack of 'conspicuity' of the lesion. Conspicuity of a lesion according to Poschen and Bisesi is the ratio between the contrast enhancement of the lesion or edge relative to the surrounding tissue. However, the phenomenon of not seeing an obvious abnormality on initial examination has not been satisfactorily explained. Anderson et al. referred to this phenomenon as *irreducible necessary fallibility emanating from uncertainties inherent in medical predictions based on human observation and laws of nature*.[9] Although all the courts have consistently held that the physician's knowledge and skill must be at least that much which is minimally acceptable but need not be perfect, the increasing expectations of the society from doctors and decreasing tolerance for errors means that the definitions of *average* and *reasonable* are not straight-forward. The Supreme Court of India has opined against the misuse of law for victimizing doctors for trivial reasons.[16] At the same time, the Supreme court has awarded humongous compensation for medical negligence.[17] Fear and uncertainty persists amongst doctors also because of the possibility of uneven outcomes for apparently similar legal issues.

■ AVOIDING LITIGATION IN RADIOLOGY

The ideal solution to avoid medicolegal conflicts would be not to make any mistakes at all, which indeed is unrealistic. Apart from being a competent radiologist, there are some other things that can help to avoid litigation in radiology:

Being Alert

A radiologist has to be observant all the time. While performing every single imaging study, a radiologist should actively search for any abnormality by keeping in mind all diagnostic possibilities, rather than just letting the abnormality makes itself obvious. Active searching always gives better results than passive observation. Similarly, while signing a typed report, a radiologist should be alert so as to pick-up any typographical error. There is always a trade-off between speed and accuracy. There are two ways of improving quality: (1) Increasing positive impact; (2) Reducing negative impact. A radiologist should ideally aim for the both.

Communication with the Referring Doctor and the Patient

According to the guidelines issued by American College of Radiology (ACR), it is a duty of the radiologist to communicate all essential findings to the patient and the treating physician, wherever necessary. Though there are no official guidelines in this regard in India, it makes ample sense to follow the ACR guidelines nevertheless. Communication with a fellow clinician helps a radiologist in two ways: (1) A rapport develops between the two, and (2) makes the radiologist, patient and clinician more confident about the diagnosis/treatment. Failure to communicate can result in an inappropriate delay in treatment, thus jeopardizing the patient's condition. These days, patients expect even radiologists to counsel them about the diagnosis. Communication with the patient helps create a healthy doctor-patient relationship and prevents misunderstanding.

Role of Informed Consent

The general theme that emerges after going through the opinions of many experts is that patients need to be *officially* informed about the scope and limitations of a diagnostic procedure *before* they undergo one.[18] No surgeon operates on a patient without taking a written informed consent. It is high time radiologists start taking written informed consent from patients before performing any imaging study. As the patients are not expected to know much about the capabilities and limitations of imaging, it is our duty to make them aware of the same. The consent should essentially include information regarding:
- Diagnostic limitations of imaging modalities.
- Possibility of a false negative study despite careful evaluation.
- Inter-observer and intra-observer variability.
- Possibility of a rare typographical/proofreading error in a printed document.

There are chances of opposition for introduction of consent forms in all the diagnostic and therapeutic services offered by radiology. Introducing a process which is not a routine to radiology practice may be perceived as an undue process that would hamper the radiology working environment. Secondly, some may look at a consent form as an attempt to avert responsibility on the part of radiologists. However, both these thoughts do not appeal to logic. It is a routine practice to take consent for CT and MRI examinations, primarily because CT/MRI may involve contrast injection and MRI may be hazardous for patients with metallic implants. It is advisable that the consent forms must be more informative and extend the process of informed consent to ultrasonography, mammography and radiography examinations in addition to CT and MRI.

An informed consent may not give a complete legal immunity to the radiologists, yet it goes a long way in minimizing misconceptions amongst the patients. Educating a patient is legally as well as medically correct step. Informed consent is surely a vital part of good clinical practice and indeed a sound defence against malpractice litigation.

Publishing Diagnostic Errors Regularly

Published literature is of immense help to a doctor while defending himself in the court of law. Regular publishing of errors reiterates the fact that errors keep occurring despite improvement in imaging machinery and the subject knowledge.[19] It is advisable that there must be a section in medical journals dedicated for reporting errors in routine practice. Isolated radiological diagnostic errors find it difficult to get published in journals either because they are repeated or they lack statistical significance. Rather than the missed finding itself, what is more important is the reason behind the missed finding. These reasons may be novel and add new information to radiological literature.

Errors in Radiology: The Way Ahead

Irrespective of whether a case is won or lost in the court of law, the mental stress and humiliation incurred by a radiologist during the process is enormous. Even if an allegedly distressed patient does not actually go to the court, the mental harassment caused to the doctor is significant. Lawsuits of medical negligence are associated with the feeling of guilt and isolation, which may even affect the health of the radiologist.[20] Medical professionals who commit a severe error are susceptible to reduction in quality of life and early burn-out.[20,21] Tension and stress caused by the error makes the doctor more prone for making more errors, thus initiating a vicious cycle.[22]

There can be no intellectual growth in an insecure environment. Hence, in a society where the chances of litigation are high, doctors are more inclined towards practicing defensive medicine. In case of radiology, defensive medicine takes the form of non-conclusive and non-committal reporting of imaging studies. Radiologists tend to keep their reports open-ended rather than trying to make diagnostic conclusions. This automatically increases the number of investigations, thus increasing the cost of healthcare.

It is unfortunate, if a radiologist is forced to practice defensive medicine because the society, he serves is ignorant. This is not to say that radiologists can never be negligent, but to highlight the fact that the nature of radiological modalities and radiology practice plays a very important role in feeding the errors. We are already in an era where radiology has become the centre point of diagnosis. If radiologists continue to get cornered for unintentional errors, one might soon see *conditions apply* rather than *clinical correlation is suggested* in the footnote of radiology reports.

■ CONCLUSION

Radiology as a specialty has come a long way since its inception. Radiological modalities have grown by leaps and bounds, and so have the responsibilities and accountability of radiologists. Radiologists today face multiple challenges. The rising expectations of patients and referring physicians coupled with the inherent nature of radiology practice, limitations of radiological modalities and fallacies of human perception sometimes put a radiologist in a spot of bother. The stringent PCPNDT Act intentioned to curb the social evil of female feticide in India is also a source of great anxiety for Indian radiologists due to the prospect of irrational implementation. Hence, in addition to being competent and honest, it is extremely essential for radiologists to implement legal safeguards in the form of adequate documentation and follow international guidelines of best practice. Doing so will help reduce the doctor-patient conflict in day-to-day practice, and also the chances of being successfully sued in the court of law.

■ ACKNOWLEDGMENT

The author's article (letter to the editor) published in Indian Journal of Radiology Imaging cited as: Sohoni CA. Medical negligence: A difficult challenge for radiology. Indian J Radiol Imaging 2013;23:110-12, has been partly reproduced in this chapter with due permission.

■ REFERENCES

1. Sir William Cecil Dampier. A History of science and its relations with philosophy and religion (1931). Available: https://www.goodreads.com/quotes/953652-great-discoveries-are-made-accidentally-less-often-than-the-populace.
2. Tuddenham WJ. Visual search, image organization, and reader error in Roentgen diagnosis: studies of the psychophysiology of Roentgen image perception. Radiology. 1962;78:694-704.
3. Smith MJ. Error and variation in diagnostic radiology. Springfield, IL: Thomas. 1967;pp. 71-104.
4. Kundel HL, Nodine CF, Carmody D. Visual scanning, pattern recognition and decision-making in pulmonary nodule detection. Invest Radiol. 1978;13:175-81.
5. Pitman AG. Perceptual error and the culture of open disclosure in Australian radiology. Australas Radiol. 2006;50(3):206-11.
6. Samuel S, Kundel HL, Nodine CF, Toto LC. Mechanism of satisfaction of search: eye position recordings in the reading of chest radiographs. Radiology. 1995;194(3):895-902.
7. Woodring JH. Review Pitfalls in the radiologic diagnosis of lung cancer. AJR. 1990;54(6): 1165-75.
8. LaBine SJ, LaBine G. Determinations of negligence and the hindsight bias. Law Hum Behav. 1996;20:501-16.
9. Berlin L. Radiologic errors and malpractice: a blurry distinction. Am J Roentgenol. 2007;189 (3):517-22.
10. Wood BP. Decision making in radiology. Radiology. 1999;211:601-03.

11. Berlin L. Defending the missed radiographic diagnosis. Am J Roentgenol. 2001;176:317-22.
12. Merry A, McCall Smith A. Errors, medicine, and the law. Cambridge, UK: Cambridge University Press. 2003;pp.162-64:194-98.
13. Berlin L. Outcome bias. AJR. 2004;183:557-60.
14. Brennan TA, Sox CM, Burstin HR. Relation between negligent adverse events and the outcomes of medical-malpractice litigation. N Engl J Med. 1996;335:1963-67.
15. Blendon RJ, DesRoches CM, Brodie M, et al. Views of practicing physicians and the public on medical errors. N Engl J Med. 2002;347: 1933-40.
16. Bhullar DS, Gargi J. Medical Negligence: Majesty of Law–Doctors. Journal of Indian Academy of Forensic Medicine. 2005;27: 196-200.
17. Mahapatra D. SC awards record Rs 6 crore for medical negligence. The Times of India. October 25, 2013. Available: http://www.articles.timesofindia.indiatimes.com/2013-10-25/india/43394791_1_medical-negligence-crore-compensation-ncdrc.
18. Alfirevic Z. Failure to diagnose a fetal anomaly on a routine ultrasound scan at 20 weeks. Ultrasound Obst Gynecol. 2005;26:797-98.
19. Berlin L, Hendrix RW. Perceptual errors and negligence. AJR. 1998;170:863-67.
20. Pinto A, Brunese L. Spectrum of diagnostic errors in radiology. World J Radiol. 2010;2(10): 377-83.
21. Gallagher TH, Waterman AD, Ebers AG, Fraser VJ, Levinson W. Patient's and physician's attitudes regarding the disclosure of medical errors. JAMA. 2003;289:1001-07.
22. West CP, Huschka MM, Novotny PJ, Sloan JA, Kolars JC, Habermann TM, Shanafelt TD. Association of perceived medical errors with resident distress and empathy: a prospective longitudinal study. JAMA. 2006;296:1071-8.

CHAPTER 27

Medicolegal Issues in Blood Transfusion Practice

Ranabir Pal, Amrita Ghosh, Debashis Sinha, Shrayan Pal

"Despite all the technological marvels that humanity is experiencing, a reliable and safe blood supply, is still out of reach for untold millions of people around the world."
—GH Brundtland, Director General, WHO[1]

■ INTRODUCTION

Blood transfusion is often needed to save lives, and there is no substitute for human blood and its components. From the collection of blood to its transfusion is an intricate process. A well built-up procedure for safe blood transfusion must be established in order to eliminate the risk of transfusion-transmitted diseases. A robust system with provision for grievance redressal mechanism needs to be in place for safe and effective blood transfusion and managing any complications which can arise. Advancement in the field of transfusion technology has further necessitated strict control over the quality of transfusion process. Blood transfusion services (BTS) in India are primarily hospital-based and are regulated under the Drugs and Cosmetic Act. India has a National Blood Transfusion program through National Blood Transfusion Council, known as NBTC, and the policy is known as "National Blood Policy." There is requirement for a specific and stringent legislation regulating all the legal aspects related to blood transfusion. In the absence of effective legal sanction, the optimal quality of non-remunerated blood donation movement will remain a mirage. Availability and proper utilization of blood and its components is extremely compromised in dearth of well-trained healthcare professionals and adequate infrastructure. Blood is an important factor, and transfusion requires care and safety which should be achieved. With the National Blood Policy, we hope to achieve nationwide improved transfusion services with greater awareness on transfusion at par with international code of ethics for blood donation and transfusion. We need Indian blood law to streamline the regulatory framework of BTS in-line with the developed countries.[2] In the real-life scenario, legal complications often pop up against the healthcare professionals in case there is any medical complication, or any undesired outcome. This chapter is to sensitize the readers toward the medicolegal aspects of BTS in India, and also to provide medicolegal tips for safe transfusion practices.

CURRENT SCENARIO IN INDIA

National Blood Policy

Government of India published in the year 2002 the "National Blood Policy" with the objective to provide safe and adequate quantity of blood, blood components and products, to procure non-remunerated regular blood donors by the blood banks. It also addresses various issues related to technical personnel, research, and development to eliminate profiteering by private blood banks. The policy also predicts that fresh licenses to stand alone blood banks in private sector shall not be granted and renewal of such blood banks shall be subjected to thorough scrutiny.

National Blood Policy was later incorporated in 2007 as part of jurisdiction of National AIDS Control Organization (NACO) activities. Thus, a need for modification and change in the BTS has necessitated formulation of a National Blood Policy and development of a National Blood Program which will also ensure implementation of the directives issued by the Supreme Court of India in 1996.[3] This policy ensured the safety of transfusion recipients by a standard operative procedure (SOP) that a doctor or qualified nurse must check all possible identifiers of donor and recipient along with their respective blood group before starting the procedures. Physicians will not be held responsible for wrong cross-matching or tests for human immunodeficiency virus (HIV), hepatitis B infection, etc., (pathologist shall be responsible). However, it is the physicians' responsibility to ensure that the blood is transfused in proper volume and at proper rate with unambiguous orders for monitoring pulse, respiratory rate, temperature, and early signs of mismatched blood transfusion.[4]

National AIDS Control Organization and NBTC are the technical bodies to frame guidelines for the practice of transfusion medicine. The National Blood Policy is an offshoot of the National AIDS Control Program. NACO together with NBTC has played a key role in improving blood safety by infrastructure development, setting up component separation units, promoting voluntary blood donation, training staff, and also laying down standards for blood banks in India.

SCENARIO OF LEGAL FRAMEWORK

In a landmark judgment of *"Common Cause vs. Union of India"* the Supreme Court of India made licensing of all blood banks mandatory. All blood banks are licensed today. The honorable court also directed that NBTC along with State Blood Transfusion Councils (SBTC) be set up for monitoring the activity of blood banks.[5]

Blood has been treated as a "drug" under the Drugs and Cosmetics Act (D and C Act), 1940 and Drugs and Cosmetics Rules, 1945.[3] With the classification of blood as a drug, the drugs controller became the regulatory authority. Human blood is covered under the definition of "Drug" under Sec. 3(b) of the Drugs and Cosmetics Act. Hence, it is imperative that blood banks need to be regulated under the Drugs and Cosmetics Act and rules thereunder. The legislation regulating the safe handling of blood products in the transfusion service are the Drugs and Cosmetics Act, 1940 and the Drugs and Cosmetics Rules, 1945 as amended from time to time as per requirements of the transfer of benefits of scientific discoveries of translational researches to the last man on the road.

Drugs and Cosmetics Rules

- *Part X-B*: Requirement for the collection, storage, processing, and disposition of whole human blood, human blood components by blood bank and manufacture of blood products:
    - *122 EA*: Provide definition of apheresis, autologous blood, blood, blood bank, blood component, blood product, donor, leukapheresis, plasmapheresis, plateletpheresis, professional donor, replacement donor. Requirement for the collection, storage, processing, and disposition of whole human blood, human blood component by blood bank and manufacture of blood product has been categorized.
    - *122 F*: Form of application for license for operation of blood bank/processing of human blood for component/manufacture of blood product for sale or distribution has been explained.
    - *122 G*: Form of license for the operation of blood bank/processing of whole human blood for component and manufacturing of blood product and the conditions for the grant or renewal of such license is expressed. Conditions of license have been expressed and explained.

In the last decade of the past century, the Supreme Court banned professional blood sellers and directed the government to formulate a national blood policy. The NBTC, with the National Blood Policy as a tool, and the Drugs Controller, with the help of the Drugs and Cosmetics Act, now aim to ensure blood safety and ethical transfusion practices in India. In this context, the office of Drugs Controller General of India made draft rules to further amend the existing law in the Drugs and Cosmetics Act, 1940 and Rules thereunder to meet the direction of Hon'ble Supreme Court in order to improve the blood banking system across the lengths and breadths of the country.

In the year 1967, Ministry of Health and Family Welfare enacted a separate provision in Schedule F Part XII-B of Drugs and Cosmetics Rules. An assorted prerequisite such as accommodation, technical staff, equipment, etc., for operation of blood bank were included in this Part. State Drugs Controllers were authorized to issue the licenses for blood banks and the standards for "whole human blood" were prescribed in Indian Pharmacopoeia.

The Ministry of Health and Family Welfare (Govt. of India) issued a notification in the year 1989 under the Drugs and Cosmetics Rules, and made the testing of HIV-1 and 2 antibodies of whole human blood as mandatory requirement before transfusion.

As trained technicians were not available in the blood banks to carry out the test for HIV-1 and 2 antibodies, the Ministry of Health and Family Welfare notified 112 surveillance centers to act as testing laboratories for the blood banks for mandatory testing blood for anti-HIV-1 and 2, anti-hepatitis C virus (anti-HCV), hepatitis B surface antigen (HBsAg), malaria and rapid plasma reagin (RPR) for syphilis before transfusion of human blood. NACO has promoted that a dedicated generator backup should be maintained in all the blood banks across the country to maintain cold chain in the BTS.

Following M/s Ferguson's Report (which brought out various deficiencies with regard to quality control of blood and blood products, etc., in the year 1990) and based on disquiet expressed in the Parliament, the D&C Rules were again amended (Rules 68A, Part X-B and Part XII-B of Schedule F) in the year 1992–93 and Drugs Controller General (India) was vested with the power of Central Licence Approving Authority (CLAA) to approve the license of notified drugs, viz. blood and blood products, intravenous fluids, and vaccines and sera.

The requirement of a blood bank is inserted in Part X-B of the Drugs and Cosmetics Rules, 1945. The rules from 122F to 122P explain the various procedures of making applications by a blood bank, fees to be paid for grant/renewal of license by the applicant and conditions of license to be followed by the applicant after grant/renewal and conditions of license to be followed by the applicant after grant/renewal of license.[6]

■ MEDICOLEGAL ASPECTS

In our country, the BTS lacks in many vital aspects, i.e., adequate infrastructure, financial resources, man power resources, etc. The usual screening tests performed cannot detect HIV and Hepatitis antibodies within 12 weeks of infection. The ultimate threat to blood safety is donation by seronegative persons during this infectious "window period" during seroconversion without being detected by available screening tests. We look forward to uniform implementation of all the processes and procedures at par with the developed countries for which stringent legislation is a must.[6,7]

Façade of Non-remunerated Blood Donation

Blood is yet to be produced in mass scale in any industry. Someone donates blood so that others get it making blood transfusion an altruistic ethical responsibility. For this the government as well as all the healthcare personnel need to be trained with behavior change communication (BCC) materials to provide both donor and recipient all necessary and updated information on blood transfusion. An updated legal system will precisely encourage more people to become regular donors. There is a wide gap in the demand and supply of blood as the annual collection is six million against the demand of nine million. Blood collection from the voluntary blood donors constitutes half and majority are first time donors due to paucity of campaign regarding regular repeat voluntary blood donation. In India there is no strong monitoring or expert donor counseling in the blood banks to stop paid illegal blood donation.

In a study done in North eastern Part of India the knowledge about blood donation was found to be significantly related with occupation and education; knowledge was greater among the higher educated. Yet only half were ready to donate blood voluntarily though one-fourth of them have ever donated. Never donors found excuse in health problems, painful procedure and post-donation morbidity. In the behavior disparities model, the people were donating blood to save friends and relatives and influenced by per capita income. The information, education, and communication system must be strengthened with the mass media approach to motivate the general public for voluntary blood donation to clear the myths and realities. The misconceptions behind the unwillingness to donate blood should be covered up with positive campaign for importance of saving life as well as health awareness about the advantages of blood donation, not only for the recipient but also for the donor himself, could possibly encourage voluntary non-remunerated donation. Nonmonetary incentives can be a motivating factor to improve voluntary blood donation.[2,8-10]

The BTS in Oman developed slowly to become self-reliant by voluntary and non-remunerated blood donors within the sultanate. A balanced expansion of blood banks was noted in each phase of blood banking including blood collection, processing and supply, use of blood components and irradiating blood products.[11]

Code of Ethics Relating to Transfusion Medicine[12,13]

In 1980 the International Society of Blood Transfusion (ISBT) validated its first formal code of ethics; later agreed by the World Health Organisation and the League of Red Crescent Societies. The ethics for blood donation and transfusion was updated in 2000, with inputs from different related organizations to encompass accountabilities of donor, collection agency and prescribing authority for patient welfare. Till the other day informed consents were not collected from donors and recipients; screening tests had high false positive rates with no confirmatory tests. The National Blood Policy of 2002 has covered up this gap. The ethical issues related to blood transfusions are essentially similar to the medical management. To ensure ethical BTS, potential ethical conflicts inherent in many medical decisions should be managed as per good moral values and ethical guidelines.

The Code of Ethics relating to Transfusion Medicine was approved in General Assembly of ISBT at Copenhagen on 20th June, 2017. This Code defines the ethical and professional principles, and identifies the ethical and professional standards for practitioners working in the field of transfusion medicine. The Code has emphasized that it is important that the contribution of the donors and their donation is respected. All reasonable steps should be taken to protect their health and safety. It should be ensured that appropriate precautions are in place so that the products derived from the donation are used appropriately and equitably for the patients. The Code outlines the responsibilities of professionals involved in the field of transfusion medicine to donors and to patients.

Ethical Principles Relating to Patients

The patient has a right to expect that her/his autonomy is respected and that a decision to transfuse is made for her/his benefit and avoids the risk of unnecessary or unreasonable harm to her/him.

Autonomy

- Specific consent must, where feasible, be obtained prior to the transfusion.
- The consent should be informed and in order to achieve this, information must be provided on the known risks and benefits of blood transfusion and any possible alternative therapies in order to enable a decision whether to accept or refuse the procedure. The information must be provided in a way that is comprehensible to the potential recipient.
- In cases where specific consent cannot be obtained, the basis for treatment by transfusion must be in the best interests of the patient.
- Any valid advance directive should be respected.

Beneficence and Nonmaleficence

- The patient has a right to be treated with dignity and therefore decisions on the need for transfusion should be based on genuine clinical need.
- Transfusion therapy must be given under the overall responsibility of a registered healthcare professional who is competent to do so.
- Patients should be informed that they have, or may have been, harmed by the transfusion (if information becomes available following a transfusion).
- Information about the patient and the treatment received by them should be managed in a confidential manner.

Justice
- Patients should be treated equitably for the same healthcare condition. Medical decisions relating to transfusion of blood should be based on the best available evidence and treatments for patients.
- The patient should, within the constraints of the local health system, receive the most appropriate blood product(s) that is (are) available. The patient should receive only those products (whole blood, cells, plasma, or plasma derivatives) that are clinically appropriate and afford optimal safety.
- There should be no financial incentive to prescribe blood.

Ethical Principles Relating to Donors
The donor should be exposed to as little harm as possible, in compliance with the principle of nonmaleficence.

Autonomy
- The donor should expressly provide consent to the donation of blood. The consent must be informed, and should include: information of all known risks associated with the donation, of the subsequent legitimate use of the donation, and of how information pertaining to the donor and donation will be treated confidentially. The consent should, where appropriate, include information on whether the donation might be used for research, quality control or any other purpose.
- Information provided by the donor and generated about the donor (i.e., test results) must be treated confidentially. The donor should be informed in advance of the release of any such information.

Dignity and Nonmaleficence
- Donor selection criteria must be applied to protect the health of recipients and donors. Donors must be made aware of their responsibility not to harm the recipient.
- Donors must be informed if they have, or may have been harmed or in the event that any results or information regarding their donation may have an impact on their health.
- The decision to administer any substance or medicine to a donor for the purpose of increasing the concentration of specific components of the blood or for any other reason should take into account that there is no benefit to the donor. This should only be considered when there is good evidence of specific benefits to the recipient, or in the context of research approved by an Ethics Committee and also ensure that the donor has been informed of all known risks and these have been reduced as far as is possible.
- Anonymity between donor and recipient should be ensured except when both donor and recipient freely and expressly consent otherwise.

Stewardship of Blood Supply
The Code includes a series of statements directed to health authorities that relate to the stewardship of the blood supply. Health authorities have a responsibility to ensure that blood services are established and progressively developed so as to assure the needs of the patients using an ethical framework encompassing the care of both donors and patients.

Dignity and Beneficence

- Donated blood should be seen as a "community good" in order to assure the dignity of the donor and not as a commodity to meet others' ends. Therefore, the establishment of a blood service should be based upon not-for-profit principles.
- Blood donation should be voluntary and non-remunerated. A donation is considered voluntary and non-remunerated if the person gives blood, of his/her own free will and receives no payment for it, either in the form of cash, or in kind which could be considered a substitute for money. Small tokens, refreshments, and reimbursements of direct travel costs are compatible with voluntary and non-remunerated donation.
- Any form of incentive that might influence the underlying reason to donate blood should be actively discouraged and must be prohibited if this will either impact on the safety of the blood, result in exploitation of the donor or lead to inequity of access for recipients.
- Blood donor selection should be based on current, accepted and regularly reviewed scientific data. The ability to donate should not be unnecessarily restricted and blood donation criteria should not be justified on the basis of gender, race, nationality, religion, sexual orientation or social class.
- Neither donor nor potential recipient has the right to require that any such discrimination be practiced.
- No coercion should be made on the donor to give blood.

Justice

- Blood and blood products should be considered as a public resource. Access to the products should be based on clinical need taking into account the overall capacity of the local health system. Discrimination based on factors such as patients' resources should be avoided.
- Wastage of blood should be avoided in order to safeguard the interests of all potential recipients and the donor.

Nonmaleficence

- All matters related to donation of blood and its clinical use should be in compliance with appropriately defined and internationally accepted standards.

A key ethical apprehension on the use of blood products is that the community perception of the related hazard is far greater than the actual risk. The sustained system for a voluntary, anonymous and not paid for the donations should be developed. Alternatively, directed donations and autologous blood transfusion will definitely reduce the risk of contamination and costs. A multipronged approach will reallocate resources to research on new medical interventions that will offer more alternatives in societal good versus the individual good. Mentally capable adults are entitled to refuse any medical treatment, including a blood transfusion. Nevertheless, in an incapable patient (underlying depression) further expert opinion is needed to confirm the refusal as truly informed and voluntary, especially in cases with life-threatening situations. In multicultural multilingual India, with unending ethnic variations, the doctors should respect the sociodemographic processes for successful public policy advocacy. The need to provide information on legal and ethical criteria is immense; to obtain consent either directly or via a trusted member of the community, doctors have to communicate with utmost empathy.[14]

All countries need a regular supply of safe blood. In low-income countries, the biggest demand is for blood transfusions to treat severe anemia in children <5 years, and to manage pregnancy related complications. In high-income countries, transfusions are most commonly used for supportive care in cardiovascular and transplant surgery, massive trauma, and cancer treatment.[15]

The Informed Consent in Blood Donation

The patient should be informed contextually and conceptually on impending risks and benefits of alternative treatments that do and do not require transfusion. All information should be explained comprehensively, giving due consideration to the essential components of valid consent:[16]
- Voluntariness
- Competence and capacity to consent, and
- Adequate knowledge.

Right to consent is supplemented by the right to refuse, and this applies even when refusal to start/continue the treatment may result in harm to the patient or death. In case of denial to blood transfusions, the religious opinions of the health seekers toward defending the right to health, intended also as freedom of choice and individual self-determination. The conflict between an ethical and legal duty to safeguard life and the constitutionally guaranteed right to decide freely about healthcare treatments continues to be an unresolved problem. As per rule, transfusion against wishes of a patient is an illegitimate act which violates the fundamental rights of a patient and in case of the violation by any government/state authority may call for remedy under Article 32 of the Constitution of India.[14]

Consent forms may provide some evidence that consent was taken, although they may not establish the participatory "process of consent" through which the physician informs the patient. In the long run, the treating physician bears the legal responsibility for obtaining informed consent. However, the physicians are privileged to treat a patient without consent in emergency life-threatening situations; the patient is incapable of giving or refusing consent; or there is no substitute decision-maker available. Regarding the substitute consent laws provide that in the case of adults who were once competent, but have become temporarily or permanently incompetent, their prior wishes regarding treatment decisions, to the extent that they are known or can be determined, should be respected; parents generally can consent for minor children, except when their rights lost due to abuse or neglect or legally.[16]

Challenges of Blood Screening

Many persons in India are suffering from HIV, Hepatitis B and C, malaria, syphilis due to faulty blood transfusion which could have been avoided by proper screening of the blood. Without proper screening, blood should not be transfused and if alternatives are available, the healthcare professionals should not be unmindful regarding the same.

In India, we have currently 2903 licensed blood banks under different administrative controls; >1 million units of collection per year; of them 77% from voluntary blood donors.[17] Since last two decades, Union Government of India is streamlining BTS across the country by introducing and updating "Policies" and "Guidelines" related to BTS, viz. Guidelines on Processing Charges for Blood and Blood Component (2018), Revised Manpower Norms for Blood Banks 2018, National Blood Policy And Guidelines 2016, National Blood Policy

(2007), Guidelines for Blood Donor Selection and Donor Referrals (2017), Guidelines for Setting up Blood Storage Centres (2007), The Drugs and Cosmetics Act (2003), MoHFW—Gazette Notification (registered). Transfer of Blood and Blood Components to other Blood Banks and Blood Donation Camps (2017), National Policy for Access to Plasma Derived Medicinal Products from Human Plasma for Clinical/Therapeutic Use (2003), Voluntary Blood Donation—Operational Guideline (2007), Regulatory requirements of blood and/or its components including blood products (2002).[18] Each unit of blood is screened for Hepatitis B and C, HIV, malaria and syphilis before transfusion as per updated rules; yet, stringent quality controls are needed in a centralized testing site to assure safety.[19-21]

In a north-east Indian study, overall seroprevalence of major blood-borne pathogens (HIV, HBV, HCV, and syphilis) was 1.63% (HIV 0.32%, HBsAg 0.78%, HCV 0.27%, and syphilis 0.27%); higher HIV, HBsAg, and anti-HCV seropositivity in voluntary donors as compared to replacement donors. However, no sample showed malarial parasites or positive for coinfection with two or more infectious agents.[22] World Health Organization has summarized most important facts for public education which clearly mentioned that, "unnecessary transfusions expose patients to needless risk." Often, transfusions are prescribed when simple and safe alternative treatments might be equally effective. As a result, such a transfusion may not be necessary. An unnecessary transfusion exposes patients to the risk of infections such as HIV and hepatitis and adverse transfusion reactions.[23]

Different developed and developing countries reported infectious disease marker in the collected blood before transfusion. In the Australian study it was estimated that the annual number of blood donations made by donors potentially infected with Creutzfeldt–Jakob disease was 1.15.[24] The median overall risks of transfusion related infections of HIV, HBV, and HCV in sub-Saharan Africa were 1, 4.3, and 2.5 infections per 1,000 units, respectively. Epidemiologic data supports the success of three cheap strategies to prevent transfusion-associated HIV transmission in sub-Saharan Africa: HIV antibody screening, avoidance of unnecessary use of blood products, and exclusion of donors at high risk of infection with health gains and saved costs.[25-27] In UK study, the expected rate of infectious donations between 1993 and 2001 the frequency of HIV-infectious donations remained unchanged; the risk from donations from new donors was 7-fold higher than donations from repeaters.[28] In the Caribbean study, research group noted high prevalence rates of HBV (10–75 per 1,000 donors) and HCV (7–19.3 per 1,000 donors); screening prevented 21 005 HCV and 22 100 HBV infections.[29] The National Heart, Lung, and Blood Institute Retrovirus Epidemiology Donor Study reported an unadjusted prevalence rates to be significantly higher for younger age groups for HIV HBsAg, and HCV; incidence rates and transmission risk estimates for HBsAg were significantly higher in <50 donor group.[30] In northern Thailand study, the prevalence of HIV-1 antibodies staggered from 0.84% in 1988 to 4.04% in 1991; maximum in paid donors. After banning of paid donation in 1993, HIV-1 antibody prevalence reduced to 3.34%; antibody prevalence in replacement donors improved from 0.56% in 1988 to 5.82% in 1991; among 44,446 donors, 7 (0.016%) were tested HIV-1 p24 antigen positive but antibody negative.[31]

Donor Screening: A Concept to be Conceptualized

Donor screening, primarily performed by using a questionnaire, needs to be implemented in letter and spirit. The American Association of Blood Banks came out with version 1.3 of the donor questionnaire and approved by the FDA as indicated. This screening includes:
- Deferrals of donors due to specific medication use with tailor-made referrals for following: Finasteride, isotretinoin, dutasteride, acitretin, etretinate, growth hormone

from human pituitary glands, prior use of bovine insulin, hepatitis B immunoglobulin, clopidogrel
- Screening of donated blood by a series of tests for the following: HBV and HCV, HIV-1 and HIV-2, human T cell leukemia virus type 1 (HTLV-1) and HTLV-2, syphilis, *Trypanosoma cruzi;* apheresis platelets are also tested for bacterial contamination.[32]

Who will Bell the Cat?

A strategic plan is required for managing the challenges faced in the practice of blood transfusion. A mindset full of empathy can help to solve the crisis and reach the horizon of a mission of safe transfusion services. Transfusion professionals must endeavor to identify and resolve the issues related to transfusion practices which have legal implications;
- Why do healthcare providers prescribe blood products?
- How much blood is to be transfused?
- Who are the beneficiaries?
- Whether the patient/relative has consented for the transfusion?

Answer to these questions is the real key to judicious and safe utilization of BTS. Further, well-maintained documents may be helpful for futuristic models. Medical practitioners should unite and raise their voice in the demand for a dedicated blood law to effectively improve the quality in transfusion practice.[2,33]

■ ALTERNATIVES TO BLOOD TRANSFUSION: NEWER RESEARCH

Stem Cell-derived Blood Cells

Exclusive dependence on voluntary blood donation may lead to shortage of transfusion products, and current practice of packing of blood products in general and red blood cells (RBCs) in particulars in liquid or semiliquid phases are associated with biochemical changes over time, branded as "the storage lesion." So, we need alternative sources of red blood cells to supplement transfusable products in conventional blood transfusion system. Extracorporeal manufacture of stem cell-derived RBCs (stem RBCs) may be considered in futuristic vision as the potential and yet unexploited source of fresh, transfusable RBCs, viz. RBC differentiation from $CD34^+$ cells. Nevertheless, we should not be complacent whether these stem RBCs mass production model might ultimately be operative substitutes for RBCs collected from voluntary blood donation due to potential differences in oxygen carrying capacity, viability, deformability, and other critical parameters like in vivo oxygen delivery potential of stem RBCs.[34]

Several ethical and legal issues related to stem cell research need a conclusive discourse with ultimate intention to resolve the hurdles in the path of research. Much of the ethical controversies relating to stem cell research derive from the fact that, until very recently, the only way to obtain human pluripotent stem cell lines was to derive them from a human embryo by a process that necessarily destroyed that embryo. One of the most controversial questions is, whether research on human embryos should be permitted and if so, what kind of research and for what purpose.

Placental Umbilical Cord Blood Transfusion

Placental umbilical cord whole blood transfusion is a safe and genuine alternative to adult whole blood transfusion. Cord blood is the blood that remains in the placenta and umbilical cord following the birth of human babies. After birth, placenta is commonly discarded. This has 80–150 mL precious whole human blood that can be used as replacement of adult whole human blood. Placental blood can be easily collected in pediatric plastic blood collection bags, and anemic babies can be transfused placental cord blood after following all SOPs of safe transfusion.[35]

■ BLOOD TRANSFUSION SAFETY

WHO Recommendation for Blood Safety and Availability[36]

The risk of transmission of serious infections, including HIV and hepatitis, through unsafe blood and chronic blood shortage brought global attention to the importance of blood safety. Through its Blood and Transfusion Safety program, WHO supports countries in developing national blood systems to ensure timely access to safe and sufficient supplies of blood and blood products and good transfusion practices to meet the patients' needs. The program provides policy guidance and technical assistance to countries for ensuring universal access to safe blood and blood products and work toward self-sufficiency in safe blood and blood products based on voluntary unpaid blood donation to achieve universal health coverage.

WHO has been at the forefront to improve blood safety and availability, and recommends the following integrated strategy for blood safety and availability:

- Establishment of a national blood system with well-organized and coordinated BTS
- Effective evidence-based and ethical national blood policies and legislation and regulation that can provide sufficient and timely supplies of safe blood and blood products to meet the transfusion needs of all patients.
- Collection of blood, plasma and other blood components from low-risk, regular, voluntary unpaid donors through the strengthening of donation systems, and effective donor management, including care and counseling.
- Quality-assured screening of all donated blood for transfusion-transmissible infections, including HIV, hepatitis B, hepatitis C and syphilis, confirmatory testing of the results of all donors screen-reactive for infection markers, blood grouping and compatibility testing, and systems for processing blood into blood products (blood components for transfusion and plasma derived-medicinal products), as appropriate, to meet healthcare needs.
- Rational use of blood and blood products to reduce unnecessary transfusions and minimize the risks associated with transfusion, the use of alternatives to transfusion where possible, and safe and good clinical transfusion practices, including patient blood management.
- Step-wise implementation of effective quality systems, including quality management, standards, good manufacturing practices, documentation, training of all staff, and quality assessment.

Guidelines for Administration of Blood and Blood Components[37]

British Committee for Standards in Haematology (BCSH) published guidelines for administration of blood and blood components and the management of transfused patients. The summary of key recommendations is as follows.

Patient Identification

- A patient identification band (or risk assessed equivalent) must be worn by all patients receiving a blood transfusion. The minimum patient identifiers are: last name, first name,

date of birth and unique patient identification number. This information must be legible and accurate. This is best done by printing the identification band directly from the organizations computerized patient administration system (PAS).
- Whenever possible, the unique patient identification number should be a national unique identification number, such as the NHS number in England and Wales, the CHI number in Scotland, or the HSC number in Northern Ireland.
- Positive patient identification is essential at all stages of the blood transfusion process:
  - Blood sampling
  - Collection of blood from storage and delivery to the clinical area
  - Administration to the patient.

  At sampling and administration, whenever possible, the patient must be asked to state their full name and date of birth. This information must match exactly the information on the patient's identification band.
- Patient identification is clearly enhanced by using robust IT systems incorporating, for example, bar-coded identification. Organizations should explore, and where appropriate, implement IT systems to control the clinical transfusion process, in particular the positive patient identification check as well as identification of samples, blood components and staff.
- The healthcare professional administering the blood component must perform the final administration check. This check must be performed at the patient's side immediately before administering the blood component by matching the patient details attached to the blood component with the details on the patient's identification band (or equivalent).

Documentation

- Full and complete documentation, governed by local policies and guidelines, is required at every stage of the blood transfusion process to provide an assured and unambiguous audit trail. All paperwork relating to the patient must include, and be identical in every detail with, the minimum patient core identifiers contained on the patient's identification band.
- Organizations should have a local policy or guideline detailing how transfusion traceability or "fate of unit" must be achieved using robust electronic or manual systems. Communication: Clear and unambiguous communications between all staff involved in the transfusion process, including all clinical and laboratory staff and any other support staff, is essential. Organizations should have local policies and guidelines to minimize the risk of misinterpretation or transcription errors in all communications relating to transfusion, whether written, verbal or electronic. Training and Competency Assessment: All staff involved in the blood transfusion process should receive regular training and be assessed as competent for the tasks they are involved in. Only staff who are trained and competent should participate in the blood transfusion process.

Communication

- Clear and unambiguous communications between all staffs involved in the transfusion process, including all clinical and laboratory staff and any other support staff, is essential.
- Organisations should have local policies and guidelines to minimise the risk of misinterpretation or transcription errors in all communications relating to transfusion, whether written, verbal or electronic.

Training and Competency Assessment

- All staff involved in the blood transfusion process should receive regular training and be assessed as competent for the tasks they are involved in.
- Only staff who are trained and competent should participate in the blood transfusion process.

Summary of key action points for administration of blood components is provided in **Table 1**.

Joint United Kingdom (UK) Blood Transfusion and Tissue Transplantation Services Professional Advisory Committee suggested following basic riders for blood transfusion

TABLE 1: The administration of blood components: Key action points.

Positive patient identification	• Positive patient identification must be worn by all patients receiving a blood transfusion. Patient core identifiers are: Last name, first name, date of birth, unique identification number • Whenever possible ask the patient to state their full name and date of birth • For patients who are unable to identify themselves (pediatric, unconscious, confused patients, and language barrier), verification of the patient's identification should be done from a parent or carer. This information must match exactly the information on the patient's identification band (or equivalent) • All paperwork relating to the patient must include and be identical to the patient core identifiers contained on the patient's identification band
Patient information and consent to transfusion	• Consent should be taken from the patient (where possible) before transfusion • The risks, benefits, and alternatives to transfusion should be explained to the patient in a timely and understandable manner
Pretransfusion documentation	Patient's clinical records should contain: • The reason for transfusion (clinical findings and laboratory data) • The information provided to the patient (risks, benefits, and alternatives to transfusion), and consent to proceed
Prescription	The prescription must contain: • The patient's core identifiers; and • The components to be transfused, date of transfusion, volume/number of units to be transfused, rate of transfusion and any other instructions, e.g., irradiated cytomegalovirus (CMV)-seronegative, blood warmer, or any concomitant drugs required
Requests for transfusion	Requests for transfusion should include the following: • Patient identifiers • Gender • Current diagnosis and any relevant significant comorbidities • Reason for the request • Type of component • Volume/number of units required • Any special requirements • Location of the patient, location where transfusion will occur (if known to be different, name and contact number of the requester)

Continued

Continued

Blood samples for pretransfusion testing	• All patients being sampled must be positively identified • The collection of the blood sample from the patient into the sample tubes and the sample labeling should be performed as one continuous, uninterrupted event, involving one patient and one trained and competent healthcare worker only. Sample tubes should not be prelabeled • The request form should be signed by the person drawing the sample
Collection and delivery of blood component to the clinical area	• Before collecting the blood component, ensure that the patient is ready to start the transfusion and has patent venous access • When collecting the blood component from the laboratory or blood refrigerator, a trained and competent healthcare worker should take authorized documentation containing the patient's core identifiers and check these with the label on the blood component • Core patient identifiers, date and time of collection and staff identification details must be recorded • The component should be delivered to the clinical area without delay
Administration	• The final administration check must be conducted next to the patient by a trained and competent healthcare professional who also administers the component • All patients receiving a transfusion must be positively identified—see above • All patient core identifiers on the patient's identification wristband (or risk assessed equivalent) must match the details on the blood component label • Transfusion should be completed within 4 h of leaving temperature-controlled storage
Monitoring of the patient	Regular visual observation throughout the transfusion episode. Minimum monitoring of the patient should include: • Pretransfusion pulse (P), blood pressure (BP), temperature (T), and respiratory rate (RR). These should be noted and recorded no >60 min before starting the transfusion • P, BP and T should be taken 15 min after the start of each component transfusion. If these measurements have changed from the baseline values, then RR should also be taken • More frequent observations may be required, e.g., rapid transfusion, or patients who are unable to complain of symptoms that would raise suspicion of a developing transfusion reaction • If the patient shows signs or symptoms of a possible transfusion reaction, P, BP, T, and RR should be monitored and recorded and appropriate action taken. • Post-transfusion P, BP, and T should be taken and recorded not >60 min after the end of the component transfusion • Patients should be observed during the subsequent 24 h for (or, if discharged, counseled about the possibility of) late adverse reactions • Organizations should ensure that systems are in place to ensure patients have 24-h access to clinical advice
Completion of transfusion	• If a further blood component unit is prescribed, repeat the administration/identity check with each unit • If no further units are prescribed, remove the blood administration set. Ensure all transfusion documentation is completed

services, viz. to reflect avoidable transfusions, minimize human error out of ABO incompatibility, stop identification errors during pretransfusion blood sampling, transporting, collecting or transfusing wrong component from the blood bank to curtail possible mistransfusions, ensure patient identification by exceptional communication and flawless documentation. A mitigation visionary national policy enactment with electronic transfusion management along with barcode system and capacity building of personnel in clinical transfusion process is the key to reduction of transfusion related emergencies. It was suggested that systems approach for safe blood administration is the call of the day based on utmost empathy for the recipient where informed consent process should be implemented in letter and spirit from patients and their caregivers.[38] Equitable access to safe and rational transfusion practices is still a global challenge even after three decades of resolution on blood safety at the first World Health Assembly (WHA28.72) particularly in developing countries due to demand and supply discrepancy in quantity and quality. Universal access to safe blood transfusion by exclusive non-remunerated donation and quality-assured systems in the transfusion chain, reinforced by the trained workforce with regular updating of infrastructure is the key to improve transfusion services.[39]

ADVERSE EFFECTS OF TRANSFUSION[40-42]

Each blood product transfused is accompanied with a risk of an acute or late adverse effect. Doctors prescribing the transfusion should carefully select the patients for transfusion therapy according to established criteria. The indication for transfusion should be documented in the medical record of the patient. The patient/attendant should be informed of the possible adverse effects that may occur. Patients should be monitored closely during the transfusion. Any adverse reaction to the transfusion of blood or blood products should be reported to the patient's treating doctor and to the hospital blood bank at the earliest, and the same should be documented in the medical records. Joint United Kingdom Blood Transfusion and Tissue Transplantation Services Professional Advisory Committee has clearly enlisted the adverse effects of blood transfusions.

Noninfectious Hazards of Transfusion

Acute Transfusion Reactions

Febrile nonhemolytic transfusion reactions—usually clinically mild, allergic transfusion reactions—ranging from mild urticaria to life-threatening angioedema or anaphylaxis, acute hemolytic transfusion reactions, e.g., ABO incompatibility, bacterial contamination of blood unit—range from mild pyrexial reactions to rapidly lethal septic shock depending on species, transfusion-associated circulatory overload (TACO), and transfusion-related acute lung injury (TRALI).

Severe and Life-threatening Reactions

Acute hemolytic reactions due to ABO-incompatible RBC which react with the patient's anti-A or anti-B antibodies; transfusion of a blood component contaminated by bacteria showing rigors, fever (usually >2°C above baseline), hypotension and rapidly developing shock and impaired consciousness.

Severe Allergic or Anaphylactic Reactions

Shock or severe hypotension associated with wheeze (bronchospasm), stridor from laryngeal edema or swelling of face, limbs or mucous membranes (angioedema) is strongly suggestive of anaphylaxis—an acute, life-threatening emergency. Other skin changes may include flushing and urticaria
- Severe allergic reactions associated with IgA deficiency:
    - Transfusion-related acute lung injury
    - Transfusion-associated circulatory overload
    - Hypotensive reactions
    - Febrile nonhemolytic transfusion reactions
    - Delayed transfusion reactions: Delayed hemolytic transfusion reactions; transfusion-associated graft-versus-host disease; post-transfusion purpura.

Infectious Hazards of Transfusion

- *Viral infections:* Hepatitis A, B, C and E, HIV-1 and 2, cytomegalovirus, human T-cell lymphotropic virus types I and II, human parvovirus B19, and West Nile virus.
- *Bacterial infections:* Syphilis, pathogenic gram-positive bacteria, such as *Staphylococcus aureus*, and gram negatives, such as *E. coli, Klebsiella* species and *Pseudomonas* species may produce life-threatening reactions.
- *Protozoal infections:* Malaria, Chagas disease.

■ DOCUMENTATION OF BLOOD TRANSFUSION PRACTICE[43-47]

Documentation is a tool to ensure quality in blood transfusion practice. The documentation should comprise the information generated during collection, testing, and disposal of unsuitable donations, storage, issue and usage. Reasonably good quality documentation ensures implementation of specified standards of a quality system from "vein-to-vein" and ensures retrieval of transfusion-related events.

Blood Collection Records

After initial counseling, credentials of prospective donors should be accurately recorded with utmost sincerity even if donation may not happen due to self-defer, temporary or permanent ineligibility and for whatever reasons. Sanctity of records of donors should be of prime importance with access only to authorized personnel only containing units and weight of pack/volume of blood, type and batch number of blood bag, batch number of local anesthetic, name of individuals involved in the process.

Laboratory Records

Before any clinical application, following collection collected blood is tested for blood grouping and cross-matching, and screened for transfusion related infections. Documentation will include calibration and maintenance of instrument used and test, sources and batch numbers of the testing kits, results, and suitability reports. Strict confidentiality is needed regarding name of donor or laboratory records with alphanumeric or superior identification codes and cross-checked by senior official. Special precautions are needed to earmark as

"Permanently excluded" to prevent lifelong from any donations for HIV-infected donor by separate, confidential and restricted file.

Blood Issue and Usage Records

Complete and accurate documentation is an integral part of good quality transfusion services regarding specific recipient who actually received the unit blood or blood component. In case of discarded units of blood, reason for discarding and evidence of safe disposal must be documented.

Storage of Records

Documents should be archived in safe custody for stipulated period depending on specific regulatory agencies till their disposal. A system of storing records with their location is needed so that relevant data can be retrieved quickly and easily confidentially with exclusive access to authorized staff. Records need to be secured from physical damage or burglary, alteration and tampering. Documentation of safe return after use regarding identity of user, reason, with in and out time information with strict cross-check will complement safety of data.

Disposal of Records

After stipulated periods documents are disposed that ensures nonaccess of confidential information by unauthorized person, ideally by incineration or instead shredding keeping a disposal log with date, index, and disposal method of records with cross-check.

■ CLINICIAN'S GUIDELINES IN CASE THE PATIENT NEEDS TRANSFUSION[48]

- Inform and explain to the patient/relatives about the benefits and risks of proposed transfusion of blood/blood products, and record the same in the patient's file.
- Ensure proper identity of the patient, and correctly complete a blood request form.
- Collect the blood sample from the right patient in the right sample tube and correctly label the sample tube.
- Order blood in advance, whenever possible.
- Provide the blood storage center with clear information on:
  - The number of units required
  - The reason for transfusion
  - The urgency of the patient's requirements for the transfusion
  - When and where the blood is required.
- Ensure correct storage of blood and blood products in the clinical area before transfusion. Formally check the identity of the patients, the product and the documentation at the patient's bedside before transfusion.
- Correctly record transfusion in the patient's notes:
  - Reason for transfusion
  - Number of units transfused
  - Time of transfusion
  - Monitoring of the patient before, during and after transfusion
  - Any adverse events.

Collecting Blood Prior to Transfusion

A common but avoidable cause of transfusion reaction is the transfusion of an incorrect unit of blood that was intended for a different patient. To avoid the mistakes while collecting blood from the blood storage center, it is important to follow the instructions provided below:
- Ensure proper identification of patient prior to transfusion.
- Check that the following details on the compatibility label attached to the blood pack, exactly match with the details on the patient's documentation:
    - Patient's name
    - Patient's hospital reference number
    - Patient's ward, operating room or clinic
    - Patient's ABO and Rh(D) group.
- Whole blood should be issued from the blood storage center in a cold box or insulated carrier (brought from the ward) which will keep the temperature between 2°C and 6°C if the ambient (room) temperature is >25°C or there is a possibility that the blood will not be transfused immediately.
- Whole blood stored in the ward refrigerator at 2-6°C until required for transfusion. The upper limit of 6°C is essential to minimize the growth of any bacterial contamination in the unit of blood. The lower limit of 2°C is essential to prevent hemolysis, which can cause fatal bleeding problems or renal failure.

Storing Blood Products Prior to Transfusion

- Once issued by the blood storage center, the transfusion of whole blood, frozen plasma should be commenced within 30 minutes. If the transfusion cannot be started within this period, they must be stored in an approved blood refrigerator at a temperature of 2°-6°C, preferably in the center shelf.
- The temperature inside every refrigerator used for blood storage in wards and operating rooms should be monitored and recorded daily, to ensure that the temperature remains between 2°C and 6°C.
- If the ward or operating room does not have a refrigerator that is appropriate for storing blood, the blood should not be released from the blood storage center until immediately before transfusion.

Administering Blood

- Staff involved in the administration of blood/blood components should ensure the FINAL IDENTITY check of the patient, the blood pack, the compatibility label and the documentation.
- For each unit of blood supplied, the blood storage center should provide documentation stating:
    - Patient's name on the requisition and that given on the sample
    - Patient's ABO and Rh-D group
    - Unique donation number of the blood pack
    - Blood group on the blood pack
    - Compatibility label: A compatibility label is attached firmly to each unit of blood, as shown in **Box 1**. This information should be checked before administering blood.

| BOX 1 | Compatibility label attached to blood bag. |

Blood Pack No. _____
- Patient's Name: _____
- Patient's hospital reference number: _____
- Patient's Ward: _____
- Patient's ABO and Rh (D) group: _____
- Expiry date if blood: _____
- Date of compatibility test along with- _____
  - Signature of the technician: _____
- Blood group of blood pack: _____

Checking the Blood Pack

- The blood pack should be inspected for signs of deterioration on arrival in the ward. However, the staff receiving the blood pack from blood storage center should check for any leakage before signing the issue register.
- Discoloration or signs of leakage may be the only warning that the blood has been contaminated by bacteria and could cause a severe or fatal reaction when transfused.

The Final Patient Identity Check

- The final identity check should be done at the patient's bedside just before the transfusion. It should be undertaken by two persons, at least one of whom should be a registered nurse or doctor.
- Ask the patient to identify himself/herself by family name, given name, date of birth and any other appropriate information.
- If the patient is unconscious, ask a relative or staff to state the patient's identity. Check the patient's identity and gender. Check the following details on the compatibility label attached to the blood pack, exactly matching the details on the patient's documentation and identity wristband:
  - Patient's family name and given name
  - Patient's hospital reference number
  - Patient's ward or operating room
  - Patient's blood group.
- Check that there are no discrepancies between the ABO and Rh (D) group on the blood pack compatibility label
- Check that there are no discrepancies between the unique donation number on the blood pack compatibility label
- Check that the expiry date on the blood pack has not been passed.

The final check at the patient's bedside is the last opportunity to detect an identification error and prevent a potentially incompatible transfusion, which may be fatal.

Documenting the Transfusion Process

- Before administering blood products, it is important to write the reason for transfusion in the patient's case-notes. The records should show who ordered the blood and why. The following information should be recorded in the patient's notes: (i) the patient and or relatives have been informed about the proposed transfusion treatment, (ii) the reason for transfusion, and (iii) signature of the prescribing clinician (**Box 2**).

Transfusion Reactions: What Every Physician Should Know

- Severe reaction mostly occurs within the first 15 minutes of the start of transfusion. So all patients should be monitored carefully during this period.
- Things to be done in case of transfusion reaction:
  - Stop the transfusion
  - Keep IV line open
  - Inform the doctor in-charge, and administer antihistaminic and steroids
  - Continuous monitoring of vitals of the patient.
- Whenever a transfusion reaction occurs, the doctor in-charge should document the following records in the patient's file:
  - Date and Time of Reaction
  - Bag No./Unit No.
  - Patient's ID No.
  - Blood group as entered in the patient file and the blood group on the bag issued
  - Check all the labels and records for any clerical error
  - Record the volume of the blood that has been transfused, and that remaining in the bag.
- *Investigation of a transfusion reaction*: The following samples are to be sent to the blood storage centre along with the reaction report:
  - Ethylenediaminetetraacetic acid (EDTA) Vial
  - Plain Vial
  - First urine sample after the transfusion reaction
  - The blood bag along with the transfusion set.

■ LITIGATION RELATED TO BLOOD TRANSFUSION PRACTICE

HIV Infection by Blood Transfusion

- The Supreme Court of India agreed to hear a petition filed by a Mumbai-based woman seeking a compensation from the doctor and blood bank as she was allegedly transfused HIV infected blood during pregnancy that led to the death of her 5-month child, 20 years

---

BOX 2 | **Pretransfusion check.**

- Patient's identity
- Blood pack
- Compatibility label
- Sign of the person performing the pretransfusion identity check
- Volume of blood transfused
- Unique donation number of each unit transfused
- Blood group of each unit transfused
- Time at which the transfusion of each unit commenced
- Signature of the person administering the blood
- Monitoring of the patient before, during and after the transfusion

ago; appealing against the National Consumer Disputes Redressal Commission for providing higher compensation as she claimed to be HIV negative before that.[49]
- M. Chinnaiyan vs. Sri Gokulam Hospital and Anr. on 25th September, 2006; Complainant's wife R. Lalitha, as seen from medical records was transfused two units of blood in December 1990 from where she acquired HIV through blood transfusion. Considering the trauma caused to the family and untimely death of the wife of the complainant due to AIDS National Consumer Disputes Redressal awarded compensation.[50]

Wrong Blood Group Transfusion

- There are many cases on mismatched blood transfusion in India; few of them are mentioned. Dr. Pankaj Mehrotra vs. Salim Ansari on 13th September, 2017 in no. 1203 of 2006 as leading appeal—wrong blood supply by private blood bank and wrong transfusion of A +ve blood by doctors in the private hospital whereas required blood group was B +ve followed by death of complainant's daughter. State consumer disputes redressal commission passed order in favor of complainant.[51]
- R.P. Sharma vs. State of Rajasthan and Anr. on 5th October, 2001—complainant's wife was transfused B +ve blood whereas the required blood group was O +ve. The State of Rajasthan was directed to pay to the petitioner as compensation for the loss of his wife due to the negligence in performance of duties by government servants at Government Medical College and Hospital, Rajasthan.[52]

■ TAKE HOME MESSAGE

- The physician should obtain the patient's informed consent before administering blood products. This includes explaining to the patient the relative benefits and risks of receiving and not receiving the blood product, as well as any reasonably viable alternatives. A competent adult is entitled to refuse or cease any treatment for any reason. Substitute consent must be obtained for incompetent patients according to provincial or territorial laws. A physician can be liable for breaches of the principle of informed consent in: by failing to seek consent, by failing to disclose properly the information required for the consent to be considered "informed" and by providing treatment in the face of an express refusal.
- Generally, in emergency situations where treatment is necessary to preserve the life or health of the patient and consent is not available (because the patient is unconscious or otherwise unable to consent) the physician may administer blood products (and any other treatment) necessary to preserve the life or health of the patient. Exact provisions will vary by province and territory. This does not apply if the patient has expressly refused the treatment before becoming incompetent.
- Parents ordinarily have the responsibility to provide consent on behalf of their young children; however, it is highly unlikely that parents can refuse life-saving treatment for their children. Physicians may not simply override a parent's refusal; recourse must be through the relevant children's aid society.
- Although it is legally clear that a mentally competent adult is entitled to refuse any medical treatment, including a blood transfusion, physicians have a responsibility to ensure that the refusal is truly informed and voluntary.
- In the case of adults who were once competent, but have become temporarily or permanently incompetent, substitute consent laws, generally, provide that their prior

wishes regarding treatment decisions should be respected to the extent that are known or can be determined.
- Always preserve records of informed consent at each step of blood transfusion. This consent should always be in writing and preferably it should be a witnessed consent and it will of great value in case there is death due to adverse reaction.
- Blood sample sent for grouping and cross-matching should be properly labeled and this fact should be recorded in the case file. Request for the blood requirement should preferably be on the proforma of the blood bank or of the institution and all the details should be filled correctly. Always keep the records that mentions from where blood for transfusion was obtained grouped and matched.
- Please see that all the required tests have been done on the blood which is being transfused.
- Check label properly for blood group to see that this is meant for that exact patient only.
- Do not administer blood and drugs through a common administration set or inject drugs into blood bag or use a small bore needle for blood transfusion.
- In case of blood transfusion reactions always treat promptly and document all the treatment of the patient. Attending clinician/nurse must be aware of the sign/symptoms of adverse blood reactions. With platelet infusion particular attention should be toward ill effects of bacterial contamination as platelets are stored at 20°–24°C.
- Always inform the blood bank in case of adverse reaction with sign and symptoms of the patient. In case of death do not panic, always inform police and keep patient record securely.
- Think positive for your rights and responsibilities as a healthcare provider.
- Blood insurance scheme may be started with a dedicated blood law with government support.

■ WORLD BLOOD DONOR DAY, 14TH JUNE 2018

Every year, on 14th June, globally "World Blood Donor Day" is observed to thank voluntary, unpaid blood donors for their life-saving gifts of blood and raise awareness of the need for regular blood donations to ensure the quality, safety, and availability of blood and blood products for the needy. Transfusion of blood and blood products helps save millions of lives every year to help patients suffering from life-threatening conditions live longer with a higher quality of life, and supports medical and surgical procedures; also has an essential life-saving role in maternal and child care and during the emergency response to man-made and natural disasters. Transfusion services give patients access to safe blood and blood products in sufficient quantity as a key component of an effective health system. An adequate supply can only be ensured through regular donations by voluntary and unpaid blood donors. However, in many countries, blood services face the challenge of making sufficient blood available, while also ensuring its quality and safety. Focus of 2018 campaign: "Be there for someone else. Give blood. Share life" to draw attention to the roles that voluntary donation systems play in encouraging people to care for one other and generate social ties and a united community in solidarity. It highlights the fundamental human values of altruism, respect, empathy, and kindness which underline and sustain voluntary unpaid blood donation systems with stories of lives saved through blood donation, to motivate regular blood donors to continue and to motivate people in good health who have never given blood to begin doing so, particularly young generation. Commemorative events, meetings, publication of relevant stories, scientific conference, publication of article in national, regional and international scientific journals, and other activities can help in promoting the themes of World Blood Donor Day. Host country for World Blood Donor Day 2018 events is Greece, through the Hellenic National Blood Centre. The global event was held in Athens on 14 June 2018.[53] The objectives of this year's campaign:

- To celebrate and thank individuals who donate blood and to encourage those who have not yet donated blood to start donating;
- To raise wider awareness that blood donation is an altruistic action that benefits all of society and that an adequate supply can only be ensured through regular donations by voluntary, unpaid blood donors;
- To highlight the need for committed, year-round blood donation, in order to maintain adequate supplies and achieve national self-sufficiency of blood;
- To focus attention on blood donation as an expression of community participation in the health system, and the importance of community participation in maintaining sufficient, safe, and sustainable blood supplies;
- To promote the community values of blood donation in enhancing community solidarity and social cohesion and in in encouraging people to care for one another and build a caring community;
- To promote international collaboration and ensure worldwide dissemination of and consensus on the principles of voluntary non-remunerated donation, while increasing blood safety and availability.

■ CONCLUSION

It requires an empathetic understanding of the apprehension and ability of the patients and their caregivers to compare the risks of receiving the blood products vis-à-vis refusing blood products. The healthcare providers should be compassionate to check and balance all the aspects before rendering any blood transfusion; yet to avoid legal complications they must be alert of lawful considerations. The SOP of procuring, issuing, and administering blood should be openly displayed for each site of service.[54] Mandatory training and retraining on transfusion for all levels of healthcare providers may ensure safe transfusion practice. Further, patient safety will be improved with the downstream effects of reduction of legal hazards.

■ REFERENCES

1. These were the Words of Dr. Brundtland GH, Director-General of the World Health Organization, at the launch of World Health Day 2000 dedicated to Blood Safety. [online] Available from: http://hinfo.humaninfo.ro/gsdl/ healthtechdocs/documents/s15376e/s15376e.pdf. [Last accessed Aug., 2019].
2. Pal R, Kar S, Zaman FA, et al. The quest for an Indian blood law as of blood transfusion services regulatory framework. Asian J Transfus Sci. 2011;5(2):171-4.
3. National Blood Policy. NACO. Ministry of Health and Family Welfare. Government of India 2007. [online] Available from: http://naco.gov.in/sites/default/files/National%20Blood%20Policy_0.pdf. [Last accessed Aug., 2019].
4. Tiwari S. Legal aspects in medical practice. Indian Pediatr. 2000;37(9):961-6.
5. Common Cause vs Union of India and Others. Case No. Writ Petition (civil) 91 of 1992. [online] Available from: https://www.indiankanoon.org/doc/1449517/. [Last accessed Aug., 2019].
6. Regulatory Requirements of Blood and/or its Components Including Blood Products. [online] Available from: http://www.cdsco.nic.in/forms/list.aspx?lid=1642&Id=1. [Last accessed Aug., 2019].
7. Viswanathan C. Are our donors safe? Indian J Pediatr. 2001;68(1):69-75.
8. Shenga N, Thankappan K, Kartha C, et al. Analyzing sociodemographic factors amongst blood donors. J Emerg Trauma Shock. 2010;3(1):21-5.

9. Shenga N, Pal R, Sengupta S. Behavior disparities towards blood donation in Sikkim, India. Asian J Transfus Sci. 2008;2(2):56-60.
10. Shenga N, Pal R, Sengupta S, et al. Correlates of voluntary blood donation among people in a hill capital in India. Int J Green Pharm. 2009;3(2):167-74.
11. Joshi SR, Shah Al-Bulushi SN, Ashraf T. Development of blood transfusion service in Sultanate of Oman. Asian J Transfus Sci. 2010;4(1):34-40.
12. Elhence P. Ethical issues in transfusion medicine. Indian J Med Ethics. 2006;3(3):87-9.
13. Code of Ethics Relating to Transfusion Medicine. [online] Available from: https://helsedirektoratet.no/Documents/Transfusjonsmedisin/Code_of_Ethics_version_June_2017_.pdf. [Last accessed Aug., 2019].
14. Molinelli A, Rocca G, Bonsignore A, et al. Legal guardians and refusal of blood transfusion. Blood Transfus. 2009;7(4):319-24.
15. Self-sufficiency in Blood Supply Based on Voluntary Unpaid Donors: An Achievable Goal. [online] Available from: http://www.who.int/features/2013/world_blood_donor_day/en/. [Last accessed Aug., 2019].
16. Chaturvedi A. Consent - Its Medico-legal Aspects. [online] Available from: http://www.apiindia.org/pdf/medicine_update_2007/153.pdf. [Last accessed Aug., 2019].
17. BTS Data 2016-17, NACO. [online] Available from: http://www.nbtc.naco.gov.in/. [Last accessed Aug., 2019].
18. Policies & Guidelines. National Blood Transfusion Council. Ministry of Health and Family Welfare, Government of India. [online] Available from: http://www.nbtc.naco.gov.in/page/policies_guidelines/. [Last accessed Aug., 2019].
19. Primer. NAT: Safe Blood, Safe India. [online] Available from: http://www.healthcare.financialexpress.com/200810/knowledge02.shtml. [Last accessed Aug., 2019].
20. Shenga N, Pal R, Sen Gupta S. Knowledge of transfusion transmitted infections among the Sikkimeese. Pan Arab Med J. 2008;2(11):11-4.
21. Guidelines for Blood Donor Selection and Blood Donor Referral National Blood Transfusion Council, National AIDS Control Organization. Government of India. 2017. [online] Available from: http://www.naco.gov.in/sites/default/files/Letter%20reg.%20%20guidelines%20for%20blood%20donor%20selection%20%26%20referral%20-2017.pdf. [Last accessed Aug., 2019].
22. Adhikari L, Bhatta D, Tsering DC, et al. Infectious disease markers in blood donors at Central Referral Hospital, Gangtok, Sikkim. Asian J Transfus Sci. 2010;4(1):41-2.
23. 10 Facts on blood transfusion. [online] Available from: http://www.who.int/features/factfiles/blood_transfusion/blood_transfusion/en/. [Last accessed Aug., 2019].
24. Correll PK, Law MG, Seed CR, et al. Variant Creutzfeldt-Jakob disease in Australian blood donors: estimation of risk and the impact of deferral strategies. Vox Sang. 2001;81(1):6-11.
25. Jayaraman S, Chalabi Z, Perel P, et al. The risk of transfusion-transmitted infections in sub-Saharan Africa. Transfusion. 2010;50(2):433-42.
26. McFarland W, Mvere D, Shandera W, et al. Epidemiology and prevention of transfusion-associated human immunodeficiency virus transmission in sub-Saharan Africa. Vox Sang. 1997;72(2):85-92.
27. van Hulst M, Smit Sibinga CT, Postma MJ. Health economics of blood transfusion safety--focus on sub-Saharan Africa. Biologicals. 2010;38(1):53-8.
28. Soldan K, Barbara JA, Ramsay ME, et al. Estimation of the risk of hepatitis B virus, hepatitis C virus and human immunodeficiency virus infectious donations entering the blood supply in England, 1993-2001. Vox Sang. 2003;84(4):274-86.
29. Cruz JR, Pérez-Rosales MD, Zicker F, et al. Safety of blood supply in the Caribbean countries: role of screening blood donors for markers of hepatitis B and C viruses. J Clin Virol. 2005;34(Suppl 2):S75-80.
30. Busch MP, Glynn SA, Schreiber GB. Potential increased risk of virus transmission due to exclusion of older donors because of concern over Creutzfeldt-Jakob disease. The National Heart, Lung, and Blood Institute Retrovirus Epidemiology Donor Study. Transfusion. 1997;37(10):996-1002.
31. Mundee Y, Kamtorn N, Chaiyaphruk S, et al. Infectious disease markers in blood donors in northern Thailand. Transfusion. 1995;35(3):264-7.
32. AABB Full-Length Blood Donor History Questionnaire, Version 2.0 May 2016 (Officially Recognized by the FDA in Guidance). American Association of Blood Banks. [online] Available from: http://www.aabb.org/tm/questionnaires/Pages/dhqaabb.aspx. [Last accessed Aug., 2019].
33. Gorea R. Medico-legal aspect of blood transfusion. J Punjab Acad Forensic Med Toxicol. 2010;10(1):5-8.
34. Shah SN, Gelderman MP, Lewis EM, et al. Evaluation of stem cell-derived red blood cells as a transfusion product using a novel animal model. PLoS One. 2016;11(12):e0166657.
35. Bhattacharya N. A study of placental umbilical cord whole blood transfusion in 72 patients with anemia and emaciation in the background of cancer. Eur J Gynaecol Oncol. 2006;27(2):155-61.

36. Fact Sheets. Blood Safety and Availability. [online] Available from: https://www.who.int/en/news-room/fact-sheets/detail/blood-safety-and-availability. [Last accessed Aug., 2019].
37. Guideline on the Administration of Blood Components. British Committee for Standards in Hematology. [online] Available from: https://www.b-s-h.org.uk/media/5152/admin_blood_components-bcsh-05012010.pdf. [Last accessed Aug., 2019].
38. Safe Transfusion—Right Blood, Right Patient, Right Time and Right Place. [online] Available from: https://www.transfusionguidelines.org/transfusion-handbook/4-safe-transfusion-right-blood-right-patient-right-time-and-right-place. [Last accessed Aug., 2019].
39. Universal Access to Safe Blood Transfusion. Blood Transfusion Safety. [online] Available from: http://www.who.int/bloodsafety/universalbts/en/. [Last accessed Aug., 2019].
40. Adverse Effects of Transfusion. [online] Available from: https://www.transfusionguidelines.org/transfusion-handbook/5-adverse-effects-of-transfusion. [Last accessed Aug., 2019].
41. Adverse Reactions to Blood Transfusion. Division of Blood Transfusion Services, Ministry of Health and Family Welfare. [online] Available from: http://www.nbtc.naco.gov.in/assets/resources/training/17.pdf. [Last accessed Aug., 2019].
42. Clinical Transfusion Practice Guidelines for Medical Interns. Geneva: WHO; [online] Available from: http://www.who.int/bloodsafety/transfusion_services/ClinicalTransfusionPracticeGuidelinesforMedicalInternsBangladesh.pdf. [Last accessed Aug., 2019].
43. Guidelines and Principles for Safe Blood Transfusion Practice. Introductory Module. Safe Blood and Blood Products. WHO. Reprint 2009 Originally Published 2002. [online] Available from: https://www.who.int/bloodsafety/transfusion_services/bts_learningmaterials/en/.[Last accessed Aug., 2019].
44. Standard Operating Procedures for Blood Transfusion. Directorate General of Health Services (BANBCT), Mohakhali. Technical Assistance by WHO and Supported by The OPEC Foundation for International Development. [online] Available from: http://www.who.int/bloodsafety/transfusion_services/sop-bts_bangladesh.pdf. [Last accessed Aug., 2019].
45. Document Control. [online] Available from: http://www.naco.gov.in/sites/default/files/pdf2_0.pdf. [Last accessed Aug., 2019].
46. Procedure Checklist. Chapter 36: Administering a Blood Transfusion. [online] Available from: http://www.people.westminstercollege.edu/students/ncb0708/Program%20Files/FA%20Davis/Fundamentals%20of%20Nursing%20ESG/proc_check/pc_ch36-01.pdf. [Last accessed Aug., 2019].
47. Blood Transfusion Services. National AIDS Control Organization. [online] Available from: http://www.naco.gov.in/blood-transfusion-services-publications. [Last accessed Aug., 2019].
48. Guidelines for Setting Up Blood Storage Centres. NACO, Ministry of Health and Family Welfare, Government of India. New Delhi 2007. [online] Available from: http://www.naco.gov.in/sites/default/files/Guidelines%20for%20Setting%20up%20Blood%20Storage%20Centres.pdf. [Last accessed Aug., 2019].
49. Supreme Court to Hear Woman's Plea on 'HIV via Transfusion'. 2019. [online] Available from: https://www.hindustantimes.com/india-news/supreme-court-to-hear-woman-s-plea-on-hiv-via-transfusion/story-DOUa5MZrbFY1kt0eKG8qlM.html. [Last accessed Aug., 2019].
50. M. Chinnaiyan vs Sri Gokulam Hospital and Anr. III (2007) CPJ 228 NC. [online] Available from https://indiankanoon.org/doc/1919829/. [Last accessed Sept., 2019].
51. Dr. Pankaj Mehrotra vs Salim Ansari. Appeal no. 1203 of 2006. [online] Available from https://indiankanoon.org/docfragment/89191502/?formInput=wrong%20blood%20transfusion. [Last accessed Sept., 2019].
52. R.P. Sharma vs State of Rajasthan and Anr. AIR 2002 Raj 104. [online] Available from https://indiankanoon.org/doc/480351/. [Last accessed Sept., 2019].
53. World Blood Donor Day 2018. [online] Available from: http://www.who.int/campaigns/world-blood-donor-day/2018/event/en/. [Last accessed Aug., 2019].
54. Guidelines for Requisition, Handling, Storage and Transfusion of Blood and Blood Components. Department of Transfusion Medicine. Chandigarh: PGIMER; [online] Available from: http://www.pgimer.edu.in/PGIMER_PORTAL/AbstractFilePath?FileType=E&FileName=GuideTranBlood24Jan2014112621.pdf&PathKey=SPOTLIGHT_PATH. [Last accessed Aug., 2019].

CHAPTER 28

Medicolegal Issues in Dentistry

Shilpa Pharande

> "Remember, Dentistry is not expensive, but Neglect is!"
>
> —**Anonymous**[1]

■ INTRODUCTION

Dentistry has been practiced in some form as a separate field of healthcare since antiquity.[2] Over the years it has developed to one of the highly advanced specialties. In addition to general practice, dentistry includes many specialties and subspecialties. The latest trend of utilizing the advanced technology and newer techniques in dental practice has resulted in ever increasing expectations of highest standards in dental care. In a new information era, convenient access to the unreliable health information has transformed the patients into *impatient patients* who demand unrealistic results from healthcare providers. Unrealistic expectations and poor communication skills are the key drivers for medical liability claims particularly if complication occurs during treatment. Dental practitioners must be aware of the legal principles applicable to the dental practice, as the risk of malpractice lawsuits is increasing.

■ MEDICOLEGAL ASPECTS OF DENTAL PRACTICE

Patient safety is one of the key medicolegal issues in the practice of dentistry. The primary goal of patient safety is to prevent the avoidable adverse events and to limit the harmful consequences of those which are unavoidable. A study analyzed 415 adverse events in dental practice in Spain during 2000–2010. The highest frequency of adverse events occurred in implant treatments (25.5%), endodontics (20.7%) and oral surgery (20.4%). Up to 44.3% of the adverse events that occurred were due to predictable and preventable errors and 55.7% adverse events were unforeseeable complications and accidents.[3]

Thorough understanding of the adverse events that are possible in each dental activity is a must for their prevention. Quality in dental care not only assures patient safety but also reduces the liability claims against the healthcare providers.

Temporomandibular Disorders

Temporomandibular disorder (TMD) is a poorly understood set of conditions characterized by symptom complex, which is assumed to be caused by multiple factors. TMD is the second most frequent cause of orofacial pain after dental pain (toothache).[4] Temporomandibular disorder is a frequent finding in cases of facial trauma. The symptoms can become chronic, and the persistent pain, psychological discomfort, and physical disability may have detrimental effect on quality of life. The exact cause of TMD is not clear, but it is believed that symptoms arise due to problems with the jaw muscles or part of the joint itself. Many other conditions can cause symptoms similar to TMD including a toothache, sinus problems, arthritis, or gum disease. The dentist should thoroughly evaluate the patient's history and physical examination to determine the cause of symptoms.

Over the years, malpractice claims for temporomandibular disorders have increased. Temporomandibular disorders assessment is complicated by the peculiarities of these disorders, whose symptoms are heterogeneous, fluctuant, and may have a multifactorial origin. Despite the medicolegal aspects of the dental practice gaining attention, there is paucity of literature dealing with patients with TMD assessment. For these reasons, evidence based knowledge in the field of TMD diagnosis and treatment is indispensable.[5]

Root Resorption

External apical root resorption is a clinical complication of orthodontic treatment that can be detected on periapical radiographs 5-6 months after the orthodontic treatment. It is characterized by reduction in length of the root from the apex. Root resorption is associated with multifactorial risk factors. Comprehensive evaluation of the predisposing factors viz personal medical history, severity of malocclusion, anterior cross bite, and past history of dental treatment due to trauma, etc., should be conducted. Orthodontic tooth movements especially intrusion and other movements like tipping, torque are also known to influence the root resorption.

Diligent evaluation is an essential *risk management practice* that helps the orthodontists in detecting the occurrence and severity of the root resorption and thereby planning the treatment effectively. Early detection of root resorption is helpful in identifying teeth at risk of severe resorption. Delayed diagnosis or improper management of root resorption may result in malpractice claims.[6,7]

■ MEDICAL EMERGENCIES IN DENTISTRY

Inhalation/Ingestion of Foreign Objects

Unfortunately orthodontic appliances or their parts may accidentally enter the airway or the gastrointestinal tract, resulting in avoidable medical emergencies. Most dental patients are treated in the supine position, enhancing the risk of accidental aspiration or swallowing of foreign objects. These avoidable medical emergencies have high-risk of malpractice litigation.

A case report of an orthodontic patient who accidentally ingested a part of orthodontic wire and coil spring from a fixed expansion device placed in the maxillary dental arch has been reported.[8] In another case, accidental swallowing of a gold cast crown that became loose after separation with brass wire for orthodontic band placement, was reported.[9] Two instances are described in which the cutting of distal sections of arch wires proved hazardous.[10] Orthodontic appliances that become dislodged can cause problems in the airway or the gastrointestinal tract. Accidental ingestion of a fractured twin-block appliance was reported due to inadequate retention. Therefore, precautions must be taken by the orthodontists to prevent such accidents.[11] Trans-palatal arch wire is commonly used in orthodontic practice.

A case of broken trans-palatal wire, swallowed and stuck to the patient's throat was reported.[12] These case reports emphasize the importance of careful examination of the appliances at each scheduled visit.

Orthodontists should follow guidelines for medical emergency management in cases of inhalation or ingestion of orthodontic objects. Most of the events of inhalation or ingestion of orthodontic appliances occurs outside the orthodontist's office.[13] Every orthodontist should also have written emergency protocols to be followed by the patients in case of *out of office events* and present them to the patients before starting the treatment.

Incidental Findings on Pretreatment Screening

Certain anomalies are discovered as incidental findings on the cephalometric radiographs obtained in the process of orthodontic treatment. Patients had severe instability of the cervical spine at the articulation between first and second cervical vertebrae that required referral to a medical specialist. Such cases emphasize the need to evaluate head and neck structures visible on cephalometric radiographs, independent of the traditional morphometric analysis routinely done by the orthodontists.[14]

Dentists routinely do X-ray examination during the dental procedures. The X-ray films might contain evidence of anatomic anomalies and pathologic findings that require dental/medical consultation. In a study, thorough screening of pretreatment orthodontic radiographs of 1354 patients was done. Total of 154 significant anomalies and pathologic findings were recorded. The findings included fractured odontoid process of the axis vertebra, os odontoideum, spondylolisthesis, fractured surgical needle in the oropharynx, unrecognized carotid artery stenosis, cystic lesions, and calcified stylo-hyoid ligaments.[15]

Pretreatment cephalometric radiographs may contain important incidental findings that require attention before orthodontic therapy. Familiarity with the appearance and prevalence of skeletal and dental anomalies and normal variants seen in cephalometric radiographs, and the ability to distinguish the case that require follow-up from those that does not need followup, is an important facet of good orthodontic practice.[16]

Developing a complete differential diagnosis might be beyond a dental professional's expertise and might be best done in consultation with a radiologist.[17] The dentist should be aware of the potential to detect anatomic anomalies and pathologic findings in pretreatment orthodontic panoramic radiographs. Missing the anomalies and pathologic findings during the pretreatment screening of orthodontic radiographs may have a significant medicolegal implication. Such pretreatment screening should be performed diligently to detect/exclude the significant anomalies and pathological findings as per the standard guidelines, even if it is presumed to be beyond orthodontic purposes.

Diagnosis of Malignancy in Dentistry

Dentists should be observant for oral premalignant and malignant diseases and head and neck involvement by the malignant disease. A patient may present in a dental clinic with oro-facial pain as a chief complaint which in fact is due to malignancy. Thorough medical and dental history along with careful examination, including inspection and palpation of the oral and extraoral structures, and the cervical lymph nodes should be done particularly in high-risk patients. History of smoking and alcohol consumption must be specifically asked.[18] If a dentist observes a suspicious finding, he should document it thoroughly in the patient's dental record and take consultation from an oncologist in writing.

Failure to diagnose or delayed diagnosis of malignancy can have a devastating effect on patient's health.[19] These issues have potential medicolegal implications and must be managed as per the standard guidelines. If a dentist fails to incorporate an oral cancer screening as part of his examination protocol, or a suspicious lesion prevails for an extended period, without proper diagnosis or referral, he may be sued by the patient for not following the standard of care.

Esthetic Dentistry

Esthetic dentistry includes the dental procedures intended to improve the patient's appearance. It includes a wide range of dental treatments including crown, veneer, orthodontic treatment, bridge and bleaching, etc. This specialized domain of dentistry has high-risk of malpractice claims due to associated high expectations of the patients. In case a patient seeks services of a dentist due to esthetic reasons, it is advisable to ascertain the exact nature of the *presenting complaint* and the *patient's expectation* from the proposed dental treatment. Detailed records of the presenting complaint, patient's expectations, dental history and pretreatment examination findings must be maintained as there may be discrepancy later on if the patient feels unsatisfied from the outcome. In performing orthodontic treatment, records that need to be maintained include pre-treatment radiographs, pretreatment dental cast, pre- and posttreatment photographs, as well as clinical notes. Poor record keeping could give rise to troubles if a claim is subsequently made by a patient. In esthetic dentistry, written informed consent has indispensable role. The dentist should provide sufficient and accurate information related to the patient's complaints, the proposed treatment, and the expected outcome. To assure that the patient understands the information properly, the dentist should consider using visual aids, such as photographs, models or diagrams, and the copy of the same must be included as part of dental records.[20]

Negligence in Dentistry

- Failure to attend an emergency is considered as negligence. Similarly a patient cannot be refused treatment on the ground that it is a medicolegal case.[21]
- Transmission of infection to the patients may lead to malpractice claims. It is the responsibility of a dentist to prevent cross infection between the patients. Endangering the health or lives of other patients can invite criminal negligence (*Sec 336 IPC*).
- All the patients have right to information about the procedure and possible outcomes. No treatment can be given to the patient without his/her informed consent. Failure to explain may be considered as invalid consent. Often, lack of informed consent or improper consent is a cause of malpractice action.[21]
- General dentists who attempt to treat beyond their level of competence and failure to refer the case to a specialist is an objectionable practice that may invite negligence claims.[22]
- Any deviation from the evidence based practice resulting in injury to the patient is prone to be sued in a court of law. However, it must be known that dentistry is not an exact science and there can always be difference of opinion between the dentists regarding the choice of treatment. Deviation from the acceptable practice is not negligence if the same is accepted as proper by a few professional colleagues, even if there is a body of opinion that takes a contrary view.

- Failure to give clear instructions to the patient resulting in any complication is also considered negligence. Dentist must give clear written advice regarding diet and postoperative care, etc.
- If the prescriptions are not clear or lack proper instructions, the dentist is deemed to be negligent.[23]
- Avoidable accidental ingestion of crowns, dental instruments, teeth, etc., can also result in medical negligence lawsuits in court of law.
- In case local anesthesia is given without test dose leading to anaphylaxis/death, the dentist will be held liable for the act of omission.
- Under Public Liability Insurance Act, a dentist can be held liable for the harm caused to the public by inadvertent exposure of harmful substances like mercury, arsenic or for those matter even radiations.[23]

'No Negligence' Occasions in Dental Practice

- Patient dissatisfaction with the progress of the treatment cannot be called as negligence. Law expects that a doctor must treat the patient with due care and skill, and with diligence. However, it is suggested that patient's dissatisfaction must not be ignored. Proper counseling and shared decision making in the process of informed consent can help a lot to educate the patient regarding realistic expectation and limitation of the dental procedure proposed to be performed.
- Not obtaining consent in an emergency is not negligence. In medical emergencies where delay caused by waiting for informed consent cannot be afforded at the cost of life of the patient, and also there is no evidence to indicate that the patient would refuse the procedure, it is legally acceptable to start the treatment without informed consent.
- Charging a fee that is considered exorbitant by the patient is not negligence. However, it is suggested that in today's world of consumerism, while taking consent for the proposed treatment, tentative cost of the treatment must also be informed to the patient.
- When patient does not follow the advice of the dentist and does not get satisfactory results, dentist cannot be held negligent or at least contributory negligence on the part of patient shall be considered by the court while deciding the liability of the treating doctor.
- Poor outcome, unexpected outcome or any complication occurring due to the procedure performed is not negligence per se. To fix the liability of a dentist, the courts apply *Bolam's rule,* which is considered *locus classica* in the field. The Bolam's rule says that:

"A doctor is not guilty of negligence if he has acted in accordance with a practice accepted as proper and responsible by a responsible body of medical men skilled in that particular art."[24]

■ PROTECTION AGAINST LITIGATION

Valid informed consent, reasonable standard of care, good communication skills and good quality medical record keeping are some of the risk management strategies that go a long way in nurturing a congenial physician-patient relationship as well as a strong armor against medical negligence litigation. In a medical negligence case, State Consumer Dispute Redressal Commission highlighted the importance of maintaining comprehensive medical records and noted that the doctor's defence against negligence was not supported by the documentary evidence. It further stated that, in the absence of case papers and documentary evidence regarding the treatment given, it would appear that the doctor had not given proper, adequate or standard treatment and was trying to cover up negligence.[25] Based on the medicolegal principles it is recommended to maintain comprehensive treatment records. Judiciary holds absence of medical records against health practitioners and considers them negligent and liable to pay compensation. Dental records might be the only permanent evidence available as a defense in case of medical negligence litigation. Therefore, it must be stressed that one of the most important risk management strategies is the maintenance of accurate, complete and up to date records of all the treatment provided.

HOW TO AVOID LITIGATION?

Steps at Personal Level

- *Qualification and Registration*: Possessing a qualification and training which is accepted by the regulatory authority (DCI) and getting himself/herself registered with the State Dental Council is a primary safeguard against any litigation. The prescription slips, signboards and advertisements should mention the qualification of the practitioner and the actual facilities available.
- *Communication*: Good communication is the key to warm doctor-patient relationship. Increasing patient volume alongwith improper communication to patient about the disease and plan of treatment, expected outcome, complications and guarantee of 100% results are the main reasons for patient's anguish against their doctor. It is desirable for the dentists to show empathy and reply all queries of their patients and always keep patient's interest as priority. The right of patient/relatives to seek explanation about the treatment expenses should not be denied.

Interpersonal Behavior

The human face of medical care decides the patient's reaction toward any complication occurring due to the treatment. The whole system of healthcare establishment should be courteous, and polite. Specialized training should be imparted to the staff about dealing with patients/relatives generally as well as specifically when the patient has any anguish against any aspect of the healthcare process. Get the patient's feedback about the services provided, healthcare establishment, staff's behavior, charges, etc., and try to fix the imbalances. It is advisable to refrain from guaranteeing 100% results.

Academic and Technical Update

To keep pace with fast changing scenario of technical advancement, one should regularly attend education programs, workshops and other academic sessions. Nursing staff and other healthcare personnel should also be encouraged to upgrade their knowledge and skills.

In a questionnaire based study conducted on awareness about the knowledge, attitude and practice regarding Consumer Protection Act in Dental professionals, Interns and Postgraduate students in a Dental Institute 65.88% of MDS staff, 48.75% BDS staff, 48.88% postgraduate students and 49.34% interns showed awareness about Consumer Protection Act. Hence there is a need to increase the level of awareness regarding Consumer Protection Act in Dental professionals at academic level.[26]

Awareness of Medical Laws

A thorough knowledge of medical laws is essential for all healthcare professionals. Unless one is aware about the medical laws regulating the dental practice, one cannot improve the practice standards.

In a questionnaire-based study conducted on awareness about the knowledge, attitude and practice of informed consent in Dental professionals, Interns and Postgraduate students in a Dental institute, it was concluded that 85% Dental professionals and 51.97% students were aware about informed consent. Hence there is a need to increase the level of awareness regarding informed consent in order to avoid litigations in future.[27]

Reasonable Skills and Care

The key steps for safe practice in dentistry are, exercising reasonable skills and care in diagnosis and treatment, proper documentation of facts and legally valid informed consent. Reasonable skill and care in practice has medical, legal as well as social relevance.

Medical Relevance of the Reasonable Skill and Care

The practice of reasonable skill and care while treating the patients is an essential component of good clinical practice. It minimizes the risk of medical mistakes and ensures the best usage of medical science in healthcare. It is imperative for every doctor to exercise reasonable skill and care expected of an average professional colleague with equivalent qualification and experience in similar circumstances.

Social Relevance of the Reasonable Skill and Care

The society expects from their healthcare providers to exercise reasonable skill and care. The reasonable skill and care provided to the patients should be evident in all the aspects of patient care; discussions, compassionate behavior, and communication with the patients and their relatives. The doctor may be very sincere and dedicated in performing his/her duties, but failure to exhibit these gestures may lead to doubts in the mind of the patients and their relatives.

Legal Relevance of the Reasonable Skill and Care

Whenever a matter regarding professional negligence is to be decided, Courts always look for whether the reasonable skill and care was provided or not. Expression of reasonable skill and care as documentary evidence (*in medical records*) is based on the medicolegal principle: "Anything which is not documented in medical records was not actually done." The reasonable skill and care provided to the patient must be palpably visible in the comprehensive clinical notes incorporating all the relevant aspects of the healthcare provided. In case the patient fails to follow instructions, refuses any investigation or does not come for the follow-up on specified date, then such facts should be documented in the medical records. These negative findings may act as crucial protective shield while defending against allegation of negligence in a Court of law. It is advisable that the handwriting must be legible, and all the entries must be properly dated and signed and in chronological order.

Professional Indemnity Insurance

Profession indemnity insurance is a tool which not only meets the claim of compensation awarded against doctor/hospital but also gives a sense of assurance that in case compensation is ordered against them, the insurance company will take care of it. Professional indemnity insurance is a contractual agreement made between two parties, in which one party agrees to pay for potential losses or damages caused by the other party. None of us are immune from medical negligence lawsuits and keeping in mind the trend of high quantum of compensation awarded by the courts, it is advisable to get financial security by getting professional indemnity insurance.

In a questionnaire based study it was found that only 58.33% Dental professionals were aware about dental indemnity insurance. Hence there is a need to increase the level of awareness regarding dental indemnity insurance to financially safeguard the dental healthcare providers.[28]

CONCLUSION

To err is human. Unfortunately in the healthcare profession errors can result in serious harm to the patients, in turn leading to civil/criminal liability against the erring/negligent doctor. A dentist who has acted in accordance with a practice accepted as proper by a reasonable body of practitioners cannot be considered negligent merely because there is a body of opinion that takes a contrary view. Although it may be desirable for a dentist to possess the highest degree of skill, it is sufficient that the practitioner exercise the ordinary skills of a reasonably competent health professional of same field. The dentists must be aware of their medicolegal duties and incorporate the risk management strategies in their daily practice of dentistry. Acting in best interest of the patient, must also be supplemented by the concept of *shared decision making* which encourages patient involvement in healthcare decisions as *partners*.

REFERENCES

1. Anonymous Quote. Available: http://www.pinterest.com/pin/286963807479716881/
2. Orland FJ. The rise of dentistry as a special field. How and why we grew up apart from the field of medicine. CDS Rev. 1978;71(7):18-21.
3. Bernardo Perea-Pérez, Elena Labajo-González, Andrés Santiago-Sáez, Elena Albarrán-Juan, Alfonso Villa-Vigil. Analysis of 415 adverse events in dental practice in Spain from 2000 to 2010. Med Oral Patol Oral Cir Bucal (2014) doi:10.4317/medoral.19601.
4. Manfredini D, Guarda NL, Winocur E, Piccotti F, Ahlberg J, Lobbezoo F. Research diagnostic criteria for temporomandibular disorders: a systematic review of axis I epidemiologic findings". Oral surgery, oral medicine, oral pathology, oral radiology, and endodontics. 2011;112(4):453-62.
5. Manfredini D, Bucci MB, Montagna F, Guarda-Nardini L. Temporomandibular disorders assessment: medicolegal considerations in the evidence-based era. J Oral Rehabil. 2011;38(2):101-19.
6. Ramanathan C, Hofman Z. Root resorption in relation to orthodontic tooth movement. Acta Medica (Hradec Kralove). 2006;49(2):91-5.
7. Pizzo G, Licata ME, Guiglia R, Giuliani G. Root resorption and orthodontic treatment. Review of the literature. Minerva Stomatol. 2007;56:31-44.
8. Quick AN, Harris AM. Accidental ingestion of a component of a fixed orthodontic appliance—a case report. SADJ. 2002;57(3):101-4.
9. Kharbanda OP, Varshney P, Dutta U. Accidental swallowing of a gold cast crown during orthodontic tooth separation. J Clin Pediatr Dent. 1995;19(4):289-92.
10. Killingback N, Stephens CD. A little distal archery. Br J Orthod. 1988;15(2):121-2.
11. Rohida NS, Bhad WA. Accidental ingestion of a fractured Twin-block appliance. Am J Orthod Dentofacial Orthop. 2011;139(1):123-5.
12. Abdel-Kader HM. Broken orthodontic trans-palatal arch wire stuck to the throat of orthodontic patient: is it strange? J Orthod. 2003;30(1):11.

13. Bilder L, Hazan MH, Aizenbud D. Medical emergencies in a dental office: inhalation and ingestion of orthodontic objects. J Am Dent Assoc. 2011;142(1):45-52.
14. Tetradis S, Kantor ML. Anomalies of the odontoid process discovered as incidental findings on cephalometric radiographs. Am J Orthod Dentofacial Orthop. 2003;124(2):184-9.
15. Abdel-Kader HM. Medicolegal perspective: interpretation of pretreatment orthodontic radiographs. World J Orthod. 2008;9(1):14-20.
16. Tetradis S, Kantor ML. Prevalence of skeletal and dental anomalies and normal variants seen in cephalometric and other radiographs of orthodontic patients. Am J Orthod Dentofacial Orthop. 1999;116(5):572-7.
17. Kuhlberg AJ, Norton LA. Pathologic findings in orthodontic radiographic images. Am J Orthod Dentofacial Orthop. 2003;123(2):182-4.
18. Marshall JA, Mahanna GK. Cancer in the differential diagnosis of orofacial pain. Dent Clin North Am. 1997;41(2):355-65.
19. Epstein JB, Sciubba JJ, Banasek TE, Hay LJ. Failure to diagnose and delayed diagnosis of cancer: medicolegal issues. J Am Dent Assoc. 2009;140(12):1494-503.
20. David K. Medicolegal aspects of aesthetic dentistry. Hong Kong Dental Journal. 2004;1:21-3.
21. D'Cruz L. Legal aspects of general dental practice. Churchill Livingstone/Elsevier. 2006.
22. Rajan Dhawan, Shivani Dhawan. Legal aspects in dentistry, Journal of Indian Soc Periodontology. 2010:14;81-4.
23. Paul G. Medical law for the dental surgeon. New Delhi: Jaypee Brothers; 2004.
24. Bolam vs. Friern Hospital Management Committee. 1957 1 WLR 582.
25. KR Trivedi vs. Dr. S Vishwakarma. 1996;3 CPR 24 (Guj).
26. Pharande SV, Toshniwal NG, Potnis SS, Sonawane RS, Patil SS, "Awareness about the Knowledge, Attitude and Practice regarding Consumer Protection Act in Dental Professionals, Interns and Post Graduate Students in a Dental Institute - A Questionnaire Based Study", International Journal of Science and Research (IJSR). 2019;8(3):718-22.
27. Pharande SV, Toshniwal NG, Potnis SS, Patil SS, Sonawane RS, "Awareness about the Knowledge, Attitude and Practice Regarding Informed Consent in Dental Professionals, Interns and Post Graduate Students in a Dental Institute - A Questionnaire Based Study", International Journal of Science and Research (IJSR). 2019;8(6):999-1004.
28. Pharande SV, Toshniwal NG, Potnis SS, Patil SS, Sonawane RS, "A Stitch in Time Saves Nine-Indemnity Insurance in Time Saves Fine: A Questionnaire based Study in a Dental Institute", International Journal of Science and Research (IJSR). 2019;8(3):735-8.

CHAPTER 29

Medicolegal Issues in Anesthesiology

Manpreet Singh, Ajay Kumar, Lakesh Anand

"Anesthesiology has played a pioneering role in the patient safety and in the establishment of standards for safe practice."
—WHO guidelines for Safe Surgery[1]

■ INTRODUCTION

In the last decade, there has been significant improvement in healthcare system, specifically the operating theaters across the India. Anesthesiologists have been leaders in drawing attention to the need for a systematic approach to improving patient safety. It all started perhaps with the ground-breaking work of anesthesiologists analyzing critical incidents. There has been an enormous amount of work put into reducing error and improving safety. However, the practice of anesthesiology has associated inherent risks and complications which may not be entirely predictable or preventable. The anesthesiologists must be well versed with the essential medicolegal principles related to day-to-day clinical practice. The basic medicolegal principles specifically related to the specialty of anesthesiology are discussed here.

■ STANDARD OF CARE

An anesthesiologist is liable only, if the care provided falls below a reasonable standard. It is not required that he should use the highest degree of skill. Each deviation from normal professional practice is not necessarily evidence of negligence. However, it is expected from anesthesiologists to regularly update their knowledge on the current practices of the specialty. If a case reaches a court, then standard of care followed will be evaluated by comparing it that of a *prudent and reasonable* anesthesiologist. In 1986, American Society of Anesthesiologists approved Standards for Basic Anesthetic Monitoring. These standards were last amended in 2010. Following are the criteria for standards of care for basic anesthetic monitoring:[2]
- Personnel should be present throughout the conduct of general and regional anesthetics and monitor anesthesia care.
- Evaluate continually oxygenation, ventilation, circulation, and temperature.
- Monitor blood oxygen level.

The anesthesiologist, as mentioned, should provide proper and continuous ventilation to the anesthetized patient. This is accomplished through four methods:
1. Continually measuring clinical signs as "chest excursion, observation of the reservoir breathing bag, and the auscultation of the breathing sounds. Also, it is encouraged to monitor the level of expired carbon dioxide unless it was restricted by the patient, procedure, or equipment
2. Ensuring the correct positioning of the endotracheal tube or laryngeal mask and identifying carbon dioxide in the expired gas, as well as performing postoperative capnography, or mass spectroscopy.
3. Attaching a device that detects whether a disconnection occurred in the breathing system when the patient's ventilation is controlled by a mechanical ventilator.
4. Observing the ventilation adequacy through continual observation of clinical signs and/or monitoring the level of expired carbon dioxide.

In 1998, the Indian Society of Anesthesiologists (ISA) taking guidelines from World Federation of Society of Anesthesiologists (WFSA) promulgated monitoring standards for anesthesia. These standards are considered as national standards, and are applicable for anesthesia services in any part of the country. There is a need to update the currently applicable guidelines.[3]

■ DUTY OF CARE AND LIABILITY

Once the anesthesiologist examines the patient preoperatively and agrees to provide anesthesia care to the patient, a duty toward the patient has been established. The choice of anesthesia is made by the anaesthetist in conjunction with the patient and surgeon. The contractual agreement of medical care imposes both joint and several liabilities. It represents a joint responsibility in that modern surgery is truly a team effort. It is several or individual in that each specialist contracts to provide his particular ostensible skills and knowledge to and for the benefit of specific patient and procedure.

■ MEDICOLEGAL ISSUES IN ANESTHESIOLOGY

Death on Operation Table

Death on operation table (DOT) is the most dreaded complication during a surgical procedure that calls for a postmortem, audit and police investigation. Death on Table (DOT) is a medicolegal case, and during investigation there is a chance that the police will seize the belongings of the deceased, broken ampoules of the drugs used, and documents of the patient and seal the operation theater after taking over the dead body for postmortem examination. In DOT cases, both the anesthesiologist and the surgeon have to share the responsibility of the event, in different measures depending upon the cause and effect of the complication. Intraoperative deaths are uncommon, but they do occur. In England, Wales and Northern Ireland, there are around 2,000 deaths on the table each year (11% of the total number of deaths within 30 days of surgery). Around 15% of these deaths are unexpected.[4,5]

Witnessed Death on Operation Table: Recommendations for Doctors[6,7]

- *Look after the deceased*: Leave all drains in situ and close catheters or cannula with a spigot. Keep endotracheal tube in situ. Cover the surgical incision site with a dressing.

Complete all the documentation. Preserve all ampoules and vials used during the surgery.
- *Equipment*: Sequester before subsequent use and check anesthetic (or other) equipment, if suspected of contributing to death.
- *Documentation*: Make accurate, full, contemporaneous record of the facts of what happened in the operation theater. Record all decisions taken on the management of the patient, and the reasons underlying those decisions. Establish timeliness correctly with the surgical team and others involved in the patient consultation and care.
- *Communication*: In the aftermath of an intraoperative death, communication with others is of vital importance. Patient's family, hospital management, police and other staff involved in patient's care need to be informed. Breaking the sad news of death is a challenging task for the doctors but has to be performed with solemn dignity by all concerned. The operating surgeon and the anesthesiologist should communicate together with the patient's family. The relatives should be given an opportunity to know the facts of the case, clear any doubts and pay their last respects to the patient. What should be communicated by doctors to the relatives should be pre-decided and should be strictly followed. At this stage, there should not be any attempt to fix the blame on any team member. The communicating member of the team should be the one who enjoys the best rapport with the relatives during the preoperative visits and has good communicating skills. The communicator may not be necessarily an anesthesiologist or a surgeon, but communication should be undertaken in the presence of the involved surgeon and anesthetist. The paramedical staff should also be briefed about the designated communicator and made to understand the suspected cause of death to prevent conflicting reports given to the patient attendant. A hospital policy should be in place to deter perpetuation of unsubstantiated statements by the staff to the relatives.
- Police should be informed as per the requirement of the law. If the anesthesiologist and surgeons informs the police without meddling with the operation theater (OT) scenario, it is generally interpreted as an honest endeavor on the part of the doctor, who does not wish to hide anything.
- *Transfer to mortuary*: The senior OT nurse should ensure that the deceased is transferred to the mortuary as soon as possible following the declaration of death.
- *Analyze and review*: It is important that the incident must be analyzed so that lessons can be learned and future practice and protocol improved, particularly, in the case of unexpected deaths. All deaths within 24 hours of admission and other unexpected deaths should be promptly reviewed in a multidisciplinary forum like mortality and morbidity meetings. The outcome of the review and lessons learnt should be formally documented. Provide counselling for individuals involved in the management of *death on table*, if needed.
- *Internal audit*: After the incident, an institutional audit of the sequence of events must be done to suggest and institute corrective measures in order to prevent future occurrences.
- *Legal implications*: In the event of the occurrence of death within the four walls of the operation theater, where relatives have no access, the onus lies on doctors to explain as to what really went wrong in the operation theater (OT) which led to the tragic death. The time limit for filing a case in the courts is calculated either from the time of event or from the date a new fact was discovered by the relative (complainant). In the consumer courts, the time limit is 2 years while in other courts, it is 3 years.
- *Prepare defence*: Doctors involved in the incident of *death on table* should make a summary of their case report and search the authentic medical literature and compile the data on

its incidence, causes and management in the similar cases from standard textbooks and journals. All the documents related to the deceased patient should be preserved in safe custody so that they are available to the doctors when required.

Anesthesia Deaths

Various reasons for deaths due to anesthesia are explained from time to time. Many times the cause death is explainable but sometimes, it remains unexplained. Several classifications have been published regarding deaths associated with anesthesia. It has been found that anesthetic deaths are declining. A systematic review of the Brazilian and worldwide studies demonstrated a decline in anesthesia related mortality rates, which amounted to less than 1 death per 10,000 anesthetics in the past two decades. Perioperative mortality rates also decreased during this period, with fewer than 20 deaths per 10,000 anesthetics in developed countries.[8]

The anesthesia related deaths may be attributed to the following factors:

Inexperience: Deaths during anesthesia may occur due to inexperience and failure to adopt precautions when clearly indicated. These include mishaps due to intubation (aspiration, kinked tubes, etc.) and bronchoscopy. Human factors involved in preventable anesthesia mishaps are like: breathing circuits disconnections, equipment failure, haste in work, etc.

Drugs: There may occur, accidental over dosage, relaxant drugs without airway management, abnormal or anaphylactic reactions to drugs. Inadvertent hypothermia, hyperpyrexia, sensitivity reactions are other possible hazards.

Technical mishaps: Incompatible blood transfusion although rare, but may cause death of the patient. The labels on the syringes or on drugs should be done by anesthetist himself. Dental anesthesia is an important aspect of anesthesia but many mishaps may occur in it. Specific hazards include inhalation of blood, teeth, mouth packs, periodontal lignocaine and hypotension due to fainting in a sitting posture. The hazards of dental operations on patients in sitting positions in dental chairs and of single handed operator anesthetists has been increasingly a matter of concern during past. Skilled nursing care during post-operative period with safe positioning of the patient is an important protection, and there should be direct observation of the patient until he recovers consciousness. If the patient is left alone even for few minutes, fatal inhalation of vomit may occur.

Deaths due to surgical mishaps: Deaths under this category are detectable at autopsy. Usually, the principal findings are massive haemorrhage, as from slipped ligatures, uncontrollable oozing, accidental perforation of a viscous such as bladder, air-embolism in special cases.

Deaths from disease: Majority of cases where death is associated with anesthesia, the cause of deaths can be due to the disease for which the surgery was being performed. On occasions, however, the death may occur due to previously unsuspected natural disease and it is in these instances, that the performance of autopsy is extremely valuable.

Awareness During Anesthesia

Intraoperative awareness is associated with postoperative psychological sequelae for the patients which include: insomnia, depression, anxiety and post-traumatic stress disorder (PTSD) with distressing flashbacks. The majority of patients who have suffered intraoperative awareness fear future surgery and anesthesia. In addition to distressing effect on patients awareness during anesthesia entails medicolegal consequences for the anesthesiologists.

Awareness occurs after 1 in 3000 anesthetics. The most frequent cause of awareness is selection of an inadequate dose of anesthetic agent. The majority of the signs of awareness involve sympathetic nervous system activation; these may be masked by drugs or co-existing pathology. In high-risk situations, the use of a monitor of depth of anesthesia is justified.[9] Studies performed in the 1970s using 60–70% nitrous oxide as the sole anesthetic agent revealed an incidence of awareness of up to 7% (1 in 14).[10] In recent times, the incidence of awareness with explicit recall of severe pain has been estimated at 0.03% of general ancsthetics (1 in 3000).[11] The risk of awareness correlates with depth of anesthesia. Light anesthetics, particularly where the patient is paralyzed by a neuromuscular blocking agent, are associated with the highest risk of awareness. The depth of anesthesia may be unduly light for several reasons. These are described here. Awareness is frequently associated with poor anesthetic technique. Errors include the omission or late commencement of a volatile agent, inadequate dosing or failure to recognize the signs of awareness. Under-dosing of anesthetic agent may occur during hypotensive episodes, when anesthetic is withheld in an attempt to maintain arterial pressure. A number of surgical scenarios are associated with a higher risk of intraoperative awareness. These include: Cardiac surgery, emergency surgery, surgery associated with significant blood loss and Cesarean section. Anesthesia awareness is a term used to describe when a patient is awake during surgery, experiencing pain, hearing conversations between doctors, yet completely unable to communicate that they are aware. Before most surgeries involving general anesthetic, individuals are given a paralyzing drug to keep them motionless during surgery. As a result, when the anesthesia is not working they can do nothing to alert the doctors. It has been estimated that between 20,000 and 40,000 people every year experience anesthesia awareness, with effects ranging from complete consciousness during surgery with feelings of pain and detailed memories, to only having vague recollections of pain, pressure, difficulty breathing or conversations during surgery. Many victims of anesthesia mistakes experience post-traumatic stress disorder, most of them never get over the trauma. Problems could include nightmares, insomnia, flashbacks, paranoia and other symptoms which are associated with other traumatic events such as rape. Anesthesia awareness can be avoided or at least greatly reduced, by the exercise of proper standards of medical care by the anesthesiologist and nurse anesthetist. Anesthesia mistakes resulting in problems during surgery could include:

- Inadequate drug dosing
- Poor monitoring
- Failure to refill the anesthetic machine's vaporizers
- Insufficient training
- Unfamiliarity with techniques used
- Machine misuse or malfunction

Codes of practice improve standards and it is for the benefit of the medical profession and the patients who place themselves in its hands that further steps are taken expeditiously to achieve this objective. If the rising tide of medical litigation and professional indemnity premiums are to be checked it is necessary for individual anesthesiologist to know and to follow the minimum standards expected of them by the public, their profession and the law. The introduction of the ASA *standards for basic intraoperative monitoring* was accompanied by a decrease in the number of anesthesia-related liability claims. Improved monitoring, especially the greater use of pulse oxymetry and capnography, has undoubtedly contributed to the decrease in severe complications and the associated large awards.

The key factors in improving the patient care and outcome include vigilance, adequate monitoring, pre and postoperative evaluation, updating the professional knowledge and skills, and following the protocols in day-to-day practice. Indian Society of Anesthesiologists must develop protocols to be followed by its members in different clinical situations. The anesthesiologists following the protocols have a better defence available against the allegation of negligence in court of law.

Every surgical operation involves risks. It would be wrong, and indeed bad law, to say that simply because a misadventure or mishap occurred, the hospital and the doctors are thereby liable. It would be disastrous to the community if it were so. It would mean that a doctor examining a patient or a surgeon operating at a table instead of getting on with his work, would be forever looking over shoulder to see, if someone was coming up with a dagger; for an action for negligence against a doctor is for him like unto a dagger. Doctor's professional reputation is as dear to him as his body, perhaps more so, and an action for negligence can wound his reputation as severely as a dagger can his body. So doctor must not, therefore, be found negligent simply because something happens to go wrong; if, for instance, one of the risk inherent in an operation actually takes place or some complication ensues which lessens or takes away the benefits that were hoped for, or if in a matter of opinion he makes an error of judgment. The doctor should only be labelled as guilty of negligence when he falls short of the standard of a reasonably *skillful medical man*.

■ ERROR OF JUDGMENT

Lord Denning said, "*We must say and say it firmly that, in a professional man, an error of judgment is not negligence.*"[12] Indian courts have also held the same view. In the medical profession, as in others, there is room for differences of opinion and practice. A doctor cannot be found negligent merely because in a matter of opinion he made an error of judgment. It is also well-settled that when there are genuinely two responsible schools of thought about management of a clinical situation, the Court could do no greater disservice to the community and the advancement of medical science than to place the hallmark of legality upon one form of treatment. What amounts to a responsible body of medical opinion cannot be determined by counting heads. It is open to a judge to decide that a small number of specialists constitute such a body; it is not necessary for the body to be substantial.[13] However, all errors of judgment are not consistent with exercise of proper care. In House of Lords, Lord Edmund Davies said "*to say that a surgeon committed an error of judgment is wholly ambiguous for while some such errors may be completely consistent with the due exercise of professional skill, other acts or omissions in the course of exercising clinical judgment may be glaringly below proper standard so as to make a finding of negligence inevitable.*"[14] The crucial test is whether the surgeon in reaching his decision displayed such a lack of clinical judgment that no surgeon exercising proper care and skill could have reached the same decision as he did.[15]

■ MISTAKE

Often, in a medical malpractice lawsuit, a plea is taken that it is a case of bonafide mistake which under certain circumstances may be excusable. A mistake that tantamount to negligence cannot be pardoned. Gross medical mistake will always result in finding of negligence. Use of a wrong drug or a wrong gas during anesthesia will frequently lead to the imposition of liability and in some situations even the principle of res ipsa loquitur may be applied. Degree of care must be proportionate with the magnitude of risk. For example, when an anesthesiologist was handling a dangerous substance which was known to be highly inflammable and he knew of the hazard arising from electrostatic sparks in an operating room, the degree of care required from him was proportionately high and he was bound to take special precaution to prevent injury to his patient. Those who engage in operations inherently dangerous must take precautions which are not required of persons engaged in ordinary routine of daily life.[16,17]

■ BURDEN OF PROOF

The burden of proving that the anesthesiologist was negligent falls on the complainant alleging negligence against the specialist. Court allows both parties to prove their case by means of producing evidence. This may include records, books, journals or expert witnesses. However, in the ordinary course of events, the plaintiff does not have to establish that a duty of care arises, for this is generally accepted where an anesthesiologist undertakes any professional service for a patient whether or not he is paid for that service.[18] As a matter of right, both the parties to a case can produce expert witness to support their claim. In many cases, the success of a suit depends primarily on the stature and believability of the expert witness. There have been a number of cases where courts have dismissed the complaints when complainant has not produced expert witness to substantiate his claim.[19,20]

If something happens which a reasonable prudent anesthesiologist could not have foreseen, the anesthesiologist will not be held negligent. Court of appeal in a case held that an act of a physician should be judged in the light of knowledge available at the time when the incidence took place. Denning LJ commented, it is so easy to be wise after the event and to condemn as negligence that which was only misadventure. We ought to always be on our guard against it, especially in cases against hospitals and doctors.[21] A reasonable man may foresee the possibility of many risk factors, but life would be almost impossible, if he were to attempt to take precautions against every risk, which he can foresee. He takes precautions against risk which are reasonably likely to happen.[22]

■ RES IPSA LOQUITUR

This legal phrase means *things speak for themselves*. It applies when the event which is complained of would not ordinarily happen in the absence of negligence. In such cases, the burden of proof shifts from the complainant to the defendant. He has to prove that he was not negligent. Use of a wrong drug or a wrong gas during anesthesia will frequently lead to the imposition of liability and in some situations even the principle of res ipsa loquitur may be applied.[16]

Applicability of the doctrine of *res ipsa loquitur* requires proving that:
- The injury is of a kind that typically would not occur in the absence of negligence.
- The injury must be caused by something under the exclusive control of the anesthesiologist.
- The injury must not be due to any contribution on the part of the patient.

Where a patient developed massive tissue emphysema due to wrong placement of needle for jet ventilation of lungs, the Anesthesiologist was held liable because if the needle had been placed correctly into the trachea, tissue emphysema would not have occurred.[23] Following an operation under general anesthesia, patient sustained hypoxic brain damage in recovery ward. The anesthesiologist was held liable.[24]

Instances where the doctrine of res ipsa loquitur was applied:
- Where an explosion occurred during the course of administering anesthetic to the patient when the technique had been frequently been used without any mishap.[25]

- Surgical mop left in the abdomen during LSCS under spinal anesthesia.[26]
- Artery forceps left in the abdomen during operation. Compensation granted by the State Commission was further enhanced by the National Commission.[27]
- Artery forceps left in the abdomen during surgery. Found at the cremation ground when relatives went to collect the last remains.[28]
- Metallic tip of suction cannula left in the abdomen during LSCS. Surgeon was held negligent.[29]
- Unexplained cardiac arrest during anesthesia leading to death is negligence.[30]
- Where surgery for the removal of a swelling from the parotid gland under general anesthetic, the plaintiff was taken to the recovery ward but sustained brain damage caused by hypoxia for a four-to five minute period, which the anesthesiologist had failed to prevent, it was held to be negligent.[24]

Doctrine of *res ipsa loquitur* was not applied in a case where globe was perforated in the course of giving a local block prior to cataract surgery.[31] Other examples where doctrine of *res ipsa loquitur* was not applied: In another case where a patient suffered permanent partial paralysis of legs following anesthesia, the court said, "Medical science has not yet reached a stage where the law ought to presume that a patient must come out of an operation as well or better than he went into it.[32] Patient developed meningitis after spinal anesthetic. Court found that anesthetic was not contaminated and the staff had taken the usual precautions to disinfect themselves before the operation, it held the hospital was responsible for some fault in sterilization procedure.[33]

■ HOW TO DECREASE THE LIKELIHOOD OF A LAWSUIT?

To decrease the likelihood of a lawsuit, anesthesiologists should adhere to the following points:
- The anesthesiologists must improve his *doctor-patient relationship*. This is accomplished by spending as much time as possible with the patient and his/her family preoperatively describing the procedure, calming nerves and building a relationship of trust. The anesthesiologist should be aware of the patient's condition, be ready to follow up actively, if any complications occur and explain it in full, if it does. He/she should project a professional image and appear as a person to be trusted[16]
- The anesthesiologist should adhere to the *standards of care* through keeping his/her knowledge bank updated, being prudent in his/her choice of agents, and maintaining the patient's vital signs within a reasonable range.[16]
- Good quality medical records must be maintained. It is advisable to always keep in mind, the legal presumption, *If it is not written, it was not done*. Always write preoperative notes, so as to distinguish the poor outcome from negligent act. The physician should include a differential diagnosis. He/she should not write notes admitting any wrong doings nor accusing others.[16]
- The anesthesiologist should respond appropriately when an incident does occur through obtaining consultations and following up on the patient until his/her services are no longer needed and document that in the medical record. The physician should avoid *vicarious liabilities*. He should diligently supervise the assistants as supervising assistants may make him liable for their actions. He should specify what equipment and techniques are to be used and not agree to supervise more cases simultaneously than he can safely handle.[16]

Liability which is incurred for, or instead of, another can be defined as vicarious liability. Every person is responsible for his own acts or omissions but there are circumstances where for the acts committed by a person, the liability comes to lie, not on that person, but on someone else. A master is liable for the acts or omissions of his servant and the principal is accountable for the acts of his.

ACCEPTED PRACTICES AND PROCEDURES

An anesthesiologist is not guilty of negligence, if he has acted in accordance with a practice accepted as proper by a responsible body of medical men skilled in that particular art. Accepted practice means practice accepted as proper by the anesthesiologist's peers. If the Anesthesiologist has complied with this practice then that is strong evidence that he is not negligent, if he does not then it is likely he will be negligent.[34] Minimum standards prescribed by the professional bodies are beneficial for improving the quality of care provided to the patients. Good quality care is also necessary to check the rising tide of medical litigation. It is necessary for individual anesthesiologists to know and to follow the minimum standards expected of them by their profession and the law.[35] Introduction of the *standards for basic intra-operative monitoring* by American Society of Anesthesiologists was accompanied by decrease in number of anesthesia related liability claims. Improved monitoring, especially the greater use of pulse oxymetry and capnography, has undoubtedly contributed to the decrease in severe complications and the associated large awards. The key factors in the prevention of patient injury are vigilance, up-to-date knowledge, and adequate monitoring.[36] Threat of law suits against anesthesiologists seems to have declined somewhat in the USA and it can be accounted for in part by greater attention to monitoring and other standards of anesthetic practice, including continuing medical education.[37] Indian Society of Anesthesiologists must also come out with protocols to be followed by its members in different clinical situations. Once this is done the courts will decide the issues of medical negligence by the fact whether the protocol was followed or not. Thus the anesthesiologists following the protocols will not be held guilty of negligence. This will also improve the patient care and the outcome.

Departure from approved practices is in itself not negligence. If an anesthesiologist departs from the approved practice, and he is able to justify his action she will not be negligent, but if he cannot justify his departure from the accepted practice, it will be easy for the complainant to establish negligence against the anesthesiologist.[34] Negligent performance of an approved practice will also constitute a departure from the accepted standards.

ACCIDENTS, MISADVENTURES, AND MISHAPS

Courts have held that it would be wrong, and indeed bad law, to say that simply because a misadventure or mishap occurred, the hospital and the doctors are thereby liable. It would be disastrous to the community, if it were so. An anesthesiologist is not an insurer; he does not warrant that his treatment will succeed or that he will perform a cure. Naturally, he will not be liable if, a treatment which in ordinary circumstances would be sound, has unforeseen results. The standard of care which the law requires is not insurance against accidental slips. It is not every slip or mistake that imparts negligence. Law recognizes the dangers, which are inherent in induction and maintenance of anesthesia. Mistakes will occur on occasions despite the exercise of reasonable skill and care.[34]

INHERENT RISKS

Every anesthesia procedure has its own risk factors. Just because one of these factors becomes manifest does not mean that the anesthesiologist is negligent and his services defective. He can be held negligent only when the standard of care exhibited by him falls below the standards expected of a reasonable prudent anesthesiologist practicing under the circumstances he is placed in.[38]

■ CHOICE OF TREATMENT

Much of the anesthesia-related problems can be managed or treated in more than one way. Anesthesiologists have the discretion to choose the line of treatment they wish to adopt and can be faulted for the same only if their choice is *palpably wrong* or *dangerous* to the patient. When there are two genuinely responsible schools of thought about the management of a clinical situation, the Courts could do no greater disservice to the community or the advancement of medical science than to place the hallmark of legality upon one form of treatment.[38] An anesthesiologist is not liable for taking one choice out of two or for favoring one school rather than another.[39] He is only liable when he falls below the standard of a reasonably competent practitioner in his field. In the realm of diagnosis and treatment, there is ample scope of genuine difference of opinion and one anesthesiologist clearly is not negligent merely because his conclusion differs from that of other professional men, nor because he has displayed less skill or knowledge than others would have shown. If an anesthesiologist has followed a course of treatment or procedures accepted by and followed by a responsible section of the profession, he would not be guilty of negligence even, if another section of the profession does not subscribe to that practice and follow a different course.[10] An anesthesiologist has discretion in choosing the treatment which he proposes to give to the patient and such discretion is wider in cases of emergency, but he must bring to his task a reasonable degree of skill and knowledge and must exercise a reasonable degree of care according to the circumstances of each case.[40]

■ KEEPING THE PROFESSIONAL KNOWLEDGE AND SKILL UP-TO-DATE

Professional practices may change over time so that what was accepted as the correct procedure may no longer considered appropriate. Once the risk associated with an old procedure becomes generally known, so that it can be said that an ordinary and reasonably competent practitioner would have changed his practice, it will be negligent to continue with that procedure. The doctor has discretion in choosing treatment which he proposes to give to the patient and such discretion is relatively ampler in cases of emergency. The obligation is to make a reasonable effort to keep up-to-date. A doctor cannot realistically be expected to read every article in every learned medical journal. But where a particular risk has been highlighted on a number of occasions the practitioner will ignore it at his peril.[41]

■ CASES TO OBSERVE

Following are some of the cases that discuss the important medicolegal issues prevailing to the anesthesiology.

Case 1: *The Woolley and Roe case: An anesthesiologist was not held negligent as the risk was not foreseeable by the prevailing scientific knowledge at the time of occurrence of incident.*[21]
Albert Woolley and Cecil Roe became paraplegic after spinal anesthesia for minor surgery in 1947. During that period phenol was commonly used to sterilize the ampoules of local anesthetic before using for spinal anesthesia. In this case, the phenol in which the ampoules of

local anesthetic had been immersed had contaminated the local anesthetic through invisible cracks in the ampoule. The court decided that doctors were not negligent as this risk was not appreciated by ordinary competent anesthesiologist in 1947. It was held that the micro-cracks were not foreseeable given the prevailing scientific knowledge of the time. Thus, since no reasonable anesthetist would have stored the anesthetic differently, it was inappropriate to hold the hospital management liable for failing to take precautions. Lord Justice Denning said, "It is so easy to be wise after the event and to condemn as negligence that which was only a misadventure. We ought to be on our guard against it, especially in cases against hospitals and doctors. Medical science has conferred great benefits on mankind but these benefits are attended by unavoidable risks. Every surgical operation is attended by risks. We cannot take the benefits without taking the risks. Every advance in technique is also attended by risks. Doctors, like the rest of us, have to learn by experience; and experience often teaches in a hard way."

Case 2: *Giving anesthesia without proper medical facility: Non-availability of defibrillator in the operation theater.*[42]

A young man sustained injury to his right arm for which surgery was performed. But he continued to have pain and deformity at operation site for which he was again operated upon by another doctor. Before the second operation, he was referred to the cardiologist. The cardiologist took ECG and declared fit for anesthesia. During surgery the patient had cardiac arrest and died after one hour. The family of the deceased filed a complaint in the court that, the amount of drugs used for anesthesia were more than maximum and death was the direct result of such use of drugs and proper monitoring of the patient was not done.

The anesthesiologist denied the charges against her but admitted that the defibrillator was not available in the OT to adequately resuscitate the patient after cardiac arrest. The state commission observed that the death had occurred in a surgery in which death usually does not occur. The complications and death of the patient had occurred in OT where patient's relatives had no access. The onus therefore was on doctors in the operation theater to explain events that happened there. The surgeon, anesthesiologist, and the cardiologist could not convincingly explain the events and the outcomes.

The court held that it was duty of the anesthesiologist to assess the patient's condition completely before anesthesia. She should have refused anesthesia, if work-up of the patient was incomplete. The expert opinion also enquired and found detachment of supply system was cause. Ultimately, decision of court was that even though the surgical part of the operation was not the cause of cardiac arrest nor had surgeon's skills had been challenged. Yet, she had to bear the responsibility of the actions of the anesthesiologist and cardiologist whom she had called for the patient (vicarious responsibility). A compensation of ₹ 4,15,000 was granted to the complainant. The liability of surgeon was fixed at 20% and that of the anesthesiologist at 60% and cardiologist at 10%.

Case 3: *Anesthesiologist did not accompany the patient being transferred from the operation theater to the tertiary hospital.*[43]

In this case Anesthesiologist was held negligent because he did not accompany the patient in ambulance which he is responsible to do. In the transit, the patient was not on oxygen. The doctor was also held negligent for not providing oxygen to a patient in emergency. Compensation of ₹ 4,10,000 was awarded, to be recovered from the anesthesiologist.

■ CONCLUSION

Safety in anesthesiology has improved much during the recent years. Still, the practice of anesthesiology entails inherent risks and complications in spite of following the approved standards of practice. Anesthesiologists are at high-risk of medicolegal challenge. To avoid negligence claims, it is imperative that anesthesiologists must take a fresh look at risk management strategies. Diligently performing pre-anesthetic check-up, taking informed consent, checking the equipment, monitors, and drugs, attending the patient till he comes out from the effect of anesthesia, adequate documentation in the medical records are some of the good clinical practices that, in addition to improving the quality of patient care also decrease the medicolegal risk. Anesthesiologists must regularly update their professional knowledge and skills, and follow the approved standards of anesthesia practice so as to improve the safety and quality in anesthesiology.

■ REFERENCES

1. WHO guidelines for safe surgery. Available: http://whqlibdoc.who.int/publications/2009/9789241598552_eng.pdf?ua=1.
2. Standards for basic anesthetic monitoring. Available: www.asahq.org.
3. Mishra LD, Agarwal A. The urgency of redifining minimum monitoring standards in Anesthesia. Indian Journal of Clinical Practice. 2013;24(2):122-4.
4. Gray D, Morris CG. Organisation and planning of anesthesia for emergency surgery. Anesthesia. 2013;68(Suppl 1):3-13.
5. Ferrari H. Medical Malpractice Litigation, Consultants and Expert Witness, American Society of Anesthesiologists Newsletter. 1997;61:6.
6. Jithoo S. Death on Table. Anesthetics. 2012. Available: http://anesthetics.ukzn.ac.za/Libraries/Documents2011/S_Jithoos_FMM_booklet.sflb.ashx.
7. Catastrophes in Anesthetic Practice—dealing with the aftermath. 2005. The Association of Anaesthetists of Great Britain and Ireland. Available: http://www.aagbi.org/sites/default/files/catastrophes05.pdf
8. Braz LG, Braz DG, Cruz DS, Fernandes LA, Modolo NP, Braz JR. Mortality in Anesthesia: A systematic review clinics. 2009;64(10):999-1006.
9. Grunshaw N. Anesthetic awareness. Br Med J. 1990;300:821.
10. Heier T, Steen PA. Awareness in anesthesia: incidence, consequences and prevention. Acta Anaesthesiol Scand. 1996; 40:1073-86.
11. Schwender D, Klasing S, Daunderer M, Madler C, Poppel E, Peter K. Awareness during general anesthesia. Definition, incidence, clinical relevance, causes, avoidance and medicolegal aspects. Anaesthetist. 1995;44:743–54.
12. Crawford vs Charing Cross Hospital. The Times. 1953:8.
13. Maynard vs West Midlands Regional Health Authority. Weekly Law Reports. 1984;1634.
14. NT Subrahmanyam and Anr vs B Krishna Rao and Anr. II (1996) CPJ 233 (NC).
15. Raj Kumar Agrawal vs B Mukhopadhyay. I (1995) CPJ 260 Bihar SCDR Commission.
16. IMA vs VP Shantha and Ors III 1995 CPJ I (Supreme Court):1995 CPR 412.
17. Lakshman Balkrishna Joshi vs Dr Trimbak Bapu Godbole, AIR 1969 SC 128.
18. Poona Medical Foundation, Ruby Hall Clinic vs Marutirao L. Titkare and ANR. I (1995) CPJ 232 (NC) NCDRC, New Delhi.
19. Manilal Natha Bhai Patel and Ors vs Dr Tushar N Shah. I (1997) CPJ 560 Gujrat SCRC.
20. Pallattu George and Anr vs Dr Thankam Punnoose and Anr III (1997) 341 Kerala SCDR Commission.
21. Roe and Wooley vs The Ministry of Health and others (1954) 2 All ER 131.
22. Md Aslam vs Ideal Nursing Home and Ors. III (1997) CPJ 81 (NC).
23. Holmes v Board of Hospital Trustees of the City of London (1977) 81 DLR (3d) 67 Ont. HC.
24. In Coyne vs Wigan Health Authority (1991) 2 Med. LR 301, QBD.
25. Lindsay vs Mid western Health Board (1993) 2 I.R. (Irish Reports) 147, 181(Supreme Court of Ireland).
26. Mrs Shantha vs. State of AP and Ors. III (1997) CPJ 481 (DB).
27. NC SauMadhuri vs Rajendra and Ors. III (1996) CPJ 75 Maharashtra SCDRC.

28. Rohini Pritam Kabadi vs Dr RT Kulkarni.III (1996) CPJ 441. Karnataka SCDRC.
29. Nihal Kaur and Ors. vs Director PGIMER and Ors. III (1996) CPJ 112. State CDRC, Chandigarh.
30. Arunaben D Kothari, Ors vs Navdeep Clinic and Ors. III (1996) CPJ 605. Gujrat SCDRC.
31. Girard vs Royal Columbian Hospital (1976) 66 DLR (3d) 676 (BCSC) (British Columbia Supreme Court).
32. Vollar vs. Portsmouth Corporation (1947) 203 LTJ (Law Times Journal) 264.
33. Bolton vs. Stone (1951) AC (Appeal Cases-Law Reports) 850,863 per Lord Oaksey.
34. Mittal AS vs. State of UP. AIR 1989 SC 1570.
35. Eyre v. Measday (1986) All ER (All England Reports) 488.
36. Lockhart P, Feldban E, Gabel R, et al. Dental complications during and after tracheal intubation. J Am Dent Assoc. 1986;112:480-3.
37. Glasgow Corporation vs. Muir (1943) AC. (Appeal Cases-Law Reports) 448, 456 (1985) 37 (South Australian State Reports) 524-42.
38. Shenoy GG. Anesthesiology and the Law. Indian J. Anaesth. 2005;49(1):20-3.
39. Hepworth vs. Kerr (1995) 6 Med LR 139.
40. Hatcher v Black (1954) Times, 2nd July 1954.
41. Nunn JF, Utting JE, Brown BR. General Anesthesia. 5th edn. Boston: Butterworths; 1989.
42. Aruna Ben D. Kothari vs Navdeep Clinic, III (1996) CPJ 605.
43. Mr Sakil Mohammed Vakil Khan vs Dr Miss Perin Irani and others 1999 (2) CPR 515 State CDRC, Maharashtra.

Index

Page numbers followed by *b* refer to box, *f* refer to figure, and *t* refer to table.

A

Abortion 15
Abscess 89
  epidural 245
Abuse
  substance 65
  verbal 61, 107
Accident 336
  aspiration, risk of 320
Accreditation Council for Graduate Medical Research 114
Acitretin 302
Acquired immunodeficiency syndrome 24
Active Surveillance Programs 96
Addressing patient's emotions 115
Adult medical service 277
Adverse drug reaction 195
Advisory committee 216
Age-related macular degeneration 272
Air conditioning
  engineers 81
  function of 81
Airborne communicable diseases 80
  prevention of 81
Airborne Infection Control Program 81
Airborne infection isolation room 80
Alcohol 186
  based preparations 213
  consumption 321
Allergic reaction
  history of 253
  severe 309
Ambulatory care 87

American Association of Blood Banks 302
American Association of Orthopedic Surgeons 262
American Board of Internal Medicine's 114
American College of Obstetricians and Gynecologists 240
American College of Radiology 75, 290
American Society of Anesthesiologists 336
American Society of Heating 81
Amikacin 97
Aminoglycoside 97, 98
Amoxicillin 98
Anaphylactic reactions, severe 309
Anesthesia 338
  awareness 331, 332
  deaths 331
  mishaps 245
  procedure 336
  refused 338
  regional 256
  related problems 337
  role of 256
Anesthesiology
  medicolegal issues in 328, 329
  safety in 339
  specialty of 328
Animal anatomical waste 219
Ankle injuries 264
Anonymity 18
Anorexia 280
Antenatal care, errors in 241
Antibiotic 43
  choice of 97
  resistant organism 88
  therapy, initial 97

Anticipate violence, signs to 65*t*
Anti-hepatitis C virus 296
Antipseudomonal cephalosporin 97
Antipseudomonal penicillin 97
Anxiety 41
Anxiousness, signs of 65
Appeal 172, 218
Arthroplasty 264
Aseptic precautions 101
Aspergillus 81
Asphyxia 195-197, 281
  birth 241
Aspiration pneumonia 97
Atomic Energy Act 213
Atomic Energy Regulatory Board 75
Authorization Committee 207
Autopsy 331

B

Back disorders 264
  lumbago 264
  sciatica 264
Balloon pumps 43
Bile duct, common 257
Bio-medical waste 212-214, 218, 224
  bags, tracking 223
  categories 219*t*
  categories of 223
  handling of 215
  management 217, 226
  and handling rules 213, 222, 225
  safe 226
  records of 225
  treatment 217
  and disposal facility 214
  and disposal of 224
  facilities, common 214
  untreated 218

Biotechnology 221
  waste 219
Birth, wrongful 241
Blood 43
  administering 311
  and blood components,
    guidelines for 304
  and transfusion safety
    program 304
  borne pathogens 302
  components, administration
    of 306t
  donate 297
  issue and usage records 310
  pack, checking 312
  pressure 149
  prior to transfusion,
    collecting 311
  safety and availability 304
  screening, challenges of 301
  storage centres 302
  supply, stewardship of 299
  test 202
  utilization 84
Blood bag 312b
  number of 309
Blood banks 295, 302
  activity of 295
Blood collection 297
  records 309
Blood donation 297
  and transfusion 294
  camps 302
  Façade of non-remunerated
    297
  informed consent in 301
  non-remunerated 294, 297,
    300
  number of 302
  regular 315
  voluntary 297
Blood donor
  selection and donor referrals,
    guidelines for 302
  unpaid 315
Blood group
  tested for 309
  transfusion, wrong 314
Blood products 140, 302, 308
  to transfusion, storing 311

Blood transfusion 140, 294, 300,
    308, 313, 315
  alternatives to 303
  mismatched 295
  practice
    documentation of 309
    litigation related to 313
    medicolegal issues in 294
  process 305
  safety 304
  services 294
  system, conventional 303
Bloodstream 200
  infection, central line-
    associated 91
Body tissues 18
Bolam's rule 165, 257
Bone marrow transplant 81
Bradycardia 245
Brain death, declaration of 206

C

Canadian Medical Protective
  Association 33
Canadian Patient Safety
  Institute 36
Canadian system, tests of 98
Candida 90
Carbapenems 97
Carbon dioxide 82
Cardiac arrest 195, 245
Cardiac surgery 332
Cardiopulmonary resuscitation
    40, 140
  event, documentation of 140
Care and liability, duty of 329
Carotid artery stenosis 321
Cataract 102
  surgery 271
Cause-effect relationship 289
Cefepime 97
Cefoperazone 98
Cefoxitin 97
Ceftazidime 97
  plus 97
    vancomycin 97
Central Licence Approving
  Authority 296
Central Pollution Control Board
  217, 218

Central Supervisory Board 230
Cephalometric radiographs,
  pretreatment 321
Cesarean section 243, 332
Chemical liquid waste 220
Chemical waste 213, 220
Children
  diseases of 277
  disorders of 277
Chlorinated plastic bags 223
Chromosomal abnormalities
  241
Ciprofloxacin 97
Civil law 176
  damages in 164
Clavulanate 98
Clindamycin 97
Clinical documentation
  guidelines 150
Clinical records 150b
Clinician satisfaction, improved
  110
Clostridioides difficile infection
  88
Clostridium difficile 99
Cognitive errors 74
Cognitive impairment 74
Communication 108, 275, 290,
    305, 330
  assessment tool 114
  barriers 74, 113, 282
  behavior change 297
  channel 108
  effective 108, 109
  good 107
  in healthcare 109
  ineffective 113
  model, basic 108f
  nonverbal 108
  openness 74
  practice good 282
  principles of good 110
  skills 62, 108, 109, 114, 115,
    282
    for doctors 109
    in healthcare 107
    lack of training in 113
    of healthcare practitioners
      107
    of healthcare workers 114

types of 108
unambiguous 305
verbal 108
with attendants 111
with referring doctor and patient 290
Community
leaders 64
role of 63
Compensation 179
Competency assessment 306
Complainant's advocate 174
Complainant's allegation 101
Complaint Under Act 225
Conception, wrongful 242
Conducting medical interview 111
Confusion 41
Consent
age for 125, 279
role of 248
Consultation, conduct in 10
Consumer court 143, 172
function 170
pecuniary jurisdictions of 187
Consumer forum, members of 172
Consumer Protection Act 141, 142, 170
complaints under 170
in dental professionals 324
Contemplating suicide 61
Corneal flap 270
Corneal thinning 270
Corporate hospitals 61, 64
Cosmetic surgery 5, 270
Counseling
improper 53
techniques 115
Court of law, expert witness in 248
Criminal case, appearing in 173
Crisis reform models 181
Crooked tree, famous engraving of 261*f*
Cylinders, storage of 83
Cystic fibrosis 241
Cystic lesions 321
Cytomegalovirus 89

D

Dalfopristin 97
Data privacy and security 134
Death
certificate, cause of 137
wrongful 242
Decision making
capacity 52
assess 54
involve patient in 111
process, document shared 253
Defence lawyer, selection of 170
Delirium 41
Dental care, quality in 319
Dental pain 320
Dental practice
medicolegal aspects of 319
no negligence' occasions in 323
Dental practitioners 319
Dentistry
diagnosis of malignancy in 321
medicolegal issues in 319
negligence in 322
Depression 41
underlying 300
Diabetes 100
Dialysis 43
Diameter indexed safety systems 82
Director General Armed Forces Medical Services 218
Directorate General of Health Services 142
Disastrous consequences 173
Disc lesions 264
Discharge against medical advice
duty of doctor in 52
predictors of 50, 51*t*
validity of 52
Discharge notes 154
Discharge process, documented 140
Disease
emotional facet of 288
severity 40
transmission, risk of 81

Disposal facilities 217
Distressing symptoms 245
District Level Monitoring Committee 217
District-wise committee 68
Doctor's defence 101, 102, 196, 198, 201, 202
Doctor-patient
bonding 70
communication 114
relationship 157, 250, 290, 335
Doctors and professional association, code of conduct for 13
Doctors for criminal
negligence, prosecution of 167
rashness, prosecution of 167
Documentation 146, 275, 305, 330
adequate 56
and informed consent 265
benefits of good quality 147
errors in 148
incomplete 54
incorrect 54
legal importance of 146
of procedures 140
Documented policies 138, 139
Documenting instructions 157
Documenting patient's refusal 157
Donor
ethical principles relating to 299
maintenance charge 206
organ transplantation, deceased 210*t*
screening 302
Drugs 331
delivery systems 99
intoxications 65
resistant bacteria 98
Drugs and Cosmetics Act 15, 295, 296
Drugs and Cosmetics Rules 295, 296
Dryness 270
Dutasteride 302
Duty of care 162
Dyspnea 41

E

Eagle's eye 237
Easy to accept cause-effect relationship 289
Ectasia 270
Ectopic pregnancy 242
Effective laws, implementation of 69
Electronic health records 133
   preservation 134
Electronic medical records 77, 144
Electronic protected health information 133
Emergency
   acute 254
   error in diagnosis during 280
   medical care 283
   surgery 332
Emergency department 50, 62, 74
   safety factors in 74t
Empathy skills 62
Empiric therapy, principles of 97
Encephalocele 241
End of life
   care 40
      decisions 40
   issues, legal aspects of 45
Endorsement 14
Endoscopy room 75
Engender litigation, complications 252
Engineering design plays 80
Enterobacter cloacae 98
Enterococcus 90
Environment Law 212
Environment Protection Act 213, 225
   penalties under 225
Epidural hematoma 245
Epithelial cells 90
Equipment 330
   disposable 101
Error and omission policy 186
Erythromycin 97
Esthetic dentistry 322
Ethics
   advisory committee 47
   law and policy 33

Etretinate 302
Euglycemia 256
Euthanasia 13, 44, 45
   active 44
   debate on 45
   nonvoluntary 44
   passive 44, 45
   voluntary 44
Evolution 122
Eye surgery, types of 270

F

Facial trauma, cases of 320
Facility management and safety committee 84
Fallopian tubes 129
Family planning operation 247
Fascia 89
Fatigue 74
Faulty surgical technique 247
Fear 41
Female feticide, prevent 234
Femtosecond laser assisted cataract surgery 271
Femur, fracture of 264
Fetal anomalies, missed diagnosis of 244
Fetal autopsy 244
Fetomaternal disorders 240
Fetomaternal physiological derangement 240
Fight against violence, essential in 67
Finasteride 302
Fingerpointing, avoid 173
Fistula formation 258
Fluid replacement, adequate 256
Fluoroquinolone 97, 98
Foreign objects
   ingestion of 320
   inhalation of 320
Fractured surgical needle 321
Future litigation, protection against 51

G

Gas cylinders rules 82
Gastrointestinal tract 88
Gene therapy 269
Generic names of drugs, use of 8

Genetic counseling center 229
Gifts 13
Glassware 221
Glaucoma 275
Glutaraldehyde 213
Good clinical records, advantages of 151t
Gossypiboma 246
Gossypium 246
Gram-negative organisms 98
   combination therapy 98
   monotherapy 98
Gram-positive organisms 98
Growth hormone 302
Gynecological causes 239
Gynecology, medicolegal issues in 245

H

Hand
   hygiene 80
   injuries 264
   washing 99
Harassment 61
Haunting nightmare 175
Hazardous chemicals rules, storage and import of 213
Hazardous waste 212
Health
   court 182
      system 183
   information
      protected 133
      technology 78
   insurance
      coverage 239
      purpose 19
   related literacy 69
      low 63
Healthcare
   commercialization of 287
   cost
      high 52
      lower 181
   delivery, aspects of 109
   documentation in 145
   establishments 212, 223
   expenditure, escalating 87
   expensive 239
   facilities, implementation of rules in 217
   organization 84, 104, 133

provider 134
research and quality, agency for 94
risk management in 83
sector 61
setting
　anticipate violence in 64
　managing violence in 65
　preventing violence in 65
standards 73
strategies for safety in 74
system 33, 151
workers, occupational safety of 225
Healthcare-associated infection 79, 87, 88, 92, 93, 95, 96, 98, 100, 101
　common 89
　documented 97
　indicators of 96
　legal provisions applicable to 103
　management of 97
　medicolegal aspects related to 99
　sources of 88
　strategies for management of 97
　type of 88
Heart disease, congenital 281
Hemolytic reactions, acute 308
Hemorrhage, postpartum 241, 246
Hemostats, application of 257
Hepatitis 302
　antibodies 297
　B 302
　　infection 295
　　surface antigen 296
　C 101, 302
　　infection, suffered 101
　　test 101
　　virus 101
Herpes simplex 89
Herpes zoster 89
Hippocratic oath 5
Home care 87
Hormone
　replacement therapy 246
　secretion 245

Hospital acquired infections, prevent 95f
Hospital administrators, preventive tips for 67
Hospital management 338
Hospital readmissions 53
Hospital waste 212
　management 212
Hospital-acquired infection
　burden of 92
　incidence, trend in 92t
　indicators to control 96t
　preventing 92
　strategies for prevention of 93t
Hospitality 13
Hospitalization, reason for 154
Human anatomical waste 219
Human blood 295
Human embryos 303
Human immunodeficiency
　virus 24, 295, 302
　infection 26, 313
　　risk of 23
　　transmission of 26
　positive 23, 25
　　right of 23
　　status, disclosure of 24
　screening 25, 26
　status 23, 25
　testing 24, 25
　　guidelines on 24
　　informed consent for 24
Human life, loss of 176
Human organ 207
Human Organ Transplantation
　Act 45
　implications to 45
Human rights 13
Humerus fracture 264
Hydrocephalus 241
Hyperbilirubinemia, management of 281
Hypochlorite 213
Hypochondria 5
Hypoglycemia, neonatal 281
Hypotension 245
　severe 309
Hypothetical considerations 179

Hypoxia 195
Hysterectomy 245

I

Ideal indemnity insurance policy 190
Imipenem 97
Immune systems 100
Incisional infection, superficial 89
Indemnity insurance policy 191
Indian Council of Medical Research 19
Indian Evidence Act 142
Indian Medical Association 217
Indian Medical Council 8
　Regulations 8
Indian Penal Code
　related to consent, sections of 126b
　relevant sections of 196
　section 269 104
　section 270 104
　section 304a 103
　section 337 103
　section 338 104
Indian Radiology and Imaging Association 228
Indian Society of Anesthesiologists 329, 336
Ineffective communication
　consequences of 113
　legal risks of 283
Infection 89, 270
　anaerobic bacterial 97
　bacterial 309
　blood and urine 200
　chain 80f
　control 79, 84
　　aspect of 77
　　committee 104
　　measures 100
　　practical guidelines for 80
　deep incisional 89
　developing 87
　exogenous 88, 102
　eye 102
　high risk of 302
　hospital 88
　organ surgical site 89

postoperative 96
prevent 80
prevention
  and control 80
  initiatives 94
protozoal 309
spread of 80, 104
surgical site 87, 89
transmission of 91
type of 102
viral 309
Infectious agent 80
Infectious diseases 81
  spread of 81
Infectious hazards of
  transfusion 309
Infectious waste 212
Inflammation 270
Influenza 81
Information
  and communication
    technology 134
  disclosure of 124
  via speech 108
Informed consent 274
  documentation of 128
  medicolegal aspects of 121
  role of 291
Injury, assessment of 162
Inpatient medical records 142
Institute of medicine 31, 32
Insulin 43
Insurance
  factors influencing amount
    of 187
  schemes 69
Intensive care units 62, 87
International Society of Blood
  Transfusion 298
Interpersonal behavior 324
Intoxicant 186
Intraocular lens implants 269
Intraocular pressure 272
Intra-operative monitoring,
  standards for basic 336
Intrauterine fetal death 243
Intrusive palliative procedures
  43
Intussusception
  case of 280
  diagnosis of 280
Irrational implementation 234
Isolation rooms 77
Isotretinoin 302

J

Jecker's modification 41
Joint
  commission 264
    national patient safety
      goals 94
  replacement 257
Judgment, error of 333
Judicial decision 25, 122
  on informed consent 129
  on radiological errors 289
Judicial precedents 195
Judicial process, lack of faith
  in 64
Justice
  administration of 19
  legal requirement of 19

K

Karmachari of hospital 155
Kidney transplant 200
Klebsiella 95
Knee ligament 264

L

Laryngeal nerve injury,
  recurrent 257
Laser assisted in situ
  keratomileusis 270
  complications 270
Laudable pus 257
Law against violence,
  strengthening 67
Lawful Act 196
Lawsuit
  claim 56
  managing risk of 274
Legal liability 186
Legal restrictions, evasion of 9
Legionella 90
Legionellosis infection 97
Life, wrongful 241
Life-prolonging interventions,
  guidelines for limiting 42b
Life-saving surgery 43
Life-support
  withdrawal of 42, 43
  withholding of 42, 43
Life-threatening
  illness 41
  reaction 308
  situations 300
Linezolid 98

Lion's heart 237
Liquid waste, disposal of 215
Listen actively 111
Litigation
  causes of 263
  in orthopaedics, causes of
    264b
  process, key role in 146
  protection against 323
  risk of 53
Living donation and
  transplantation,
    medicolegal aspects of 207
Loneliness 41

M

Macula 272
Malaria 296, 302
  parasite 202
Malpractice
  crisis reform, part of 182
  liability crisis 180
  litigation 269
Malpractice lawsuits 169, 249
  obstetric cases vulnerable
    to 240
  prevent risk of 123
  risk of 319
  vulnerable to 281
Measles 80, 81
Media
  in preventing violence, role
    of 69
  role of 64
Medical acts 8
Medical advice
  cases of Discharge against 52
  causes of discharge against
    50, 50b
  compliance with 109
  consequences of discharge
    against 52
  discharge against 49, 51, 52,
    55, 55b, 56, 57t
  leave against 49, 51, 56, 140
  legal status of discharge
    against 51
  managing discharge against
    54
  medicolegal aspects of
    discharge against 49
  reason for discharge against
    53
  risk of discharge against 50

Medical air 82
Medical and legal implications 241
Medical care 132
   continuity of 146
Medical certificate 155*b*
   issuing 155
   of cause of death 137
Medical condition 74
   complex 74
Medical confidentiality 4, 23, 25
   guidelines on 20
Medical Council for Issuance of Medical Certificate 156*b*
Medical Council of India 115, 138, 155*b*
   guidelines 136, 150
   regulations 20, 143
Medical decision 6
   making 18
Medical Defense Union 270
Medical documentation 145, 147
   critical issues in 154
   good 152
   illegible 149
   quality of 146
Medical documents, cases compelling 147
Medical education, competency-based 116
Medical emergencies 128, 320
Medical errors 31-33, 113
   consequences of disclosing 33
   disclosure of 32, 33
   guidelines on disclosing 34
   types of 32*b*
Medical establishments 186
Medical ethics 3, 6
   code of 8
Medical futility 41, 44
Medical gases 82
   safety measures related to 82
Medical Injury Compensation Reform Act 181
Medical interview
   prior to start of 110
   with patient 110
Medical jousting 266
Medical laws, awareness of 325
Medical liability 180
   crisis 183

Medical literature, basis of 5
Medical maloccurrence 249
Medical malpractice
   insurance 180, 183
   liability crisis 180
   litigation 107, 169
Medical negligence 157, 161, 163, 165, 176-179, 183, 185, 253, 270
   allegations of 190
   burden of proof of 164
   cases 68, 101, 142, 176, 182
   compensation in 176
   crime 163
   essential components of 161
   guilty of 201
   issue of 143
   lawsuits of 170, 291
   liability lawsuits, cases of 190
   types of 163
   vital issues in 164
Medical practice
   confidentiality in 18
   disclosure in 18
   ethics of 3
   part of good 17
Medical practitioner 5, 53, 175
   benefits of disclosure to 34
   care required by 200
   complaints against 169
   ethical guidelines for 8
   feels 15
   harms of disclosure to 34
Medical profession, values of 7
Medical professionals 291
   criminal liability of 167
   for criminal negligence 198
   landmark judgments related to 195
Medical Protection Society 270
Medical record 77, 132, 135, 144
   categories of 135
   complete and accurate 137
   component of 132
   confidentiality of 135
   department 137
   destruction of 173
   guidelines on 136
   judicial decision related to 143
   maintenance of 8
   medicolegal aspects of 132, 141

   reflects continuity 137
   regulation governing 147
   review of 138
Medical research 13, 19
Medical science and technology, recent advancement in 85
Medical specialty 66
Medical Teaching Program, integral part of 115
Medical termination of pregnancy, incomplete 241
Medical vacuum 82
Medication
   confusion 74
   errors 283
   management of 141
Medicine 3, 285
   branches of 240
   defensive 180-183
   discarded 220
   expired 220
   incorporate philosophy of 66
   neonatal 281
   practice of 3, 121
   safe practice of 203
   tradition of 60
Medicolegal
   aspects 208, 297
   autopsy 258
   awareness 239
   cases 138, 208
   claims against gynaecologists, survey of 240
   conflicts 287
      in orthopedics 264*b*
      preventing 265
   donations 206
   examination 125
   implications 253
   issues 237, 245, 283
      recent trends of 3
   risk factors 252
   safety 71
Meningitis 281
Meningomyelocele 241
Meniscal injuries 264
Meropenem 97
Metallic body implants 221
Metronidazole 97
Microbiological examination 102
Microbiology 221

Micro-chip implants 269
Microorganism
    infecting 87
    source of 91
Ministry of Environment, Forest and Climate Change 217, 218
Ministry of Health and Family Welfare 78, 215, 296
Ministry of Urban Development 79
Misadventures 336
Misconduct 14
    adultery 14
    conviction by court of law 14
    improper conduct 14
    sex determination tests 14
    violation of regulations 14
Mishaps 336
Missed ectopic pregnancy 241
Missed test results 74
Modern medicine 73
Morbidity, high 53
Morphine, high dose of 5
Mortality 53
Motor Accident Claim Tribunal Act 142
Motor Vehicles Act 219
Multidrug-resistant organisms 96
Multiple anecdotal reports 60
Multiple gestation 241
Myomectomy 246

N

Nasal septum, margin of 195
National Academy of Sciences 31
National Accreditation Board for Hospitals and Healthcare providers 136
    guidelines 136
National Acquired Immunodeficiency Syndrome Control Organization 295
    guidelines 23
National Blood Policy 294-296, 298, 301
    and guidelines 301
National Blood Program, development of 295

National Blood Transfusion Council 294
    Program 294
National Commission 129, 143, 173
National Consumer Dispute Redressal Commission 179, 278
National Healthcare Safety Network 88
National Patient Safety
    agency 264
    goals 95
Nature of disease, diagnosis and 127
Nature, multidisciplinary in 139
Nausea 41
Negligence 197, 199
    by professionals 199
    causing death by 103, 196
    per se 164
    test for establishing 166
Negligible health impacts 224
Neonatal intensive care 281
Neonatal resuscitation 281
Neuromuscular blocking agent 332
Nitrogen 82
Nitrous oxide 82
No objection certificate 207
No-fault compensation 182
Non-hazardous waste 212
Non-heart-beat donors 45
Noninjurious assault 61
Nonmonetary incentives 297
Nonseasonal perspiration 65
Nontransplant organ retrieval centers 206
Normothermia, maintaining 256
Nosocomial infection 88
Numerous medicolegal issues 259

O

Obstetric
    case, engagement for 10
    medicolegal issues in 240
    regional anesthesia, complications of 245
    ultrasonography in 244

Obstetric anesthesia 244
    practice of 244
Obstetrics and gynecology
    medicolegal issues in 239
    practice 239
Ocular diseases 269
Ocular trauma 272
Offence
    and penalties 230
    cognizance of 68
    penalties for 225
Omission, allegation of 286
Oncology 81
Oopherectomy 245
Operation table, death on 329
Operation theater 330
Ophthalmic practice, vulnerable domains in 270
Ophthalmology 269
    medicolegal issues in 269, 270
Oral care 41
Oral cavity 90
Organ donation 209, 273
    and transplantation 208
    programme 211
    counseling for 206
    deceased 209
Organ failure, number of 211
Organ retrieval
    centers 209
    charge 206
Organ transplant 204
    surgery 257
Organization
    policy 139
    services of 139
Original complainant 202
Oropharynx 321
Orthodontic
    practice 320
    therapy 321
    treatment, complication of 320
Orthodontists 321
Orthopedia 261
Orthopedic
    medicolegal issues in 261
    medicolegal risks in 262
    practice evidence-based 266
    scope of consent in 263

surgeons, reasons of litigation against 263
surgery 261
Orthopedist in court of law 267
Osteoarthritis 264
Ovaries 129
Oxygen 82

P

Pacemakers 43
Pain
   and suffering 181
      component 181
   persistent 320
   treatment of 41
Palliative care
   at end of life 40
   wards 41
Paraverbal communication 108
Parental permission 279
Parental refusal to medical treatment 282
Parenteral and enteral fluids 43
Patent and copyrights 12
Paternalism 5, 6
   versus autonomy 5
Paternalistic philosophy 6
Patient burden 113
Patient centered documentation and record keeping 152
Patient handling and movement assessment 79
Patient related factors 62
Patient safety
   and risk management 73
   in pediatrics 280
   initiatives 71
Patient's allegation 102, 196, 198, 201, 202
Patient's interest 19
Patient-doctor relationship 267
Patient-physician relationship 107
PC-PNDT Act 227, 229, 230, 234, 292
Pediatrician 278
Pediatrics, medicolegal issues in 277, 278
Pelvic
   hemorrhage, uncontrolled 246
   inflamatory disease 246
   pain syndrome 246

Penalty and compensation 68
Permanent vegetative state 46
Personal document 135
Personal information 134
Persons with Disabilities Act 79
Persons with Disabilities, rights of 79
Phacoemulsification 271
Phagocytes 98
Phenolic derivatives 213
Physical assault causing injury 61
Physician
   duties of 9
   in consultation, duties of 10
   preventive tips for 65
   related factors 62
   responsibilities of 10
   to public and paramedical profession, duties of 11
Piperacillin 97, 98
Placenta
   adherent 241
   microscopic examination of 244
   previa, undiagnosed 241
Placental umbilical cord blood transfusion 303
Plaintiff sought damages 129
Planned surgery, deviation from 254
Plasma
   pyrolysis 224
   regain, rapid 296
Plasmodium falciparum 202
Pneumonia
   atypical 97
   ventilator associated 90
Poddar's treatment 23
Pollution Control Committee 216, 219
Poor clinical records, disadvantages of 151*t*
Poor insurance claim settlement 53
Postanalysis disclosure 36
Post-traumatic stress
   disorder 331
   syndrome 61
Pre-anesthesia assessment 140
Preconception and Prenatal Diagnostic Techniques Act 227, 285

Preconception and Prenatal Diagnostic Test Act 142
Pregnancy
   high-risk 243
   hypotensive syndrome of 245
   medical disorder in 243
Premature baby 242
Prenatal Diagnostic Techniques (Prohibition of Sex Selection) Act 147, 227
Pretransfusion blood sampling 308
Pretreatment screening, incidental findings on 321
Professional indemnity 185
   insurance 185, 325
   policy 190
Professional practices 337
Professional services, payment of 9
Proliferative diabetic retinopathy, stage 272
Proliferative vitreoretinopathy 272
Proxy, consent by 279
Pseudomonas aeruginosa 97, 98
   infection 98
Public and community health 20
Public health authorities 15
Public hospitals, problems of 63
Public lectures 15
Public safety 19
Publishing diagnostic errors regularly 291
Punishment and disciplinary action 16
Pyrexia 280

Q

Quality healthcare 180, 283
Quasi-judicial courts 170
Quinupristin 97

R

Radiation dose 76
Radioactive waste 213
Radiological errors, types of 286
Radiological negligence 289
Radiologist's rapport 288
Radiology

average diagnostic standard in 287
avoiding litigation in 290
errors in 285, 291
limitations of 288
medicolegal issues in 285
Radius and ulna, fractures of 264
Reaction, severe 308
Reasonable care 166
Reasonable skill and care 325
legal relevance of 325
social relevance of 325
Rebates and commission 12
Record
disposal of 310
keeping 228
preservation of 141
storage of 310
Recording information, process of 145
Red blood cells 303
sources of 303
Red Crescent Societies, league of 298
Registered medical practitioner 207
Registration numbers, display of 8
Rejoinder and affidavits 171
Renal failure, acute 149
Res ipsa loquitor 165, 247, 334
doctrine of 335
Resident doctor 112
Respiratory rate 295
Respiratory suppression 5
Respiratory syndrome, severe acute 81
Respiratory trouble 202
Retina 272
artificial 269
Retinal conditions 272
Rheumatic fever, acute 149
Rhythm abnormalities 140
Rifampicin 97, 98
Right to Information Act
and medical confidentiality 21
and medicolegal cases 22
Risk identification 84
sources of 84
Risk management 83

activities, evaluation of 84, 85
practice 320
process of 83
programs, implementation of 85
strategy
development of 84
implementation of 84
Robust system 294
Root resorption 320
Rubbing hands, frequently 65
Rubella 89
Rupture uterus 246

S

Sadness 41
Safe blood administration 308
Safe handling of treated wastes 224
Safe operation theater setup 266
Safe transfer, methodology of 139
Safer healthcare system 182
Safety encourages teamwork 74
Safety habits, certain 66
Sands of Sahara syndrome 270
Scope and legal interpretation 161
Secrecy and data security 18
Sedation, consent for 140
Seizures, neonatal 281
Sensitive personal information 134
Sepsis 281
Serratia marcescens 98
Sex determination tests 20
Sex ratio, declining 234
Sex, prenatal determination of 231
Sexual harassment 61
Sexual offenses 162
Sexual violence, victims of 279
Shock 309
Sick, obligations to 9
Single photon emission 75
Skill and care, medical
relevance of reasonable 325
Skin 258
incision 89
problems 41
Smoking

habits 100
history of 321
Soiled waste 219
Solicit patient assent 279
Spondylolisthesis 321
Standard operative procedure 295
Staphylococcus 90, 200
aureus 95, 98
State blood transfusion councils 295
State Commission 173
State Consumer Dispute Redressal Commission 323
State Pollution Control Board 216, 218, 219
Stem cell 269
derived blood cells 303
Sterilization operation, cases of 248
Stillbirths 243
Streptococcus pneumoniae 98
Strong and effective laws 67
Strong paternalism 6
Stylohyoid ligaments 321
Suboptimal visual outcome 270
Suicide, physician assisted 45
Sulbactam 98
Summoning medical records by courts 142
Supreme Court's observation 201
on criminal negligence 197
on expert medical opinion 203
on negligence 199
Surgery
consent in 256
medicolegal issues in 252
never events' in 258
preoperative period in 253
wrong site 258, 259, 264
wrong-procedure 265t
Surgical complications 248, 256
Surgical items, retained 258
Surgical mishaps 245
deaths due to 331
Surgical objects, retained 246
Surgical procedure, documentation before 141
Surrogate decision-maker 54

Susbequent and postanalysis disclosure 38
Sword of Damocles 263
Syphilis 89, 302, 303
Systemic diseases, missing serious 273
Systemic lupus erythematosus 273

T

Tapping hands 65
Tarasoff case 23
Tay-Sachs disease 241
Tazobactam 98
Teaching communication skill 115
Technical mishaps 331
Teicoplanin 98
Temporomandibular disorder 319, 320
  cause of 320
Testis, torsion of 280
Therapeutic interventions 87
Therapeutic privilege 128
Therapeutic relationship, dissolution of 51
Threatening behavior 61
Tibia, fracture of 264
Tonsils, removal of large 280
Toothache 320
Tort system 183
Total hip replacement 263
Total knee replacement 263
Toxic waste 213
Toxoplasmosis 89
Transfusion 310
  adverse effects of 308
  associated circulatory overload 308
  medicine
    code of ethics relating to 298
    practice of 295
  noninfectious hazards of 308
  process, documenting 312
  reaction 313
    acute 308
    adverse 302
    investigation of 313
  technology 294
  transmitted diseases, risk of 294
Transient neurologic complications 245
Transmission 80, 92
Transplant coordinators in hospitals 206
Transplantation of Human Organ Act 204, 273
Transplantation of Human Organ and Tissues Rules 204
Treatment after consultation 10
Treatment and disposal 218
Trisomy 21 241
Trypanosoma cruzi 303
Tuberculosis 80, 81, 89

U

Ultrasound machine, registration of 227
Unethical Acts 11
Unethical conduct, exposure of 9
Unipolar electrocautery 257
Unique hospital identity number 137
Upper respiratory tract 90
Urinary tract infection, catheter-associated 91
Urticaria 309
Uterine bleeding, dysfunctional 246
Uterus 129

V

Vaccine injury 283
Vaginal birth after cesarean 240, 243
Valid consent, conditions for 125
Vancomycin 97, 98
  resistant enterococci 95
Vasopressors 43
Venereal disease 25
Ventilation, function of 81
Ventilator 43
Vertebra 321
Violations, penalties for 231*t*
Violence
  against doctors 60
  factors predisposing to 61
  prohibition of 68
Vis-à-vis parenteral nutrition 281
Vis-à-vis surgery 280
Vision, lost 102
Vitreoretinal surgeons 272
Voluntariness 124, 125
Vomiting 280

W

Waste
  clinical laboratory 221
  contaminated 221
  management rules 225
  pharmaceutical 213
Water (Prevention and Control of Pollution) Act 215
Weak and ineffective laws 63
White blood cell 90
Wisconsin Department of Regulation and Licensing 289
Wisconsin radiologist 289
Witness
  death on operation table 329
  examination of 172
World Blood Donor Day 315, 316
World Federation of Society of Anesthesiologists 329
World Health Assembly 308
World Health Organization 41, 79, 94, 215, 258, 298, 302